CRC SERIES IN ENGINEERING IN MEDICINE AND BIOLOGY

Editors-in-Chief

Barry N. Feinberg, Ph.D., P.E., C.C.E.

Associate Professor, Electrical Engineering
Clinical Engineering Program
Purdue University
West Lafayette, Indiana

David G. Fleming, Ph.D., M.D.

Professor, Biomedical Engineering in Pediatrics
Case Western Reserve University
Cleveland, Ohio

Handbook of Engineering in Medicine and Biology

Volume I

General Data

Volume II

Instruments and Measurements

Editors:

Barry N. Feinberg

David G. Fleming

Handbook of Clinical Engineering

Volume I

General Principles

Editor:

Barry N. Feinberg

Handbook of Hospital Safety

Editor:

Paul E. Stanley

CRC Handbook of Hospital Safety

Editor

Paul E. Stanley
Professor Emeritus
School of Engineering
Purdue University
West Lafayette, Indiana

CRC Series in Engineering in Medicine and Biology

Editors-in-Chief

David Fleming
Department of Biomedical Engineering
Case Western Reserve University
Cleveland, Ohio

Barry Feinberg
Department of Electrical Engineering
Purdue University
West Lafayette, Indiana

CRC Press, Inc.
Boca Raton, Florida

Library of Congress Cataloging in Publication Data

Main entry under title:

CRC handbook of hospital safety.

Bibliography: p.
Includes index.
1. Hospitals--Safety measures. I. Stanley, Paul E. II. Chemical Rubber Company. III. Title: Handbook of hospital safety. [DNLM: 1. Accident prevention. 2. Hospital administration. WX185 C105]
RA969.9.C17 363.1'5 80-20950
ISBN 0-8493-0751-1.

Direct all inquiries to CRC Press, Inc., 2000 N.W. 24th Street, Boca Raton, Florida 33431.

International Standard Book Number 0-8493-0751-1

Library of Congress Card Number 80-20950
Printed in the United States

FOREWORD

Professional dedication to health and safety would seem implicit in the job functions of all safety and health professionals. However, something more is needed than just professional dedication, sincere intentions, honest efforts, general knowledge, and some kind of native intelligence. To be effective, there must be some specific understanding of what to do and how to do it. Good intentions must be supplemented by specialized skills, relevant knowledge, and useful technical information. This book provides some understanding of the objectives, methods, scope of activities, hazards and risks, preventive and corrective remedies, and loss control procedures necessary for safety in the modern hospital environment and health care delivery system.

Hospitals have become more complex and sophisticated in terms of medical instrumentation and diagnostic devices; the facilities for health care have expanded in size and bureaucracy; responsibility and accountability has become shared and blurred; and technical detail is proliferating faster than even the growth of specialization. The emergent man-machine environment seems to require some kind of systematic analysis and positive assurance that effective efforts are being made to minimize any unnecessary, avoidable harm to patients, professionals, staff, visitors, or bystanders. What seemed like a good record for the past half century may not prevail as such in an era of rising consumer expectations for physicians, nurses, technicians, and administrators. Certainly, attempts to achieve higher standards of care seem warranted, if only to avoid the specter of allegations of professional malpractice, claims of hospital negligence, and legal actions involving medical device strict liability.

Higher expectations and demands for hospital safety may or may not be the result of a combination of better educated consumers, the creation of mass media, God-like medical stereotypes who should never fail in their mission, more prospective plaintiffs alerted and sensitized by newspaper accounts of large court verdicts for alleged wrongdoing, heavy-handed legislative attempts to correct perceived inadequacies by governmental regulatory overkill, and the increasing complexity of the medical enterprise. It might be the result of the transgressions of the minority of careless or uninformed persons found in any occupation. It could reflect the possibility that something better might be achieved with the application of new knowledge and past lessons learned. It could be argued that certain statistical risks are now outweighed by benefits or remedies that are technically feasible, economically cost effective, and produce no significant penalties or undesired consequences. There is a widespread belief that no risk of death or serious bodily injury is acceptable if reasonable accident prevention measures could have prevented it from occurring.

Whatever the reasons, it has become obvious that considerable attention is being focused on the subject of hospital safety. A safety assurance program now seems essential for the well-managed hospital or health care facility. This Handbook of Hospital Safety should prove useful in the formulation and implementation of a hospital safety assurance and loss prevention effort. Of greater importance is that it could serve to improve the overall level of hospital safety, and any such improvement conceivably could directly affect and benefit each of us. Certainly, it is well worth the time and effort to read this handbook, thoughtfully consider its messages, adapt or extend the contents as necessary, and take whatever appropriate personal actions are indicated where a new resultant awareness or perception suggests that there is excessive preventable danger. Fatalistic and unconcerned attitudes should not be the hallmark of a hospital safety program. They prevail only in the darkness of an ignorance that has not been illuminated by books such as the Handbook of Hospital Safety. Let us hope that this book will have its intended and foreseeable effect in adding further laurels to those already achieved by health care professionals.

George A. Peters

PREFACE

This handbook consists of sections written by recognized authorities in the fields covered. General guidelines are given, but sufficient detail is presented in several areas to make it usable by the practitioner in many of the special disciplines found within the hospital. Its objective is to provide a single-volume handbook for day-to-day use throughout the facility. It is appropriate as a textbook for hospital safety workshops and programs.

Introductory sections give the *raison d'etre* for hospital safety. The first section describes briefly and somewhat randomly some of the problems the hospital safety officer must work with every day. The second and third sections evaluate the psychology of the hospital population — patients, staff, and visitors — and the human factors which affect safety within the hospital. A guide to the organization, function, and authority of the hospital safety committee, its membership as required by the Joint Commission on Accreditation of Hospitals, and the importance of record keeping are among the topics of the fourth section. It is intended to aid the hospital administration in establishing a safety or risk management program.

Activities in which most, if not all, personnel, patients, and visitors are involved are discussed in the next two sections. Paramount in this topic are sanitation and infection control. On an almost equal level is fire prevention and what to do in case of a fire.

A series of "how to" sections for special activities and parts of the hospital follow. Of concern to the engineering staff, and especially the clinical engineer, is the seventh section — safety in the electromedical instrumentation system. Emergency room, operating room, and special care unit safety are discussed in the next three sections. The more specialized safety problems of the pharmacy, laboratory and radiological facilities of the hospital follow, respectively. Some duplication of material will be obvious in sections 5 through 13, but it is presented with enough variation to provide the proper emphasis.

Safety practices such as body mechanics, peculiar to the portion of the hospital staff concerned with patient handling or moving of equipment, are covered in the fourteenth section. The hazards and their prevention with which housekeeping and the facility staff are concerned, as well as facility security, are the topics of the proceeding two sections. The last points out some of the legal aspects of malpractice as the term extends to the entire hospital staff and administration, reviews the need for a risk management program, and suggests some steps in implementing such a program.

The editor is deeply indebted to all of the contributing authors for their considerable effort in preparing the manuscripts for this handbook. Encouragement from the members of the advisory board, the editor's colleagues at Purdue University, and others at hospitals throughout the country is gratefully acknowledged. Special recognition is due Linda Flack, Sandy Stewart, and the numerous unnamed secretaries who were responsible for the typing and art work which made the manuscript possible. Finally, the editor's thanks go to the numerous friends and acquaintances in the health care industry whose contributions have led to the concept of a Handbook of Hospital Safety, but whose specific suggestions are no longer identifiable.

Paul E. Stanley

THE EDITOR

Paul E. Stanley holds a Ph.D. degree from Ohio State University. He taught Physics at Wheaton College in Illinois from 1936 to 1943, then joined the Department of Aeronautics at Purdue University. Since 1960 Stanley has engaged in engineering in health care specializing in electrical and instrumentation safety. He served as associate director of the Biomedical Engineering Center at Purdue, 1971 to 1976, becoming Professor Emeritus, Engineering in 1976. He is certified in Clinical Engineering and was for many years a member of the National Fire Protection Association Technical Committee on the Safe Use of Electricity in Patient Care Areas. He has been a frequent contributor of papers on electrical safety in health care, and on engineering education for health care at national conferences and in various publications.

ADVISORY BOARD

CONTRIBUTORS

James D. Barger
Chairman
Department of Laboratory Medicine
Sunrise Hospital
Las Vegas, Nevada

Ruth J. Barnes
Personnel Manager
City of Orlando
Orlando, Florida

Robert H. Bartels
Vice President
Camplin, Bartels and Associates
Safety and Security Consultants
Chicago, Illinois

Steven O. Beaudoin
Director
Safety Surveillance
Rush-Presbyterian-St. Luke's Medical Center
Chicago, Illinois

William C. Beck
President
Donald Guthrie Foundation for Medical Research
Sayre, Pennsylvania

C. Roger Camplin
President
Camplin, Bartels and Associates
Safety and Security Consultants
Chicago, Illinois

Bruce C. Carlstedt
Associate Professor
Clinical Pharmacy
Purdue University
West Lafayette, Indiana

David H. Gordon
Director
Environmental and Engineering Services
Johns Hopkins Hospital
Baltimore, Maryland

Robert A. Howells
Department of Psychological Sciences
Purdue University
West Lafayette, Indiana

James L. Knight, Jr.
Assistant Professor
School of Industrial Engineering
Purdue University
West Lafayette, Indiana

Warren Kramer
Director of Pharmacy
American International Hospital
Zion, Illinois

Allan J. McLean
Environmental Safety and Health Officer
Rush-Presbyterian-St. Luke's Medical Center
Chicago, Illinois

James H. Moore
Director
Facilities Engineering
Methodist Hospital of Indiana
Indianapolis, Indiana

Alan L. Orvis
Radiation Safety Officer
Mayo Clinic
Rochester, Minnesota

Paul R. Seidlitz
Director
Environmental Services
St. Elizabeth's Hospital
Chicago, Illinois

Earle P. Shoub
Consultant
Safety Products Division
American Optical Corporation
Southbridge, Massachusetts

Paul E. Stanley
Professor Emeritus
School of Engineering
Purdue University
West Lafayette, Indiana

Eleanor R. Wagner
Director
Division of Legal Affairs
Joint Commission on Accreditation of Hospitals
Chicago, Illinois

Barbara L. Webb
Operating Room Supervisor
Methodist Hospital of Indiana
Indianapolis, Indiana

Paul L. Ziemer
Professor and Associate Head
School of Health Sciences
Purdue University
West Lafayette, Indiana

The safety of the people shall be their highest law.

Cicero, 51 B.C.

TABLE OF CONTENTS

General Safety Principles

HOSPITAL SAFETY — AN OVERVIEW

Paul R. Seidlitz

INTRODUCTION

It has been said that the past is prologue. It has also been said there is no new history, just the same events in a different time and place with other people performing the same actions. Both of these statements are true. The past is prologue as can be seen in the study of medicine, and there is no new history as can be seen when we study the safety movement.

HISTORY OF MEDICINE

Since man's beginning, he has been attempting to conquer disease. His early efforts were based on superstition and later empiric remedies. The knowledge of rites and rituals was passed on from generation to generation. When man learned to write and was able to record his observation, knowledge gained through experience could be passed on to others. Medicine in the 20th century is now restudying and reassessing many of these early writings because it appears that early man may have had the solutions to some of our present medical problems.

There are many examples to illustrate this. The early Egyptians describe the importance of blood and encourage warriors to drink the blood of fallen soldiers so that they might have courage. The Egyptian writings also describe the interdependence of the cardiac system and the respiratory system to sustain life. These writings include the description of a procedure to "bring back to life." In the 1950s, this procedure was restudied, the techniques refined, and instrumentation added. The result is a procedure that is almost taken for granted — cardiopulmonary resuscitation.

The first known attempt at a blood transfusion occurred in 1492. Pope Innocent VIII received the blood of four college students. Since nothing was known about typing and cross-matching, the Pope died as did the students. The physician who administered the blood would have died as well but he "removed himself from Rome without delay".

Health care prior to the 17th century was very limited. Physicians could only guess at the diagnosis and experiment with different treatments. If the patient survived the treatments and was declared "cured", the physician would report his findings to fellow physicians who would use his treatment for the same disease process. This empiric approach was not scientific nor could it be because there were no means to measure the results.

One of the first instruments used to assist in the evaluation of a patient's condition was invented by Sanctorius in 1602. It was called a pulsimeter (see Figure 1). It consisted of a simple pendulum and a length of suspended string which was adjusted until the beat of the pendulum coincided with that of the pulse. The measurement observed was the length of the pendulum. This was an instrument that would permit the comparison of rates.

In 1612, Sanctorius described a thermometer to measure body temperature and in 1625, he explained how the thermometer was to be used in studying disease in human patients. The thermometer described by Sanctorius is an adaption of the thermometer invented by Galileo. These may well be the first two instruments used to assess the patient's condition.

In 1707, Sir John Floyer introduced what is considered the first efficient instrument

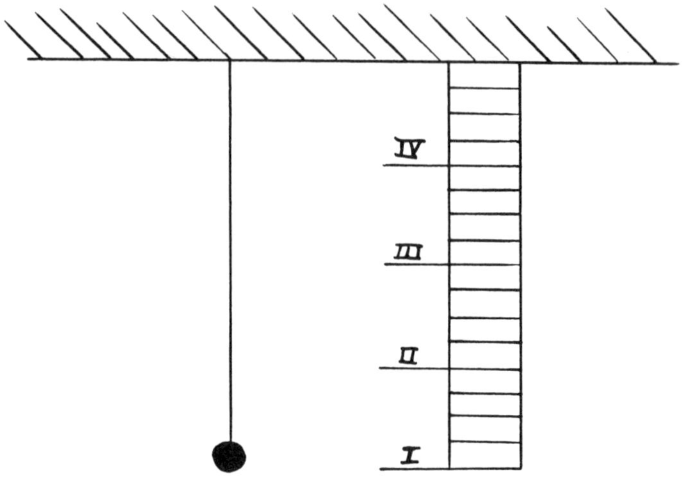

FIGURE 1. The pulsimeter of Sanctorius.

of precision to merit clinical adoption — the physician's pulse watch. In 1761, Auenbrugger invented the stethoscope, and in 1819, Laennec introduced a variation of the stethoscope. The stethoscope as we know it today was introduced about 1840. Some other instruments that were introduced prior to the 20th century were the sphygmomanometer in 1896, the opthalmoscope in 1847, and the syringe in 1855.

As with all new procedures and instruments, there was a great deal of reluctance to use them, which caused unnecessary delays in the treatment of illness. Hospitals, by today's standards, were primitive, overcrowded, and filthy. Patients often recovered in spite of the treatments. The addition of instrumentation permitted more accurate assessment of the patient's condition but the treatments were often more horrible than the disease itself.

One of the sad commentaries that can be made is that war has advanced medical science. Approximately 400 B.C., Hippocrates said "War is the only proper school for the surgeon." Florence Nightingale is credited with improving the quality of medical care during the Crimean War. After the war, a movement was started to continue this higher quality of medical care and find ways to improve it even more.

HISTORY OF SAFETY

In the last half of the 19th century American factories were expanding. It was the time of the industrial revolution. While the factories were superior in terms of production, they were often inferior in terms of human values, health, and safety. In large industrial centers, the ugly results of accidents and poor industrial health conditions became more obvious. Voices of protest were raised.

In 1867, Massachusetts used factory inspectors to assess the quality of the work environment and in 1877, a state law was enacted requiring the guarding of dangerous machinery. Beginning in 1898 there were various attempts to make employers financially liable for injuries received while working, that is, for on-the-job accidents. The first effective workman's compensation act was passed in Wisconsin in 1911 and in 1912, the first national workman's compensation act became law.

War, too, had its effect on the safety movement. Wars, especially those in the 20th century, created labor shortages, and in World War II, these labor shortages dramatically brought home the seriousness of both on- and off-the-job accidents.

This brief history is not meant to encompass all of the advances in medicine and safety but to serve to illustrate that the past is prologue and there is no new history. In medicine, we have been building upon the discoveries of others while in safety, we have not. We still have very serious accidents, the cause of which has not really changed.

To correct this, standards have been and still are being written and adopted. Standards are not new to the health care industry. In 2000 B.C. the code of Hammurabi set up a standard of professional ethics and established a penalty for wrong doing: "If he (the physician) has treated a nobleman for a severe wound and has caused him to die — the physicians hands shall be cut off." The code of Hammurabi also set the fees a physician could charge for services.

Today, the health care delivery system is regulated by many agencies:

State and local departments of health
Occupational Safety and Health Administration (OSHA)
Health, Education and Welfare
Various licensing agencies
Joint Commission on Accreditation of Hospitals (JCAH)

This listing is not all encompassing. Many of these agencies use consensus standards as the basis for their regulations. Many health care workers think the inspection process is new for hospitals; however, the American College of Surgeons had been doing inspections for many years prior to the formation of the JCAH.

In 1953, the JCAH published its first report on hospitals which showed most hospitals had fire hazards of all types. The recommendation made at the time was that hospitals should eliminate hazards and correct fire "problems".

In 1954, the Bureau of Labor Statistics conducted a study of the work-injury experiences hospitals were having. This study showed hospitals sadly trailing industry in recognizing the need for a coordinated safety program, although this study reviewed only work-injury experience and did not study the physical plant.

The JCAH moved into the area of safety slowly. In August 1957, the first radiology standards were adopted and in December of the same year, dietary standards were adopted. Infection control was stressed in March and August of 1958. In 1968, the 1967 Life Safety Code was adopted, and in October of the same year, the National Fire Protection Association Standard Use of Flammable Anesthetics was adopted. The present accreditation manual has been expanded to include all of the above mentioned standards including electrical safety, construction, medical staff, and quality assurance to name just a few. A most interesting aspect of the present accreditation manual is the requirement that the hospital have a safety director who shall have the time to coordinate the safety program of the facility.

In 1970, an independent study showed hospitals were still trailing industry in recognizing the need for coordinated safety programs. Some of the findings were

1. Little or no administrative interest in safety
2. Badly fragmented programs
3. No specific budget
4. Programs geared to incidents — not accident prevention
5. Concern of most programs was employee on-the-job accidents while other injuries were given only occasional interest

The study concluded with, "It appears that hospitals by and large pay lip service to safety and safety-related activities and do so insofar as forced by circumstances."

Hospitals in the 18th and 19th century were single-story structures. The typical ward had beds along the wall and a large coal stove in the center of the room. Lighting was by oil lamps and the nurse had — in addition to her duties to care for patients — the responsibility to fill the oil lamp, trim the wicks of these lamps, empty the ashes from the stove, and fill the stove with coal. The nurse mopped the floors and generally cleaned the ward.

One of the most significant inventions that had a profound effect on health care and safety was the invention of the elevator. Hospitals were no longer required to be single-story structures and with "high rise" buildings came the need for trained personnel to maintain equipment, deliver supplies, etc. The nurse was free to spend more time with the patient. With the addition of personnel came the need for supervision and training. As more instrumentation was added and as technology expanded, the number of people required to maintain the health care delivery system also expanded. This brought entirely new dimensions never before conceived of — supervision of nonmedical personnel. In industry, the role of the supervisor was recognized. Consider this passage from Gardiner's *Practical Foremanship* in 1925:[1]

> If safety work is properly done, it will more than pay its own way. Experience has proven that it has actually increased the output, reduced workers' fears, increased their interest in their jobs, and reduced labor turnover.
>
> From 67 to 75% of all industrial accidents can be prevented. One third of the preventable accidents can be prevented by the mechanical guarding of dangerous machines and equipment. The other two thirds can be prevented by the education of workmen in safe habits, practices, and thoughts.
>
> No one is in a better position to teach the men in the ranks than the foreman. In fact, he must be depended upon to teach safety in the shop. The dollars and cents saved by reducing accidents amount to an immense sum. The values represented in the better spirit in the working force, the prevention of human misery, and the reduction of fear are of even greater importance.[1]

The greatest impact on safety occurred on December 29, 1970 when President Richard Nixon signed the Occupational Safety and Health Act (OSHA) into law. The law went into effect on July 1, 1971 and mandated safe and healthful working conditions for the American worker. The law mandated guarding of machinery. Nothing new here: remember the Massachusetts law passed in 1877 requiring the guarding of dangerous machinery and the passage from Practical Foremanship, "One third of preventable accidents can be prevented by the mechanical guarding of dangerous equipment." OSHA mandated that guarding be accomplished under penalty of law. OSHA mandated training, protective devices, and healthful conditions in the workplace — all designed to reduce accidents. Please note another passage from *Practical Foremanship:*

> In general, the causes of accidents are similar in all plants. Accidents may be due to mechanical hazards, the physical condition of the worker, or the mental condition of the worker. By mechanical hazards is meant the dangers connected with the operating of machinery, the use of unsafe ladders, working without goggles on jobs where chips are apt to fly into the eyes, slippery floors, stairs without handrails, and open elevators. By the physical condition of the worker is meant his condition as a result of the ventilation in the shop, the temperature, the pureness of the air, the light he has to work by, the sanitary condition of the shop, and how tired he may be. These things all have a bearing on how liable a man is to have an accident. By the mental condition of the worker is meant his attitude as a result of ignorance, carelessness, indifference, recklessness, or willful disobedience. Foremen have a responsibility in the prevention of accidents from all the causes mentioned above.

The role of the supervisor is stressed in most articles on management or supervision, or in supervisory workshops. The supervisor sets the example, the supervisor sets the pace, and the supervisor represents management. This is as true now as it was in 1925. This is not new but a restatement of the past.

HOW TO HAVE SAFETY

In the September 1976 issue of the Textile Section newsletter of the National Safety Council, Corporate Director Ralph L. Clark, Safety and Health, Enka, N. C. presented an article "Elements of a Good Safety Program." He described seven basic elements:[2]

Management's responsibilities — Management must understand its responsibility for the safety effort.

Safety director or coordinator — This is generally a staff position and some of the responsibilities are training accident investigation and analysis, and maintenance of progress reports.

Safety committee — This committee is essential to the program because one of its main purposes is to maintain interest in the safety effort.

Supervisor — The supervisor is the key man in accident prevention. The supervisor is involved with daily inspection of the workplace, training and retraining of the employee, and accident investigation. The supervisor implements management's decision regarding safety.

Plant inspections — The inspections are essential to determine accident causes before the fact. The inspection effort should also include employee conduct.

Accident investigation — The purpose is to determine cause and effect relationships so prevention can be accomplished.

Employee responsibility — The employee is essential to the operation and must feel he is responsible for his own safety as well as the safety of his co-workers. The employee should report unsafe conditions to his supervisor and report all accidents, no matter how minor.

There are some individuals who feel that compliance with the standards set by OSHA, JCAH, and others will mean an effective safety program. Nothing could be further from the truth. Compliance with the standards can assure very little if the worker is not motivated to do the job in the prescribed manner. Accidents are caused, and the cause is people.

How many times have you, as a supervisor, observed improper lifting techniques, seen guards removed from dangerous machinery, seen other careless acts, and done nothing to correct the situation? This is not only unhealthful, but will lead to an accident.

Discipline is essential to the safety program but discipline must be consistent. You should also remember that discipline is "corrective training". If the individual supervisor will take this attitude, discipline will take on a whole new meaning. Discipline then will not imply a "chewing out" but will mean an action to correct undesirable behavior.

Todays health care institution is highly complex. We have equipment and technology rarely dreamed of just 20 years ago. With this technology and equipment, the active participation of the supervisor in the safety program is a must. If the supervisor does not exercise the responsibility, the safety program will be weak and, eventually, the price will be paid in accidents. I believe very strongly in the law of averages: an unsafe

Table 1
PROPERTY LOSS AND FIRE

	Number of fires	Estimated property loss
Nursing home	9,300	$6,400,000.00
Hospitals	15,700	$22,200,000.00
Other	5,200	$11,500,000.00
Total	30,200	$40,100,000.00

After National Fire Protection Association Publications, 1975.

act may occur 999 times without an accident, but the 1000th time a serious accident occurs. A good example to illustrate this is the receipt of a traffic ticket. How many times have you broken the law by exceeding the speed limit, not coming to a complete stop, running a yellow signal — and not getting caught? When you finally are apprehended, "the law of averages" has just reached your level of carelessness.

The health care supervisor is involved at a number of different levels with the facilities safety program. As you read on in this book, you, the supervisor, will gain insights into a number of different areas.

Electrical safety has become a great concern in the past several years. As our technology expanded, so did the types of electrical equipment, clinical and nonclinical, and the realization that we have a potential hazard.

Electrical power was newly discovered in 1743 when Krueger predicted that electricity would play a very important role in health care. He could scarcely have imagined just how much a role electricity does play in the health care system today.

We know a great deal about electricity and the potential for harm it can cause. In 1791, Luigi Galvani demonstrated that muscle action could be induced with electricity, and in 1800, Alessandro Volta demonstrated that a muscle could be placed in a state of continuous contraction by repeated electrical stimulation. We take such information for granted today but we forget that we have instruments that can be applied directly to the heart and only a very small amount of electric current can produce the effect described by Volta. If the supervisor can understand this and convey this message to others, electrical safety need not be a problem.

The supervisor must be ever watchful to insure employees and patients follow the electrical safety programs of the facility. Shortcuts, makeshift equipment, and home repairs to electrical equipment must not be tolerated.

Smoking is another problem area. In 1975 the National Fire Protection Association (NFPA) reported the fire statistics for health care facilities shown in Table 1. Some authorities have expressed the opinion that these losses could have been reduced by at least 50% had the supervisor enforced the smoking regulations of the facility. In the same report, the NFPA reports that in 1975 there were 137,800 smoking-related fires out of 1,264,400 building fires reported. There are efforts in many states to forbid smoking in hospitals but I feel this effort, like many others, will not correct the problem. Effective supervision of employees and patients to insure compliance with the smoking policy of the facility appears to be the only answer. Another law alone will not stop smoking.

In one facility, smoking was forbidden and the rule was enforced. But people being what they are, were hiding in bathrooms and closets to have that cigarette. The number of fire experiences increased. On the other hand, as soon as an authorized smoking area was designated and the "no smoking" rule was strictly enforced in other posted areas, the number of fires was reduced. To be effective, regulations must be enforced, but unrealistic regulations will not and cannot be enforced. Much of what has been discussed so far relates to the employee and the supervisor. A health care facility has one more element — the patient.

Our concern for the safety and well-being of the patient has been recognized for many years. Whenever there is a discussion about the patient safety, we quote from Florence Nightingale: "It may seem a strange principle to enunciate as the very first requirement in a hospital is that it should do the sick no harm."

In recent years we have become very concerned about patient safety. Some of this concern is the result of the JCAH activity, increased malpractice experience, and a better-informed public.

As was previously mentioned, the Joint Commission Accreditation Manual stresses safety.[3] The concerns for the patient, however, are not all in the section entitled "Functional Safety and Sanitation". There are standards covering the medical and nursing audit to ensure that the ordered treatment, medications, and procedures were carried out in accordance with the physician's orders and without adverse effect to the patient. There are medical staff committees that review the quality of care delivered, review drugs, including new and experimental drugs, blood transfusions, and reactions. There are medical and hospital staff committees that review infection control and the policies relating thereto. A credentials committee reviews the qualifications of a proposed medical staff appointment. Everything that is going on is subject to a review, all aimed at ensuring that the patient is receiving the best possible care. But even with all of this emphasis, the incidence of malpractice litigation has increased dramatically.

SOME CASE HISTORIES

One of the most famous malpractice cases occurred in Illinois in 1960. A young man, 18 years old, fractured his leg while playing football. He was taken to the emergency room where a physician, with the assistance of the hospital staff, applied traction to reduce the fracture and applied a plaster cast. A heat cradle was applied to assist in the drying of the cast. Not long after the application of the cast, the patient complained of pain in his toes, which protruded from the cast. The toes became swollen and dark and eventually, cold and insensitive. The day after the cast was applied and these symptoms appeared, the physician who had applied the cast "notched" the cast around the toes, and the next day cut the cast 3 in. above the foot. The physician split the sides of the cast within three days of application. While cutting the cast, the patient's leg was cut on both sides. Blood and other seepage was observed and a great stench was noted. Fourteen days after admission, the patient was transferred to a large medical center and placed in the care of an orthopedic specialist. The specialist removed the cast and found the broken limb had a considerable amount of dead tissue which, in his opinion, resulted from the interference of circulation of blood in the limb caused by swelling of the leg against the cast. Several efforts were made to save the leg, but ultimately it had to be amputated 8 in. below the knee. The young man sued.

Among other things, the young man (now the plaintiff) contended that in a case such as this it was the duty of the nurses to watch the protruding toes constantly for changes of color, temperature, and movement and to check circulation every 10 to 20 min. The evidence in the case showed that these things were done only a few times a day. The plaintiff argued that the hospital was negligent. They had failed to have at all times a sufficient number of trained nurses for bedside care of all patients, capable of recognizing the progressive gangrenous condition of the plaintiff's right leg and of bringing it to the attention of the hospital administration and the medical staff so that adequate consultation could have been secured and the condition rectified.

The court said that on the basis of the evidence before the jury, it could reasonably have concluded that the nurses did not test for circulation in the leg as frequently as necessary and that skilled nurses would have promptly recognized the conditions that signal a dangerous impairment of circulation in the plaintiff's leg, and would have known that the condition would become irreversible in a matter of hours. At that point, the court said, it became the nurses' duty to inform the attending physician, and if he failed to act, to advise the hospital authorities so that appropriate action might be taken.

As this case illustrates, reasonable care must be taken. Follow all accepted procedures and documents. It may be that his leg was checked and the physician was called, but it was not documented. Had we been doing medical and nursing audits, training the staff (both medical and nursing), and assuring good documentation, this incident could have been prevented. When one reviews current litigation, one sees the same type of cases described. The awards are very high and this results in higher premiums and great concern for the patient's welfare.

Another area of concern is medication safety. There are more and more drugs being introduced every year. There are the generic equivalents with strange-sounding names. We have medications that can be administered by more than one route and this can lead to medication errors. For example, a registered nurse received a written order from a physician calling for the administration of 3 cc of Lanoxin® to an infant patient. The nurse, thinking the drug was to be administered by an injection and not realizing that it could be administered orally, questioned the order by approaching two other physicians in the hospital at the time. The physicians, believing that the nurse knew the drug was to be administered orally, told her the dosage was not too great and advised her to follow the order. The nurse did not attempt to contact the physician who had written the order. The nurse administered 3 cc of Lanoxin® by injection, and the infant died as a result of drug overdose. As more drugs are introduced, a new problem has been introduced — incompatibility. The physician and nurse must have drug-compatibility information available. A drug profile should be maintained on each patient to assure a ready reference to the drugs the patient has received and is now receiving.

There is an information explosion, not only for medicine but for the general public. As our technology advances, the public often has the data before the professionals and asks for the latest treatments, medications, etc. The patient is not aware of procedures; he is sick and wants to be cured.

DETERRENTS TO SAFETY

Television has had a great influence on safety. The medical programs often are shown in prime time. These programs have led the public to believe there is a very high quality of medical care and that we will be able to cure them — no matter what the affliction. Some of these programs have described malpractice and what a physician was alleged to have done wrong. This has exerted, I am sure, a great influence on the entire malpractice problem.

The public has access to a great deal of medical information. In any good bookstore you can find whole sections with material on health, case histories, and medical textbooks. There are popular magazines with medical information, some of which can be very misleading. In one magazine, an article described an individual with a brain tumor and her symptoms. A statement appeared that people with similar symptoms could have a brain tumor. The article described her treatment by the hospital staff — some of it quite bad. How many patients have had similar treatment and filed a suit, and how much influence did this article have?

The patients can also be dangerous to members of the hospital staff. The individual who is using chemicals, i.e., alcohol or drugs, is the greatest danger to all members of the hospital staff. In years past, many of these patients were admitted under some other diagnosis. This still happens today but, I am happy to say, not as frequently.

Several years ago, when I was working as a staff nurse, a patient was admitted with a diagnosis of "acute gastritis". The patient became confused, disoriented, and highly combative 36 hr after admission. The patient injured two employees, one seriously enough to require hospitalization. This is one instance of how a physician created a hazard. Absolute truth about the patient's condition is necessary so that incidents such as this can be prevented.

When a patient is admitted, he is confronted with all sorts of rules and regulations, many of which are not heard. The patient is concerned about his health, the disease, the family, and of course, the prognosis. This can lead to all sorts of unusual behavior which is manifested by failure to adhere to "the rules", and this creates problems for the medical and nursing staff. One of the most frequent and more serious problems is falls — from beds, from chairs, and on the floor. To prevent falls on the floor, keep the floors dry and in good repair. To prevent falls from chairs, insure the patient is "secured" in the chair and has the signal cord readily accessible. Falls from beds, however, are more complicated. The most frequent cause of falls from bed is overreaching. To prevent these falls, keep commonly used items within easy reach and keep the signal cord readily accessible. Another cause is getting in and out of bed without assistance. Constant surveillance, educational reinforcement, and keeping the signal cord within easy reach can help prevent this type of incident. Patients do crawl over side rails and fall. In many cases, these patients are confused and the best solution to prevent these falls is to place the patient near the nursing station so that he can be watched more frequently.

Another patient safety problem previously alluded to is smoking. There are no easy solutions to this issue. Patients who smoke will do so, no matter what the restrictions. The JCAH does have some standards, but how these can be enforced effectively has not been determined.

THE ANSWER

The answer to many of our patient safety problems appears to be in proper education. As indicated earlier, a great deal of information is available to the public, some of it erroneous. The public schools are doing a great deal to properly educate the students and this same effort must be extended to the adult population. Many hospitals have initiated comprehensive patient education programs. While this effort is good, the "bedside nurse" is in the best position to educate and teach the patient. It must be remembered that patients do not act or react like "normal" people. Patients require constant reinforcement of all information. This includes rules, regulations, policies, and procedures. The staff should not only explain the what, but also the why. If the reasons are understood, gaining cooperation should be easier.

Care of children in our modern health care facility presents quite a challenge. While we may have problems with adult patients, these are nothing compared to the difficulties encountered when treating children. Care of the pediatric patient requires constant attention to detail and the entire staff must be watchful. Children are extremely active and the most likely to fall from bed. Children like to climb and crawl and they dislike anything that impedes this freedom. Children can create hazards for themselves, their peers, and the hospital staff. Toys are the frequent cause of problems. Well-meaning parents, aunts, uncles, and grandparents bring all sorts of toys to entertain the child. Many of these toys may be safe at home but are very dangerous in the health care environment. A few years ago, in a hospital in one of the Chicago suburbs, a child in a croupette was given a friction-operated toy. The croupette was flooded with oxygen and when the child played with the toy, the heat from the toy caused the bed liners to ignite and within a few seconds, the entire bed was engulfed in flames. The child died as a result of the fire.

Other factors that must be considered when selecting toys are (1) small pieces, (2) breakability, (3) sharp edges, and (4) washability. In addition, community education programs are a must in all levels of health care for the prevention of accidents.

Through this overview, I have attempted to describe briefly, and somewhat randomly, some of the problems the hospital safety officer must work with every day. There must be a hospital-wide team effort to reduce the possibility of accidents to the patient, the visitor, and the employee. Safety is a serious responsibility. Many of the problems described have existed as long as we have had medical practice. Some of the religious rituals are based on the belief that following them will prevent disease and injury. The origin of these rituals were based on fact, but in our modern times we have lost sight of this. However, since some of the same problems are recurring, we are in the process of reassuring these values. Since man's earliest beginnings, he has been interacting with his environment, and when machines were added, his life became more complex. Today, we add new machines which create many of the same problems primitive man was faced with; we "create" hazardous conditions. We should learn from our past. The information is there and we must seek it out and apply what we have learned. You, the reader, can take the collective thoughts of the authors of the various sections of this book and apply their knowledge to create hazard-free hospitals. To paraphrase Florence Nightingale again: "The very first requirement in a hospital is that it should do the sick and staff no harm."

REFERENCES

1. **Gardiner, G. L.,** *Practical Foremanship,* McGraw-Hill, New York, 1925.
2. **Clarke, R. L.,** Elements of a good safety program, in National Safety Council News Letter, Textile Section, Chicago, September 1976.
3. Accreditation Manual for Hospitals, Joint Commission on Accreditation of Hospitals, Chicago, 1979.

SAFETY CONSIDERATIONS FOR HOSPITAL POPULATIONS

Robert A. Howells and James L. Knight, Jr.*

INTRODUCTION

The modern hospital represents a dynamic and complex environment that is utilized by several different and distinct groups that constitute the overall user population. Behavioral scientists have long known that certain aspects of groups, such as their size, homogeneity, mean age, and psychological limitations, are related to group behavior. One of the most often cited examples of the relationship between the composition of a group and its behavioral propensities is found in experiments concerning the willingness of bystanders to lend assistance at crime and accident scenes. In general, the results of such research indicate that group size and homogeneity are strong determiners, within limits, of the behavior of individuals in the group of bystanders. In large groups, a diffusion of responsibility for rendering assistance develops between group members to the extent that few, if any, individuals feel compelled to act. In small groups, where responsibility can be spread among only a few individuals, the probability that an individual in the group will exhibit helping behavior is high. Helping behavior is even more likely when the group is homogeneous. For example, a group composed of college students who know each other would be more likely to exhibit helping behavior at an accident than a heterogeneous group composed of strangers.

Bryan and Test provided an illustration of the relationship between psychological limitations, such as the amount of exposure to positive role models, and the behavior of individuals in a group of motorists. Group members were more likely to lend assistance to a stranded motorist when they were previously exposed to examples of other motorists who served as role models engaged in helping behavior.[3]

Although the relationship between the physical or psychological characteristics of a group and the behavior of its individual members cannot be precisely specified, the above examples clearly illustrate that it is important to consider these and other group properties before attempting to predict group member behavior. Modern hospitals are designed to provide patients, staff, and visitors with a safe and protective recovery or work environment, free from accidental injury or death.[4] A hospital or related health care facility should, in order to fulfill this mandate, be designed in such a manner that the safety behavior of the users of the facility will be promoted. Because the overall hospital-user populations have traditionally been partitioned into distinct groups, it is important that hospital designers, administrators, and all employees associated with safety program implementation consider these groups with respect to any characteristics that might influence the safety-related behavior of their members.[5-8]

The purpose of this chapter is to provide a logical partitioning of the hospital-user population into distinct groups, define and describe the general physical, psychological, or cognitive factors influencing each group with respect to its safety behavior, and to describe the special considerations that must be applied to certain groups. Finally, a list of interesting, timely, and relevant resources is provided for the further study of the safety requirements and considerations of groups within the overall hospital-user population.

* Currently at Bell Telephone Laboratories, Holmdel, New Jersey.

FACTORS THAT INFLUENCE SAFETY BEHAVIOR

The purpose of this section is to provide a general and somewhat hospital-oriented definition and introductory description of the various factors that influence the safety-related behavior of group members. In the following section, these factors will be discussed with respect to specific groups within the overall hospital-user population.

Cognitive Factors

The term "cognitive" refers to a general psychological concept encompassing all forms of knowing and includes the processes of perceiving, imagining, reasoning, judging, and remembering.[9] Several important factors that influence the safety-related behavior of the members of a group follow directly from this definition and are thus labeled "cognitive factors".

Knowledge

Knowledge forms the basis for understanding and developing desirable attitudes concerning safe behavior. Ideally, each member of a group should learn and respect safety rules and procedures. This ideal situation, however, is rarely, if ever, realized. The dramatic reduction in industrial accidents in recent years is the direct result of safety programs that educate workers and develop positive safety habits and attitudes.[10,11] Adequate knowledge is important because it enables individuals to recognize and evaluate dangerous situations, avoid hazardous situations, and react appropriately when confronted by a hazard.

In order for a group member to perform some function safely, that individual must possess an adequate knowledge about the environment of interest. This environmental knowledge must include a description of the environment in terms of its objects and locations, a description of what is to be achieved, and a description of the operating characteristics of the objects or devices that the individual will manipulate, operate, or interact with. Finally, the knowledge must include a description of how the desired task may be accomplished. For example, the laboratory technician running various chemical tests must have an adequate knowledge of the physical layout of the workspace and the locations of all equipment and supplies that will be used. The technician must also know what tests are to be performed and the method by which the tasks may be accomplished correctly and safely. Finally, the individual must be able to properly operate the machinery or equipment that will be used to perform the tests.

A knowledge of specific hazards in the environment of interest is a specialized form of environmental knowledge that must be possessed by group members if they are to maintain safe performance. Hospitals, as will be illustrated later, contain a large number of very specific safety hazards including toxic chemicals, explosive gases, radioactive isotopes and devices, steam sterilizers, slippery floors and stairways, infectious materials and wastes, and various mechanical devices. For example, if the laboratory technician knows that a highly toxic or volatile liquid will be generated during a test procedure, the proper precautions may be taken to keep the chemical under safe containment so that safety will not be compromised. If the individual does not understand that a specific hazard situation is created by the test being performed, the risk of accidental injury is obviously increased.

A knowledge of remedial procedures is required in the event that some problem, which must be corrected in order to maintain a safe and satisfactory environment with respect to the task being performed, develops. If an individual does not have adequate knowledge of the correct remedial procedure, an attempt to rectify a problem can be more hazardous or costly than a failure to take any corrective action. Suppose that the laboratory technician, in the above example, is present when a volatile liquid spills and ignites. If the individual attempts to extinguish the fire using inappropriate procedures or equipment, the fire might be spread to a larger area and thus become even more hazardous than it would have been if no attempt to extinguish it had been made.

A knowledge of the procedures for reporting hazards is important for the preservation of safety through accident prevention. According to the psychological principle of least effort, an individual would be more likely to report a potential safety hazard such as a gas leak or frayed electrical cord if the reporting procedures were understood rather than if the procedures were disorganized, unclear, complex, or inaccessible.[9] In this example, the technician would be more likely to report a defective piece of laboratory apparatus as a potential safety hazard (thus facilitating repairs and avoiding a future accident), if the procedures for reporting safety hazards were well publicized, simple, and clearly explained. It should be noted that the same principles apply to accident incident reporting procedures.

Attitudes

An attitude is a relatively stable and enduring predisposition to behave or react in a certain way toward persons, objects, institutions, or issues.[12] Attitudes are tendencies to respond to people, institutions, issues, or events either positively or negatively. The sources of attitudes are cultural, familial, and personal; individuals tend to assume the attitudes which prevail in the culture in which they are raised.[13] Some attitudes are passed from generation to generation through the family structure, but many attitudes are developed through both formal learning and everyday experience.[14] It is important to realize, however, that attitudes may be directly manipulated through various propaganda and persuasion techniques, many of which can be effectively implemented in the development and promotion of hospital safety programs.[15-17]

It is clear that if the members of a group have negative attitudes concerning safety, the group will not be predisposed to perform safely. Thus, it is imperative that positive attitudes are established and maintained in the hospital-user population. Perhaps the most important set of positive safety-related attitudes are those concerning the prevention of accidents. The reason why this particular set of attitudes is so important is that an optimally effective safety program is difficult, if not impossible, to establish unless the majority of the individuals who will be affected by the program are actively predisposed to cooperate. Heyd and Eader and Surry noted that recent trends in safety management have focused upon both the removal of the notion that "safety is the responsibility of the safety committee" and the need to instill the attitude that "safety is everybody's business".[18,19]

A second important set of safety-related attitudes concerns the learning of safety procedures. In order for a group to exhibit safe behavior, its members must do more than cooperate with safety programs for accident prevention. Each individual should be encouraged to maintain an attitude of interest by actively contributing to the success of accident prevention. People with such active interests in accident prevention will probably devote more time and attention to the learning of safety procedures that prevent accidents, as well as to those that should be undertaken after an accident has occurred. If individuals devote insufficient time or attention to the development of a thorough understanding of these safety procedures, their ability to contribute to the safety of a group would be, at best, doubtful.

A third noteworthy set of safety-related attitudes concerns the reporting of accidents or safety incidents. The importance of accident- and safety incident reporting in formally organized safety programs has often been demonstrated.[4,18,20-22] The data concerning breaches in safety permit an ongoing evaluation of a safety program when properly utilized and serve as a valuable tool for assessing the effectiveness of safety program policy, personnel, hardware, or training modifications. If potential safety hazards are not reported promptly, unambiguously, and to the proper authority, it is possible that the hazard may not be removed and an accident may occur. If accidents are not reported, the hazard that caused the accident may be ignored and will, therefore, remain the potential cause of further accidents. Accident and hazard reports thus serve to prevent future accidents and, when properly analyzed, can provide information about the success of safety management programs.

A number of methods exist for the establishment and manipulation of the attitudes and opinions of group members. Persuasion and motivational techniques tend to be specific to particular situations and contexts, and must be selected and implemented accordingly.[2] Some very general and relevant psychological concepts should be noted, however, with respect to the sets of safety attitudes currently under discussion. Desirable safety attitudes can be fostered through the careful use of rewards. Group members can be rewarded for displaying attitudes and behavior consistent with the goals of a safety program. In addition, rewards can be used to develop and maintain an interest in learning safety procedures and in reporting accidents. Reward systems may be established in several ways including the use of such rewards as money, prizes, promotions, extra vacation days, privileges, and social status. Punishment — the counterpart of reward — should be used only with great caution. Indeed, care must be taken that certain aversive or punishing factors are not inherent in various safety program procedures. Accident reporting, for example, may include such factors when an individual faces disciplinary action if accused of negligence or responsibility for an accident. Similarly, if a friend or co-worker may be fired or disciplined when charged with unsafe behavior, an individual may find the notion of filing an accident report to be aversive. Tedious, difficult, or excessively complex reporting procedures, as well as procedures that interfere with routine duties, may also be punishing. Since the effect of punishment is the suppression of behavior, the punishment factors inherent in some forms of accident or hazard reporting may serve to increase the probability that attitudes concerning accident reports will be undesirable and, therefore, decrease the likelihood that a report will be made. Thus, reporting procedures and policies must be structured in such a manner that reward factors are maximized while punishment factors are minimized.

Another psychological concept relevant to the development of desirable safety attitudes is known as cognitive dissonance-reduction. This involves the notion that when an individual's attitudes and behavior are not consistent with each other, an attitude shift occurs in the direction of the behavior.[23] Brehm et al. have provided convincing demonstrations of this phenomenon.[24] The dissonance-reduction effect may be applied in cases where the strengthening of positive safety attitudes in specific groups or individuals is desired. For example, individuals who exhibit poor safety attitudes should show an improvement after they participate in various safety-related activities. A related concept that is useful in influencing the development of appropriate safety attitudes involves the acceptance of persuasive messages.[16] Once an individual accepts a persuasive message slightly, the probability of later full acceptance increases. Thus, if a safety supervisor desires to persuade an individual or group to adopt a more active attitude concerning accident prevention, it may be advisable to ask the group for a small commitment during an initial persuasion attempt. Such an approach is likely to result in the acceptance of a larger commitment that will be required in the future.

Another concept that is relevant to the development of appropriate safety attitudes in groups is known as locus-of-control. People who believe themselves to be internally (self) controlled respond differently to persuasion attempts than do those individuals who perceive themselves as controlled by external factors. Biondo and MacDonald demonstrated that individuals who are external in their perceived locus-of-control are responsive to both strong and weak persuasion attempts.[15] Internal individuals, however, tend to resist strong persuasion attempts but often respond to moderate efforts.

A further psychological concept of interest here might be termed "acceptance of performance responsibility". If an individual fails to exhibit appropriate safety attitudes and behavior or is involved in numerous accidents, safety-related attitudes and performance might be improved if the indiviual is taught to take the responsibility for accident involvement. The individual might believe that his or her actions and attitudes have nothing to do with successful and unsuccessful safety performance. If such a person is taught that successful safety performance is a matter of appropriate attitudes and effort, a more appropriate safety potential may be realized. This phenomenon has been demonstrated in the context of remedial education programs.[25]

Role Homogeneity and Communications Structure

The effects of the homogeneity of roles played by the member of a group, as well as its communications structure, have somewhat obvious and related effects upon safety-related behavior. These effects may be of particular importance with respect to safety training and accident reporting.

Role homogeneity refers to the relationship between an individual's behavior and the behavior of other group members. When a group is homogeneous with respect to safety goals, procedures, plans for action, and personal responsibilities, there are few obstacles to impede the flow of information within the group. For example, all group members are aware of safety plans and procedures for a specific hazard. In a specialized group, it is likely that all members will understand the relevant technical jargon and equipment operation procedures that may be required to prevent accidents or to deal with problems after they have occurred. In heterogeneous groups, the ease of information flow might be impeded by the different educational backgrounds, technical jargons, individual responsibilities, and safety experiences of the group members. Indeed, the gap between these group members may be large enough that some individuals may avoid communication with people in other roles. A similar effect can be noted in that employees are often reluctant to contact their supervisors or other supervisors, especially if the communication involves negative information such as the news that an accident occurred. These problems have been tacitly addressed in various hospital safety programs.[5,8]

Homogeneous groups may have an additional advantage over heterogeneous groups with respect to the loss of an individual's services. If an individual is absent or injured, others in the group can easily serve as replacements. In a heterogeneous group, individuals may possess distinctly different roles and training experiences, and thus might not serve as effective replacements for each other. The problem would be greatest, of course, if the individual to be replaced serves a critical safety function requiring specialized training such as radiation or toxic substance control.

Communication structure refers to the provisions for the flow of information between different individuals, departments, and management levels. Lateral information flow within a group of employees from a small department (for example, intensive care unit nurses) should rarely present a problem. Comprehensive hospital-wide safety programs are complex and involve virtually the whole management hierarchy. A hierarchical management structure must meet at least two important information-flow requirements with respect to effective safety programs. First, there must be a downward flow of information that will specify program goals, summarize present performance, and specify major corrective actions that need to be taken in order to achieve the goals. This information must descend to the lower levels in a form that preserves the intent and meaning. In addition, care should to taken to ensure that the flow of information is not impeded at any particular level. If the information concerning what is desired does not reach all those who must accomplish the necessary tasks, the safety program will not be successful. Second, an upward information flow from the lowest to the highest management levels is necessary for the establishment and maintenance of a successful safety program. Information about specific hazards, worker performance, procedure effectiveness, morale, accident events, and recommendations for change must flow upward in an unimpeded fashion, for it serves as a valuable feedback source which, among other things, allows upper management to determine whether or not program goals are being met. If goals are not being met, then the proper analysis of the upward flow of information should reveal the nature of the required changes.

The upward- and downward information-flow requirements can influence safety training as well as program management. In order for successful training to be accomplished, trainees must be aware of performance goals or behavioral objectives that are to be attained, and the means by which the goals will be achieved. If a trainee (or teacher) is not made aware of what should be learned (or taught) or of how the skill will be developed, the training experience will be less than optimal. Trainee performance serves as an upward flow of information to the instructor in that it specifies whether or not further instruction is needed and often dictates the nature of any further training. The level of performance at the conclusion of training also serves as upward information flow to upper management, which may play a role in future personnel decisions with respect to particular safety responsibilities that can be fulfilled by employees of various training levels. In addition, performance-level information can be used in the evaluation and modification of training programs. For example, if training in patient-accident prevention does not reduce the actual patient-accident incidence, the training program may be inappropriate or require various changes.

The free flow of information is vital to the success of large scale safety programs. In general, where busy employees are charged with the implementation of safety communications, such as reporting a hazard or an accident occurrence, the procedures involved should not be so complex or time-consuming that an individual is reluctant to follow them. Communication barriers between departments or management levels should be minimized. One department or level should not be hesitant to contact another for reasons such as the fear of criticism or a reluctance to endure complex bureaucratic procedures. An effort should be made in all instances of safety communications, to encourage information-sharing. A constructive attitude to establish is that the report of a safety problem is appreciated and welcomed because everyone in the organization will benefit when someone makes an effort to provide a safe environment.

Relative Authority and Social Position

Because a hospital environment requires the interaction of several distinct user groups, it is natural to consider the effects of the relative authority and social position of each group on safety-related behaviors. Although little, if any, research has been undertaken with respect to such effects in hospital safety situations, several interesting hypotheses may be offered.

First, relative authority and social position will affect the degree of safety-related motivation and stress experienced by the members of a group. Consider, for example, the differential authority and social positions held by members of different groups within a hospital. The average visitor experiences little, if any, motivation or stress related to accident prevention or other safety issues beyond those that directly impinge upon his or her personal welfare. A nurse, however, should be highly motivated to prevent accidents — a potential hazard should represent a source of stress. These effects will be due largely to the awareness of the importance of safety that has been instilled through professional experiences, safety training, and formal safety-motivation programs. Thus, one form of the relative authority and social position effect can be termed a knowledge or training-based motivation/stress differential. Another form of this effect is rooted in the individual's tendency to avoid punishment or aversive experiences and can be termed an avoidance effect. This phenomenon may be illustrated by comparing the authority differential between, for example, an experienced physician and a maintenance worker. If the worker makes a minor safety-related error, the experience may be quite stressful because the consequences of the error may be aversive. Thus, the worker will be motivated to perform safely. A physician, however, is unlikely to be dealt with in a manner that would be perceived as very aversive, in a relative sense, when a minor safety error occurs. A physician would be less likely to be disciplined for creating a wet floor hazard than a custodian. In this case, therefore, the physician is not as likely as the custodian to perceive routine safety problems as sources of stress and is thus not as motivated to avoid such stress through safe performance. It should be noted, however, that other forms of motivation for safe performance, such as altruistic motives, may influence the behavior of group members. According to the classic Yerkes-Dodson law, motivation affects performance in a positive sense only when the level of motivation is at some optimum value.[26,27] This value varies with the specific tasks, performance environment, and individuals involved.

A second hypothesis that may be offered is that relative authority and social position effects will influence individual risk-taking behavior. In a manner similar to that expressed for the previous hypothesis, employees who perceive a safety performance oversight as potentially aversive in its consequences will be less likely to risk violating safety policies. If all other motivational and stress factors are equal, it is likely that as the individual's relative authority and social position in a group or institution increases, the degree of personal risk-taking behavior acceptable to the individual also increases.

A third hypothesis that may be proposed is that relative authority and social position effects will influence individual accident- or hazard-reporting behavior. For example, a visitor might be less likely to report a potential hazard if hospital employees were present. The employees may be perceived by the visitor as apparent authorities who are charged with the responsibility of detecting and removing potential hazards. In this case, the perceived authority and role differential between visitor and employee group members creates what may be termed a responsibility transfer, where the responsibility for reporting a safety hazard is shifted to a member of a group possessing more authority. This effect would be especially strong for visitors or patients in the presence of hospital employees but might also exist between various employee groups. For example, if a nurse discovers a hazard in a piece of surgical equipment she may assume that the doctor who uses the equipment has the responsibility of tagging the equipment as defective and arranging for its repair. These employee intergroup effects may also operate in a reverse fashion. Suppose that a nurse discovers a pool of water in a heavily traveled hallway. If the nurse knows that a janitor is on duty in the area, the responsibility for detecting and removing the hazard may be transferred from nurse to janitor. Here, the responsibility shift is not from a lower to higher authority or social position, but to a person in a position of more relevance to the removal of the particular hazard. The safety management problem in such cases can be reduced to the need for all members of the hospital-user population to be made aware that safety is everyone's concern.

Stress

Each of the various groups that constitute the hospital-user population can be subject to characteristic sources and levels of stress. The particular stress sources which concern each specific group will be considered in the following section. At present, however, it is important to define and understand the nature of stress and stress phenomena which may affect safety-related behaviors.

Stress is defined as pressure from an adverse force or influence that imposes unusual demands on an organism.[2] Stress is a response to stress-producing stimuli called stressors. Examples of stressor stimuli are physical injury, emotional crises, extreme temperatures, pain, infection, and various stimuli that impose unusual psychological demands. An individual's response to stress, called the stress reaction, involves an interruption of the body's homeostatic balance. Typically, an increase in the pituitary secretion of ACTH results in an excess of adrenal corticoids. After this disturbance occurs, the individual usually attempts to remove the stressor and/or recover from the effects of stress reaction itself. The disrupting effect of long-term stress upon behavior and both physical and mental health has received much attention.[28-31] Research has shown, in general, that prolonged stress can produce psychological disorders, damage to the gastrointestinal system, heart disease, other physical damage, and even death. Several subjective factors that can influence the severity of the stress reaction have been identified. When a stressor is familiar and predictable to the extent that an individual may anticipate its occurrence, the stress response will be less extreme than when the stressor is unfamiliar and unpredictable.[29,32] The stress and anxiety levels associated with some stress-producing tasks can be reduced when the individual learns that it is possible to successfully cope with such tasks and their accompanying stress.[33]

The process of coping with stress is complex and has several interesting aspects. When the individual must cope with several continuous, nonspecific, and long-lasting stressors, the response is a three stage process called the general adaptation syndrome. The first stage is an alarm reaction and involves both vascular and nervous depression which are later followed by the previously described ACTH production. The second stage is a stress-resistance process in which a specific stressor receives increased resistance, while the resistance to the other stressors is decreased. The final stage is typified by exhaustion and an inability to maintain adaptation to stress. If the stress continues, or if a new source of stress is introduced, the death of the now defenseless individual may occur.[28] Thus, it is apparent that stress caused by continuous, nonspecific stressors that are of sufficient duration to drive an individual into the exhaustion stage will radically affect the ability to cope with stress and maintain safe performance.

Another source of interference with the ability to cope with stress is called learned helplessness. This phenomenon concerns the effect of repeated exposure to moderate stressors over which the individual has no control. Such experiences can be almost as devastating as exposure to overwhelming stressors because when an individual lives in an uncontrollable and stressful environment, the ability to cope with future stress diminishes.[34] An important point to note is that the individual can, in fact, learn through experience that future stress cannot be dealt with successfully. This learning ability implies that the individual must be capable of learning to cope with stress, and this has been demonstrated in the previously mentioned research of Ruff and Korchin.[33]

Safety programs should be designed in such a manner that the stress imposed by the work load, management, tools and equipment, co-workers, specific task demands, and other sources of pressure is minimized. It is also important to consider the individual's state of health as a source of stress — a fact of particular importance in the context of hospital patient safety.

Group Control Time

The time interval during which the members of a group are in contact with a formally organized and administered safety program may have a large impact upon important processes such as safety training, safety motivation, and the enforcement of safety policies. Transient groups within the hospital-user population, such as visitors and patients, are generally available neither for a sufficient time interval nor in a suitable capacity for safety training or motivation. However, some effective degree of safety training, motivation, and awareness may be possible through the use of aggressive in-house or local community safety promotion and motivation programs.[5]

Hospital employees are generally available for a sufficient period of time to permit the implementation of appropriate, effective, and efficient safety training, motivation, and enforcement procedures. Possible exceptions to this statement, however, might include physicians with hospital privileges who are in the hospital only on a limited basis for patient contact and staff meetings. Such personnel should be both included in safety programs and encouraged to actively participate in safety meetings and activities since they often utilize specialized and potentially dangerous equipment and must be aware of relevant safety procedures. Further, these staff members, due to their social and authority positions within the hospital, represent a group that will potentially serve an important resource and leadership function during routine daily safety activity as positive role models, and as team leaders and safety managers during acute safety emergencies.

Accountability Degree and Consequence Domain

The effects specified here are closely related to those of the relative authority and social position factors previously discussed. Here, however, the topics of interest are the degree of a group's accountability for safety performance and the set of possible consequences that its members must suffer when safety performance errors are committed. These factors can affect several processes that are essential to the maintenance of safe performance in a hospital.

Safety training is one important process that is affected by a group's accountability degree or consequence domain. When a group is highly accountable or liable for safety violations, or the potential consequences of an accident are grave, the amount of training in safety policies and procedures is likely to be increased, and/or the performance criteria to be achieved in training might be raised. Such training measures, when coupled with appropriate group member selection and motivational procedures, can serve to increase the precision of safety performance.

Safety enforcement is an important process that operates in a similar fashion. When safety liability is high and the consequences of an accident are serious, safety policy enforcement must typically be more strict than in a low liability-low risk environment. If the consequences of safety errors to be faced by an individual are those which have been established by hospital management rather than by the laws of physics, good management policy dictates that the severity of the consequences be related to the degree of risk or liability that was incurred as a result of the errors.

Risk-taking behavior represents another process that is affected by the accountability degree and consequence domain factors. When safety accountability and/or accident consequences are high (within limits), the degree of risk that is tolerable in safety-related tasks is likely to be low. It is likely that the decision-making processes used by a safety-motivated individual are based upon the desire to achieve a specified level of safe performance and thus constitute approach behaviors. However, as the degree of accountability and/or consequence possibilities become more severe, it is likely that decision making would be converted to a more avoidance-oriented process in which the goals underlying behavior would involve the avoidance of aversive experience. Because the arousal levels in approach behaviors tend to be lower than the extreme levels often observed in avoidance behaviors motivated by fear, and because efficient skilled performance requires an optimum level of arousal, it is more likely that avoidance behaviors will be performed with a somewhat lower level of precision.[26,27,35,36] Therefore, where skilled performance is required during critical safety activities (for example, in handling radioactive material spills, explosives, or unstable chemicals), and must be accomplished with maximum precision, it is probably advisable, where possible, to establish and maintain an approach-oriented task environment for the duration of the critical performance.

The event or signal-detection sensitivity of the individual is a further safety-related process (actually, signal detection is a multicomponent process) that is affected by the factors currently under discussion. The event or signal-detection ability possessed by an individual is of special importance when the individual is charged with the responsibility of detecting potential safety hazards, violators of safety policies, and accident incidents or events. A potential safety hazard, for example, can be considered an event in the work environment that must be detected and removed. The theory of signal-detection concerns the ability of an observer to determine that an event has occurred in a noisy environment.[37-39] Following the detection of the event, its special significance (if any) must be determined. If the event is significant, some response may be required. The detectability of a signal is influenced by the observer's sensitivity (d') to the signal and his response bias or decision criterion (β). For a concise and introductory overview of signal-detection theory, refer to Thorndike and Yost.[40]

The hospital environment can be considered as a noise background in which safety hazards — that must be detected and removed — are embedded. An individual's sensitivity to safety hazards may be manipulated to the advantage of safety through imaginative training techniques. The decision criterion or response bias may be manipulated through the use of instructions, various incentives or payoffs, as well as by the manipulation of the observer's expectations about the occurrence of hazards (for example, the probability of encountering a specific hazard in a specific area may serve as important information to convey in the manipulation of expectancy). If the consequences for failing to detect a safety hazard are serious, or if the observer is highly accountable for such errors, the decision criterion is likely to be such that it will result in a high incidence of false detections (false alarms) and a low incidence of detection failures (misses). A low degree of accountability or mild consequences for unsatisfactory hazard-detection performance is likely to result in a low incidence of false alarms and a large number of misses. Thus, if the hospital safety program is viewed within a signal-detection context, the accountability and consequence factor for each individual should be considered as a means of setting a payoff level for the detection of safety errors. The manipulation of this factor may permit the adjustment of the decision criterion for an individual such that safety hazard-detection performance is optimized.

Group Size

The number of individuals that belong to a group influences the propensity of an individual group member to express helping behavior. As discussed in the introduction, large groups provide many individuals over which the responsibility for failing to provide help can be diffused. This diffusion of responsibility can be an important factor in explaining why visitors, for example, not only fail to report fires and other safety hazards, but also refuse to help accident victims or report accident victims who may be in need of assistance.[1] It should be noted again that this effect can be modified by the presence of positive role models who provide examples of desirable behavior.[3]

The number of people involved in a decision process may affect the nature of the decision that is made. The risky-shift phenomenon refers to the observation that in groups, individuals will make decisions that involve a higher degree of risk than the individuals in the group would make alone.[41] Thus, a safety policy committee may make a policy decision that tolerates higher accident-risk levels in some environment than any of the committee members, acting alone, may deem advisable. A somewhat contradictory effect has also been noted. The cautious-shift phenomenon refers to the observation that when groups make decisions involving popular values favoring caution, the group members acting together tend to demonstrate more conservative decision-making behavior than the average member.[42] Therefore, under the proper circumstances, a safety-related group decision may tend to be overly cautious. The implications of the risky- and cautious-shift phenomena in safety-related group decision making are somewhat unclear and appear to center around the problem of determining whether excessive caution or excessive risk is least acceptable under given environmental conditions.

Behavioral Factors

The term "behavioral" here refers to the characteristics of safety-related behaviors that are identifiable in terms of the activities of an individual or a group rather than in terms of the subjective or mentalistic processes of any individual or group members.

Prevailing Safety Habits

The various groups that constitute the hospital-user population can be expected to exhibit widely different prevailing safety habits. Because these habits depend upon the previously discussed cognitive factors — the physical environment in which safe performance must be maintained, and other influences such as the physical capabilities and health of group members — it is difficult to precisely specify the expected prevailing habits for a particular group. It is necessary to systematically examine both the actual safety-related performance and the accident occurrence/incidence statistics that are relevant to the group of interest. Through such analysis one might determine that a particular group requires the strengthening of its safety habits, and the specific habits to be strengthened may be identified. For example, if a particular hospital facility suffers an unacceptably large number of accidents involving falls on wet floors by visitors (indicated by the study of statistics and reports), behavior observation and report analysis might reveal that the housekeeping staff has developed poor habits concerning the erection of the proper wet floor warning signs. A careful analysis of prevailing safety habits should be made before a safety program is implemented for any group. Once this analysis has been performed, the safety goals, training methods, and specific procedures can be more rationally specified for the program that is to be implemented. Periodic safety-habit analyses should be performed in order to determine whether or not modifications in safety goals, procedures, training, or supervision should be made so that safe habits are maintained at maximum strength.

Behavior Stereotyping

Modes of behavior that are relatively inflexible and uniform are called stereotyped behaviors. Stereotyped behaviors can play an important role in reducing safety performance because they interfere with an individual's active involvement in accident prevention. Stereotyped behaviors discourage the production of safety-expansive behaviors in which an individual would go beyond the usual behavior repertoire and role responsibilities to, for example, report a potential hazard observed in a work area other than his own. Stereotyped behaviors that are related to hospital-safety contexts tend to be of two fundamental origins. The first source of stereotyped behavior may be termed the role or psychological source. In this case, the role that is fulfilled by an individual imposes certain psychological limitations and demands that produce stereotyping. For example, an electrician making a wiring repair in an ambulatory patient lounge may fail to respond to a safety hazard (in the form of a large water spill from a drinking fountain) because such a response is not required under the role demands of an electrician as perceived by this individual. Ideally, safety training and motivational programs should remove such role-required stereotyping with respect to safety-related behaviors. Again, it is crucial to the success of any safety program that all individuals of interest to the program take as active a role as possible in accident prevention.

A second source of behavior stereotyping may be termed the physical source. Here, stereotyped behaviors are the result of the physical nature of the task environment. For example, a kitchen employee may be engaged in repetitive and stereotyped arm/hand motions during the process of loading a large dishwashing machine. Certain aspects of this behavior may be inherently hazardous given the nature of the task and machinery used, or may serve to distract the employee from monitoring other safety-related events in the task environment. Such stereotyping should be avoided when possible. If unsafe conditions or an unacceptable number of safety incidents are produced by physical stereotyping, the task environment should be carefully examined and modified. If modifications are not practical, the problem may be resolved through the development of more effective safety procedures or further safety training.

Environmental Factors

The term ''environmental'' refers to the totality or any aspect of the physical world that surrounds or affects an individual. A number of aspects of the hospital environment have an impact upon the safety-related behavior of individuals or groups.

Exposure to Specific Hazards

When a specific potential hazard is present within the environment, the group that is exposed to the hazard must adopt the appropriate safety-related behaviors in order to maintain safety. The fact that certain groups within the hospital-user population tend to be exposed to particular kinds of specific work hazards becomes apparent during the examination of accident statistics relevant to each group. For example, kitchen employees are subject to burns from stoves, steam tables, and grill surfaces, while nurses are more likely to suffer a back injury caused by lifting a patient. It is clear that the way to deal with the specific hazard problem is through the careful assessment of hospital work/living environments in terms of the specific hazards that each contains. The appropriate hazard-specific accident prevention or safety procedure training must then be administered to each group. The specific hazards to which particular hospital-user groups are exposed will be discussed in more detail in the following section.

Size of Hospital

The size of the industrial facility where an individual is employed has been shown to have an influence upon safety-related behaviors. Surry demonstrated that larger organizations tend to have lower accident rates than smaller ones, and explained this size-safety relationship in terms of differential management concern for the preservation of safety.[19] Some institutions tend to produce a weak personal involvement by management with respect to safety. For example, in a firm hiring 30 employees and experiencing an injury rate of 12.8 injuries per 1 million work hours, only 1 disabling injury per year should occur. In a firm hiring 1000 employees with the same injury rate, about 30 disabling injuries will be witnessed. Thus, this differential in accident frequency between large and small organizations (even when the accident rates are identical) might produce a stronger awareness of accidents and, therefore, a greater concern for safety by the management of the larger institution. Clague, however, reported different results in a study of hospital work injuries.[43] Larger hospitals exhibited a higher work-injury rate than smaller ones, and there was a difference between types of institutions. Table 1 illustrates Clague's findings. The discrepancy between the reports of Surry and Clague may be accounted for in terms of different accident rates and patterns between industrial and hospital-user populations, sampling differ-

Table 1
WORK-INJURY FREQUENCY RATES BY TYPE AND SIZE OF HOSPITAL[19,43]

Hospital type	Number of employees								
	<10	10—19	20—49	50—99	100—249	250—499	500—999	1000—2499	>2500
General	2.5	2.5	4.1	4.5	5.3	6.2	7.4	8.4	10.3
Tuberculosis	—	—	9.1	7.4	8.0	12.6	16.4	13.8	—
Special	—	—	9.3	6.7	8.6	9.6	13.4	25.5	—
Mental	—	—	—	8.1	7.6	8.7	15.4	21.0	—

Note: Mean rates — general, 6.5; tuberculosis, 11.7; special, 11.3; mental, 15.3.

ences, and the changes in safety-related knowledge and safety programs that occurred between the two studies.

Behavioral scientists have long understood that humans are limited in their ability to attend to and process information about the events in their environment.[44,45] Thus, an important environmental influence on safety is the amount of information processing the environment demands. If the environment overloads the individual with information that must be processed or interferes with ongoing information processing, by distraction, for example, then safety performance can be expected to suffer. The implications here are that the safety responsibilities assigned to an individual may only be carried out to a degree that is in part determined by the nature of the individual's environment and its information demands, plus the demands imposed by work or personal responsibilities. For example, a nurse cannot be expected to care for several critically ill patients, write reports, answer telephones, carry out several other duties simultaneously, and also perform in strict accord with complicated safety policies and accident-reporting procedures. The information-processing demands here may exceed the individual's ability, and should be appropriately adjusted.

In addition to excessive information processing loads imposed by a particular task environment, physical work demands can also serve as an important detriment to safe performance. Fatigue, physical discomfort, and stress produced by excessive work loads can directly contribute to an individual's loss of ability to maintain safe performance. Therefore, in critical safety situations where the cost of less-than-maximum safe performance is unacceptably high, the undesirable effects of excessive work loads should be minimized by the careful study of job responsibilities, performance requirements, and the thoughtful allocation of individual resources such that all relevant requirements will be met.

SPECIFIC GROUPS IN THE HOSPITAL POPULATION

The purpose of the present section is to examine the identifiable groups that constitute the overall hospital-user population. Table 2 illustrates the population partitioning most appropriate for the purposes of the present discussion. The groups selected for discussion here were chosen on the basis of several criteria including the specific kind of duty and work responsibility pursued by individual group members, the psychological demands and requirements imposed upon individuals by their physical and social role within the group, and the specific safety hazards to which they are exposed during the fulfillment of their roles within the hospital environment. Also important were both the clustering of certain types of accidents within specific segments of the overall user population and the selection and representation of a specific group in various surveys of hospital-accident statistics.

Table 2
PARTITIONING THE HOSPITAL-USER POPULATION

Employees	Patients	Visitors
Medical professionals/support	Ambulatory	Visitors of patients
Physicians	Male	Visitors attending classes or hospital events
Nurses	Female	Service visitors
Medical/surgical technicians	Elderly	Salesmen
Laboratory technicians	Youth	Vendor delivery
Administration	Nonambulatory	Repairs
Medically trained	Male	Construction
Nonmedical training	Female	Volunteers/clergy
Clerical/secretarial	Elderly	
Facility support	Youth	
Housekeeping		
Laundry		
Kitchen/food service		
Building craftsmen		
Security		

Following the identification of each group, available data concerning the types and frequency of accidents common to the members of the groups will be reviewed. A review of the factors influencing safety-related behavior discussed in the preceding section is provided and places a special emphasis upon the particular ways in which they are relevant to safety considerations for each group. Finally, the unique problems faced by each group — which represent special points of interest with respect to the preservation and promotion of the group's safety — are discussed.

Employees

Safety Problems

As may be expected, certain classes of hospital employees experience a higher accident and injury rate than others. Table 3 illustrates the the typical accident rates observed in the medical profession. Table 4 shows accident rates of the hospital administration and the facility support employees. These tables were compiled on the basis of several sources.[6,7,10,43] These statistics are useful in establishing the priorities for the development of a safety program because attention is directed toward employees who are subject to the highest accident rates. However, as Clague warned, other activities with low accident rates should not be neglected, and detailed statistical analyses of safety problems involving any employee activity or role are useful in the development and maintenance of a comprehensive safety program.[43]

The nature of the injuries received by hospital employees somewhat parallels the general pattern observed in U.S. industry. Table 5 lists hospital work injuries both by injury type and the part of the body involved. Table 6 describes the various types of accidents in terms of the dynamics of the accident cause.

It is useful to note the types of accidents that are common to specific employee groups because the information can serve to direct attention to specific environmental hazards to which an employee's attention should be directed, or against which they should be protected. Table 7 lists the causes or agents involved in accidents commonly experienced by various hospital employee groups.

Important Safety-Related Factors and Special Safety Considerations

In the previous section, several cognitive, behavioral, and environmental factors important to safety-related behavior were discussed. Several of these are of special importance when considering the safety behavior of hospital employees.

Table 3
TYPICAL RATES OF WORK INJURIES TO EMPLOYEES IN THE MEDICAL PROFESSIONAL AND MEDICAL SUPPORT GROUP[6,7,10,43]

Occupation/area	Work-injury rate[a]
Nursing services	9.1
LPN	8.1
RN	6.9
Student nurses	2.3
Aides	7.5
Orderlies	7.5
Physical/occupational therapy	6.4
Laboratory	4.5
Pharmacy	2.8
Radiology	2.5
Social services	2.5
EEG/ECG technicians	1.9
Inhalation/respiratory therapy	6.4
Anesthesiology	2.1
Surgical assistants	2.5
Physicians	2.5

[a] Average number of disabling injuries per million work hours.

Table 4
TYPICAL WORK-INJURY RATES FOR EMPLOYEES IN THE ADMINISTRATION AND THE FACILITY SUPPORT GROUPS[6,7,10,43]

Occupation/area	Accident rate[a]
Administration	
Purchasing and issuing	5.7
Clerical/secretarial	2.1
Administrators	2.1
Special services	3.4
Facility support	
Housekeeping	8.5
Kitchen/food service	13.4
Security	10.3
Laundry	6.8
Transportation services	24.0
Building craftsmen	19.1

[a] Mean number of disabling injuries per million work hours.

Knowledge of the environment and its special hazards, remedial procedures, and accident-reporting procedures should be deeply instilled in every hospital employee. Positive attitudes concerning accident prevention, the learning of safety and remedial procedures, and accident reporting are of obvious importance. Desirable attitudes and adequate knowledge may be developed through the effective use of training methods,

Table 5
TYPES OF DISABLING INJURY[10,43]

A. Nature of Injury

Injury[a]	Average work days lost	Percent of injuries
Strain, Sprain	20	33.4
Bruises	19	25.2
Cuts, Lacerations	12	12.0
Fractures	80	10.6
Job-Related Disease	441	8.0
Burns, Scalds	21	6.4
Hernias	50	2.6

[a] All other injury types each represent less than 1% of total injuries.

B. Part of Body Injured

	Percent of injuries	
Part of body	Hospitals	U.S. industry
Eye	2.6	5.0
Head (except eye)	6.3	7.0
Arms	5.8	9.0
Trunk (except back)	16.2	26.0
Back	18.7	19.0
Hands and fingers	22.0	24.0
Legs	9.9	13.0
Feet and toes	14.0	10.0
General body	4.5	6.0

motivational programs, and the appropriate manipulation of incentives. These efforts should be especially concentrated upon high accident frequency groups, areas where accidents may have extremely high associated human, monetary, legal, or public relations costs,or where employees have probably not received intensive training or motivation during the course of their professional education.

The role homogeneity and communication structure of each employee group or department should be carefully considered when safety programs are under modification or development because some groups may suffer the negative effects of this factor more than others. For example, housekeeping employees (who may be relatively inarticulate or uneducated when compared with nurses, physicians, and administrators) may show a reluctance to communicate with other groups in matters of safety due to fears of intellectual inequality, jargon differences, social and role differences, etc. In a similar way, relative authority and social position effects may establish further barriers to safety cooperation, communication, and accident reporting. Safety training and motivational programs should make a special effort to reduce or remove such communication and cooperation barriers. Group size may affect the safety policy decisions or behavior of various committees or groups. In the case of an employee's willingness to participate during a safety incident or in accident prevention, positive role models, proper safety incentives, and motivational techniques can be of benefit in encouraging behavior in favor of safety. Control time and the accountability and consequence factors should be manipulated for each group of employees such that safe performance is maximized. The hospital management staff and safety policy makers are generally free to determine what percentage of the employees' work hours shall be

Table 6
ACCIDENT TYPES IN TERMS OF INJURY AGENT DYNAMICS[46]

Dynamics of major injury agent	Percent of accidents
Struck by object	8.2
Struck against object	16.0
Caught in or between objects	5.0
Fall on same level	16.7
Fall to different level	5.5
Slip	39.0
Temperature extremes	3.3
Inhalation, absorbtion, ingestion	4.7
Continual occupational activity	Less than 1%

devoted to safety training or other safety-related activities. A possible exception might include physicians who are somewhat independent, share responsibilities between several hospitals and perhaps a private practice, or have only occasional or very limited contact hours with the hospital.

The degree of accountability and the possible consequences for unsafe behavior are — like control time — largely the control of hospital management. The manipulation of the accountability and consequence factor for the achievement of maximum safety performance can involve several aspects. First, all employees could be held equally accountable for accident prevention. In this way, the deleterious effects of relative authority, social position, and role homogeneity factors might be minimized. The consequences of unsafe performance should be appropriately set with respect to a number of variables. For example, if the unsafe performance placed several people in danger, it might be dealt with more severely than if only one person was threatened. The type of injury that was inflicted or threatened may likewise be considered. The authority position and degree of training could also be used as a guideline for establishing consequence severity; a highly trained safety instructor may be treated more severely than a new or untrained employee. The circumstances under which safety was not maintained may also be considered, For example, a nurse assisting a physician during a cardiac emergency might be treated less severely for creating a minor water spill hazard and failing to report or remove it than he or she would be if not so engaged.

Specific hazards to which employees are exposed obviously affect their safety. Almost two thirds of all injuries to hospital employees are caused by slips, falls, and the improper lifting of heavy objects, while the rest are largely due to electricity, moving machinery, tools and equipment, transportation, and explosive gases and dangerous chemicals (Tables 5, 6, and 7).[5]

Nurses are subject to a high frequency of work injuries probably because they have more direct patient contact than other employees and because they are exposed to more working surface hazards as they move from room to room.[6,7] Strain or overexertion, usually suffered during patient handling, accounts for the largest percentage of accidents to nurses in typical accident surveys. Nurses are also subject to slip and fall hazards from spilled powders and liquids, as well as from carts and equipment found in hallways and patient areas. In the California study cited above, 15% of all nursing staff injuries involved such hazards. The same study showed that the patient represents a significant hazard to nurses and that more than one half of the nurses' injuries involved being struck by a patient either directly or as the result of some form of patient contact.

Housekeeping employees, like nurses, suffer a substantial number of accidents from typical hazards in their work environment. More than one third of housekeeping em-

Table 7
CAUSES OF ACCIDENTS COMMON TO VARIOUS HOSPITAL EMPLOYEE GROUPS[6,7]

Employee group[a]	Injury agent	Percent of injuries
Nurses	Patient	42
	Working surfaces	20
	Beds, furniture	8
	Infectious materials	6
	Chemicals (hot or injurious)	4
	Hospital equipment	4
	Vehicles, carts	3
	Hand tools	2
	Containers	2
	Repeated or awkward motion	3
	Other	6
Housekeeping	Working surfaces	25
	Containers	18
	Furniture	15
	Chemicals (hot or injurious)	9
	Hand tools	7
	Vehicles, carts	5
	Other	21
Kitchen/food service	Working surfaces	23
	Substances (hot or injurious)	16
	Containers	10
	Kitchen machinery	10
	Dishes, pans, cutlery	8
	Vehicles, carts	6
	Knives	4
	Trays	4
	Other	19

[a] Information was not available in the above form for other groups.

ployee injuries reported in the California study were the result of strain or overexertion that occurred when heavy containers, furniture, or cleaning machines were being handled. A substantial number of falls on wet floors were noted. In addition, a large percentage of injuries to this group were the result of being struck by or struck against furniture, carts, and containers that were being moved.

The California study (and others) revealed that the kitchen represents one of the most dangerous areas in the hospital because here the employees are subject to many potential hazards such as wet and greasy floors, dangerous kitchen equipment and utensils, and hot surfaces and substances. About one fourth of kitchen injuries were the result of being struck by or struck against kitchen appliances, utensils, and containers. An equal number of accidents were the result of falls on wet or greasy floors. Slightly less than one fourth of the kitchen accidents were related to strain or overexertion suffered while carrying food supplies or pushing food carts. In addition, meat grinders, slicers, and hot substances were involved in a substantial number of accidents.

Because the administrative personnel and physicians are subject to relatively few injuries, few statistical surveys of these groups are available. These employees, however, have some special responsibilities that are imposed by their social roles, individual authority, and degree of education. These groups should be especially careful to serve as positive role models for other employees. The members of the groups are generally responsible for the decision to develop and implement safety programs and thus tend

Table 8
INCIDENCE OF PATIENT ACCIDENTS BY AGE AND SEX

Fagin and Vita[20]		Pablo[4]	
Age group	Accidents/1000 admissions	Age/sex	Percent of total
Newborn	0.36	40 or less	8
1 week—1 year	5.49	41—60	11
1—10	12.1	61—80	46
11—20	11.9	81 or more	35
21—30	4.99		
31—40	7.95		
41—50	12.1	All males	36
51—60	21.8	All females	64
61—70	39.6		
71—80	62.0		
80 or more	41.9		

to be self-motivated to safe performance. Such individuals should attempt to serve as effective communication channels, and should strive to spread their interest and concern for safety (as well as information concerning safety policies and procedures) throughout the hospital. Administrators, in particular, are responsible for safety enforcement. Although this responsibility may, at times, serve as a source of stress, it is important to the success of the safety program.

Physicians tend to be under some degree of stress, and have extremely heavy work loads as well as many demands upon their time. Upon occasion, such as during medical or work-related crises, normal safety procedures may be circumvented, faulty equipment may not be reported, repair logs may be neglected, or "quick fixes" may be attempted. Such actions and behaviors tend to present hazards to those using the equipment later and also serve as negative examples for other hospital employees. Unless such actions are absolutely necessary, they should be avoided. When such actions are required, however, care should be taken to remedy unsafe conditions as soon as possible.

Patients

Safety Problems

Although the hospital staff is charged with the responsibility of establishing and maintaining a healthful and safe environment, injuries to patients occur with a somewhat startling frequency. Table 2 illustrates the types of patient groups that form the patient population. Table 8 shows that the typical patient injured in the hospital is a female over 60 years of age. Table 9 demonstrates that most accidents occur during the day and evening shifts, when the largest number of people are using the facility. Few accidents appear to occur during weekends — especially on Sunday — probably because the hospital-user population declines on these days.

Table 10 illustrates that patient accidents usually occur in the patient's own room or in bathrooms. This pattern is probably best explained both in terms of the large percentage of time that patients spend in these areas and the fact that patients are often free to engage in risky and unsupervised activities in private rooms and bathrooms. Table 11 reveals that the vast majority of patient accidents involve falls or slips. The most frequent forms of these accidents involve falls from beds where side rails are in the up position. The best explanation for such accidents is probably that weak or confused patients who are left improperly restrained or unattended, attempt

Table 9
WHEN ACCIDENTS OCCUR: TIME OF DAY, DAY OF WEEK, AND SEASON

Time/day/season	Percent of total: Pablo[4]	Percent of total: Fagin and Vita[20]
7—3 p.m.	51	41
3—11 p.m.	44	29
11—7 a.m.	5	27
Sunday	13	10
Monday	15	17
Tuesday	14	14
Wednesday	13	14
Thursday	14	17
Friday	16	17
Saturday	15	11
Summer	27	—
Fall	24	—
Winter	23	—
Spring	26	—

Table 10
LOCATION OF PATIENT AT THE TIME OF ACCIDENT OCCURRENCE

Location of accident[a]	Percent of total accidents: Pablo[4]	Percent of total accidents: Fagin and Vita[20]
Patient's room	58	60
Bathroom	23	12
Corridor	8	5
Physiotherapy	5	Less than 1
Surgical and recovery areas	—	7
Radiology	—	14

[a] All others account for less than 1% each.

to climb over the side rails of the bed. A fall occurs because such patients are not capable of performing such physical maneuvers properly. Table 12 shows that when a patient is injured, the injury usually takes the form of a cut, laceration, or bruise. Most of these injuries will involve the upper extremeties and the head.

Table 13 depicts some of the frequently involved agents or activities that contribute to patient injuries. Most accidents involve insufficient supervision, improper restraint, or improper safety warnings given to patients. Further, unsafe positions assumed by the patient, plus the improper use of body parts, account for a large percentage of injuries. Patients most often involved in accidents are disturbed in some manner — confused, restless, anxious, depressed, or weak. Normal and alert patients, however, are involved in a large percentage of accidents. The accident agents most often involved in patient injuries are hospital beds and furniture, medications, wheelchairs, floors, doors, and bathroom equipment.

Information concerning patient accident patterns is readily obtained from many

Table 11
TYPES OF PATIENT ACCIDENTS

Study	Type of accident	Percent of total accidents
Pablo[4]		
	Falls, slips	75
	Struck against object	10
	Caught in, under	5
	Temperature extreme	2
	Struck by object	2
	Noxious substance (contact with)	1
	Bodily reaction	1
	Other	4
Fagin and Vita[20]		
	Falls (total)	68
	Side rails up	28
	Side rails down	15
	From wheelchair	11
	In room (not in bed)	13
	Bathroom	9
	Hallway	4
	Struck by object	7
	Medication error	7
	Injured by equipment	7
	Burned	3
	Cut by sharp object	2
	Self-inflicted	1

sources.[4,5,20-22] Major forms of patient accidents that are not disclosed in the above tables include injuries caused by explosions of anesthesia gases in surgical or special treatment areas, and electrical shock, which occurs in special treatment areas and the patient's room. The primary causes of such accidents are inexperienced or untrained operators of newly developed medical devices and the improper testing or grounding of equipment before it is utilized.[5]

Important Safety-Related Factors and Special Safety Considerations

Knowledge of the hospital environment and its specific safety hazards and safety procedures, as well as hazard and accident reporting procedures, can be of utmost importance to the patient's ability to exhibit safe behavior. Proper attitudes concerning the need to learn safety rules, perform safely, and report safety hazards and accidents are as important as sufficient knowledge. Anyone being hospitalized can become confused or disturbed by the experience. Too often, unusual and stress-producing procedures are viewed by the hospital staff as routine, rather than from the discomfort, stress, and fear-oriented perspective of the patient. In order that such effects be minimized, the patient should be oriented to the importance of bedrails, the use of signaling devices, the dangers of falls from bed and in bathrooms, smoking regulations, fire drill procedures, and the need to report safety hazards to nurses or other hospital personnel. Desirable attitudes and knowledge can be established during the admission procedure or depending upon the patient's condition, on some later occasion. The American Hospital Association has described such a patient safety orientation plan in detail.[5]

Knowledge possessed by the nursing services personnel and other patient contact groups can affect a patient's safety in a manner that seems most appropriate for consideration. Many new and sophisticated medical devices are finding use in the hospital

Table 12
TYPES OF INJURIES SUSTAINED IN PATIENT ACCIDENTS[4]

Injury	Percent of total injuries
Cuts, lacerations	48
Bruises	36
Burns, scalds	3
Sprains, strains	2
Others	10
Part of body	
Upper extremeties	52
Head	22
Trunk	13
Lower extremeties	13

environment. Frequently, the individuals operating these devices have received improper, insufficient, or no training at all. Although such personnel may appear to understand the purpose and operation of the device (for example, a volume ventilator or a heat lamp), the limitations and hazards of the device may not be appreciated. When personnel are given the responsibility of operating mechanical or electrical devices such as aspirators, oxygen equipment, monitors, nebulizers, traction apparatus, lighting and heating equipment, or motorized beds, they should be thoroughly familiar with safe operation procedures and potential hazards associated not only with each device, but with various, commonly used combinations. In addition to a knowledge of proper use, an employee must possess a knowledge of proper device-maintenance procedures, and defective-device reporting and tagging techniques.

Relative authority and social role effects may also influence patient safety. Patients may hesitate to "bother the busy nurse or doctor" when they should request assistance. For example, a patient wishing to get out of bed may not use a call button to request a nurse's help because nurses or other staff members have established patterns of behavior that discourage a patient's request for assistance. For example, excessive waits for help to arrive, the appearance of being imposed upon, and excessive authoritarian behavior can suppress a patient's willingness to ask for help. This leads to frustration and excessive risk-taking. The stronger the consumer-oriented attitude the patient establishes during safety orientation, the more able he or she becomes in resisting such effects. Patients may also suffer certain safety impairments because they engage in stereotyped behaviors dictated by the role of "patient". Such behaviors do not constitute sham performance, but are related to placebo effects and psychosomatic illnesses. Examples of such behaviors include a shuffling or sliding gate and walking with head lowered rather than with eyes ahead. These behaviors can lead to a patient injury through falls or collisions with moving equipment. Role-played behaviors should not be confused with symptoms or the effects of illness and drugs, and this should be dealt with only by the professional medical staff.

Patients, because of their role in the hospital, place their trust in hospital employees. The combination of attentive care administered to the patient and the trust that the patient has in the hospital staff may lead to a patient's overdependence upon the employee's decision-making capabilities. This overdependence may result in carelessness by the patient, since he expects that the hospital staff will make all required safety-related decisions and insure protection from injury. Patients should be made aware during safety orientation, that their participation in the maintenance of hospital safety

Table 13
CONTRIBUTIONS TO PATIENT ACCIDENTS

Fagin and Vita[20]

Activity contributing	% Total
Unsafe position, restraint, warning	29
Improper use of body	21
Unsupervised activity	19
Inattention, carelessness	11
Environmental problem	8
Unnecessary delays	5
Other	7

Major injury agent	% Total
Bed	10
Siderails	7
Chair	7
Medication	5
Wheelchair	4
Floor	4
Doors	3
Toilets	3
Tubing	3
Radiator	2
Tables	1
Other[a]	51

Pablo[4]

Condition of patient before accident	% Total
Alert, rational	40
Disturbed	54
Confused	16
Restless, anxious	10
Weak, dizzy	6
Anesthetized	6
Asleep	6
Fainted	5
Uncooperative	4
Drugged	1
Senile	1
Other (not adequately described)	6

[a] This group includes agents that are not normally directly available to unsupervised patients, e.g., X-ray machines.

is essential and that they have a responsibility to protect and preserve the safety of everyone in the hospital. Stress and its effects will be suffered by patients because infection and injury are both stressors. The techniques by which stress can be manipulated and coped with were discussed in the previous section, and should be utilized, where possible, to minimize the stress imposed upon the patients.

Because patients are the consumers of the medical care offered by the hospital, they are not subject to the same control time effects as employees. Patients are generally not available for large amounts of safety training and motivation. Their accountability for accidents or unsafe performance is questionable, and consequences for unsafe performance by patients are neither well defined nor often under the control of management. The most severe consequence that a patient can suffer is his or her own injury. Probably the only effective control time that is available for safety-related matters is that which is set aside for formal orientation. Informal control opportunities may exist when a safety-interested hospital employee (such as a nurse) is in contact with a patient. Group size will affect the safety hazard reporting behavior of patients as previously described. For example, if a large number of patients are gathered in a television lounge, it is less likely that a hazard will be reported or corrected because the responsibility for such activity can diffuse, unless counteracted, among a large number of people.

Patient safety becomes a special problem when the patient is either elderly or extremely young. Elderly patients should be carefully supervised or restrained to prevent falls from beds because more than 70% of such falls are fatal when the patient is over 65 years of age.[5] The usual causes of such falls are unassisted bed entries or exits, faulty side rails, faulty bed casters, and overreaching for trays, tables, drawers, signal devices, bed controls, personal items, and theraputic devices. Elderly patients should be closely supervised during ambulatory activities and baths or showers. Extremely young patients are also subject to falls from bed. Further, smothering hazards exist in the form of excessively soft pillows and plastic mattress and pillow covers. Children are also subject to injuries inflicted by broken toys or improperly designed toys. They should be removed. Young children should be closely supervised while eating because the child may either choke or insert small food objects, such as candy or nuts, into the nose or ears.

Patients are susceptible to a number of specific burn hazards. Hot water bottles, heating pads, heat lamps and cradles, hot foods, and steam vaporizers are but a few of the many specific burn hazards in the patient environment. Personnel and patients using these devices should be carefully instructed in their use, and such patients should be kept under close supervision. Patients' smoking behaviors may also represent another burn hazard. Because it is impossible to completely control patient smoking behavior, it is important to minimize the associated hazards to the greatest degree possible.[5] During the safety orientation, the patient must be made aware that violations of smoking policies can endanger everyone in the hospital.

Personal appliances such as televisions, radios, and hair dryers can serve as shock hazards and facilitate trips over cords, tempt overreach falls, and may strike or fall on patients. Restrictions on such devices should be carefully explained during safety orientation. Better compliance with such rules, in addition to good public relations, can be achieved if both the rules and their underlying reasons are explained to the patient and other interested parties.

The safety of patients is often threatened by nurses and staff members who commit medication errors and cause injuries to the mouth and teeth when temperatures are measured or endotrachial tubes are inserted.[4,20] Standards and policy recommendations for reducing the incidence of such injuries are given by the American Hospital Association.[5]

Visitors

Safety Problems

Table 2 shows the types of visitors that constitute the visitor population. In spite of previous complaints such as that by Morris, data concerning accidents to visitors are not as abundant as employee and patient information.[47] Few large-scale surveys have been conducted for the purpose of analyzing visitor-accident patterns and available

Table 14
TYPES AND LOCATIONS OF HOSPITAL VISITOR ACCIDENTS[a]

Accident	Percent of total accidents
Falls, slips	68
Collision (with moving object)	7
Collision (with stationary object)	5
Cuts, burns, lacerations	5
Other	15
Location	
Outdoor walks, parking lots	15
Halls, entryways, stairs	50
Lobbys, lounges, food areas	20
Patient rooms	10
Other	5

[a] Survey of central Indiana hospitals.

surveys tend to be unreliable or of narrow scope. Several small-scale general surveys, taken together, indicate that visitors' accident patterns somewhat parallel those of employees and patients.[5] Visitors are involved in accidents 24 hr/day but the vast majority occur between 3 p.m. and 11 p.m., probably due to the large influx of patients' visitors during this interval. Although visitors' accidents take many forms, the most common types of accidents appear to be slips and falls on wet indoor floors, outdoor walkways, parking lots, and building entryways. Stairwell falls, trips over carts, carpets, and electrical cords also account for a large percentage of visitor accidents. Falls and slips appear to account for about 70% of all injuries to hospital visitors, and the majority of the remainder involve collisions with objects such as glass panels, doors, and windows, and cuts from broken or chipped food service glassware and other sharp objects and furniture edges. Table 14 shows some results of an informal survey of three hospitals in the central Indiana area. The accident pattern here is typical of those observed elsewhere (see resource list for several general statistical sources).

Important Safety-Related Factors and Special Considerations

The hospital management staff has no control time during which to indoctrinate visitors, with the possible exception of visitors performing a service such as salesmen, deliverymen, and construction workers. When possible, these visitors should be advised of hospital safety policies, whose enforcement can be linked to the service relationship that exists between the visitors, employees, and the hospital. Thus, some visitors can be held accountable for unsafe behavior and the consequences that they must face for safety violations are somewhat under the control of the hospital management structure. Most visitors, however, are not subject to such manipulation. Visitor attitudes towards safety are important. Motivational programs such as that presented by the American Hospital Association should be implemented for visitors in an effort to establish positive safety attitudes, especially with respect to accident prevention and hazard reporting.[5] Poster and personnel badge programs can be used to promote visitors' awareness of the importance of safety and the presence of specific hazards. For example, signs, badges, and posters can draw attention to slippery surface or walkway hazards during hospital expansion or other construction. Visitors must be made aware of such hazards because they generally possess only a limited knowledge of the hospital environment and its particular safety hazards, safety policies and procedures, and methods for hazard and accident reporting. Visitors suffer the effects of the relative authority and social position factors in much the same manner as patients. Unless encouraged, visitors may hesitate to contact hospital employees, especially the medical and professional staff, regarding the presence of minor safety hazards. Like the patient in the previous discussion, the visitor, who while reporting a hazard is forced to wait, or is subject to other forms of abuse or hostility by busy employees, may become frustrated, accept the risk that the hazard may cause an accident, and refuse to complete a hazard report. Group size, in the form of the diffusion of responsibility effect, can further reduce the likelihood that visitors will report hazards. The larger the group of visitors in the lobby, for example, the less likely it becomes that any particular visitor will report a hazard. Many hospital visitors are under the effects of stress related to the emotional crises associated with the illness of the patient they are visiting. The effects of this stress can be to reduce the individual's ability to maintain safe performance. If visitors become extremely agitated or grief-stricken (for example, as when the patient they are visiting expires), they should be closely supervised or escorted by hospital staff members until it is assured that they are capable of safe negotiation of stairs, hallways, parking lots, or other hazards.

Visitors present a serious hazard to the entire hospital-user population when smoking regulations are violated. All hospital employees should be aware that they have a responsibility to help supervise the safe behavior of visitors and must respond to their violations of safety policies. For example, if a housekeeping employee sees a visitor violating smoking regulations, the employee should politely explain the rules and ask for the visitor's compliance. Procedures and suggestions for such intervention can be established and discussed during employee safety training, motivation, and enforcement programs.

CONCLUDING REMARKS

In an earlier section of this chapter, various cognitive, behavioral, and environmental factors of potential importance to safety-related behavior were defined and discussed in general. Later, the hospital-user population was partitioned into various groups, and the accident patterns of selected groups were described upon the basis of existing accident data. Various special problems and psychological aspects of respective accident patterns and safety behavior were discussed for each group. The perspective of the present chapter has been largely psychological. It should also be noted that the level of detail and complexity of each discussion can be substantially increased and the applications of the psychological principles discussed here can be greatly expanded. Such complexity and expansion is, however, beyond the scope of this single chapter. Other chapters in this volume provide a detailed discussion of some of the safety considerations and safety hazards alluded to in the present chapter. For example, other chapters consider human factors problems in safety, explosion and fire hazards, shock hazards, medication accidents, and other safety-related topics. A better understanding of all of these aspects of hospital safety can enhance safety planning, management, enforcement, and performance. In this manner, the safety of the hospital-user population can be better assured and the mandate that hospitals provide safe and protective environments for all those who use them can be fulfilled.

ACKNOWLEDGMENT

The authors are grateful to Stuart M. Weiss, of the Purdue University Department of Industrial Engineering for his assistance in the preparation of this section.

GENERAL REFERENCES

The following references are supplied as an aid to those who seek starting points for the further study of the safety of hospital-user populations. These materials consider various aspects of the safety of hospital patients, employees, and visitors. National Safety Council (444 N. Michigan Ave., Chicago, Ill.) library document numbers are supplied when articles are of limited distribution.

Albert, B. W., Impact of a hospital safety committee, *Nurs. Homes,* 13, 5, 1964.

Allen, J. E., Study of attitudes of laboratory workers toward accident prevention, *J. Chem. Educ.,* 43, 861, 1966.

Althouse, H. L., How OSHA affects hospitals and nursing homes, *Am. J. Nurs.,* 75, 450, 1975.

Hospital Safety Manual, American Hospital Association, Chicago, 1968, 1.

Bakko, O. E., Employee safety program, *J. Am. Hosp. Assoc. (Hospitals),* 44, 52, 1970.

Barclay, W. A., Occupational health and safety in hospitals. Proc. New South Wales Health Commission, Sydney, Australia, 1974.

Bringman, M., Safety action sheet keys program, *J. Am. Hosp. Assoc. (Hospitals),* 48, 85, 1974.

Buehrle, R., Where, when, how, and why of accidents among patients, *Hosp. Top.,* 48, 21, 1970.

Work Injuries in California, California Department of Industrial Relations, Sacramento, 1967, 1.

Work injuries in private hospitals. I. Registered nurses, in Work Injuries in California, California Department of Industrial Relations, Sacramento, 1975 1.

Work injuries in private hospitals. II. Employees other than registered nurses, in Work Injuries in California, California Department of Industrial Relations, Sacramento, 1975, 1.

Disabling Work Injuries to Employees of California Department of Mental Hygiene, California Division of Labor Statistics and Research, Sacramento, 1965 1.

Cliff, K. S., Accidents at work, *Occup. Saf. Health,* 13, 1973.

Cook, E. B., Data being collected on product related accidents, *Hosp. Manage.,* 109, 26, 1970.

Dornette, W. H., Safety in hospitals and nursing homes, *Fire J.,* p. 23, 1970.

Douglass, B. E., Health problems of hospital employees, *J. Occup. Med.,* p. 555, 1971.

Durant, R. B., Explosive hazards in hospitals, *Lifeline,* p. 13, 1977.

Farmer, D., Hospitals, *Health and Safety at Work,* p. 23, June 1979.

Firebriefs, *Natl. Saf. News,* 100, 10, 1969.

Freese, A. S., Danger in the hospital, *Popular Mechanics,* 135, 80, February 1971.

George, A., Occupational health hazards of women: a synoptic view, Advisory Council on the Status of Women, 1976.

Greene, J., Keeping tabs on product injuries, Food and Drug Administration Consumer, U.S. Food and Drug Administration, 1977, 14.

Hochberg, H. M., Hazards from electrical equipment, *Hosp. Top.,* 48, 93, 1970.

Hopps, J. A., Electric shock hazard in hospitals, *J. Can. Med. Assoc.,* 108, 1002, 1968.

Hospital laboratories are unhealthy, *New Scientist,* p. 399, November 17, 1977.

Horty, J. F., Night's special hazards create hospital liabilities, *Mod. Hosp.,* 116, 48, 1968.

Howe, H. F., Organization and operation of occupational health program, *J. Occup. Med.,* p. 528, 1975.

Iskrant, A. P., Falls in public places, *National Safety Council Transactions,* 27, 6, 1971.

Jupiter, R. M., Hospital safety during civil disorder, *Safety,* p. 2, 1968.

Keene, J., Safety: another cap for nurses, *Natl. Saf. News,* 117, 65, 1978.

Koren, H., Environmental hazards in hospitals, *J. Environ. Health,* 36, 122, 1974.

Lee, D. C., Promoting safety, *Hosp. Prog.,* 55, 32, 1974.

Lubin, D., Electrical safety, *J. Am. Hosp. Assoc. (Hospitals),* 43, 57, 1969.

Lunn, J. A., Hospital electrical safety, *National Safety Council Transactions,* 18, 29, 1973.

Lunn, J. A., Hospital hazards, *Practitioner,* 210, 490, 1973.

Manella, B., Electronic dangers cited where oxygen is used, *J. Environ. Health,* 34, 509, 1972.

Mann, K. J., Work injuries in a medical organization, *Arch. Environ. Health,* 13, 554, 1967.

McFarland, R. A., Accidental injuries and deaths in the U.S., U.S. House Committee on Appropriations, Washington, D.C., 1960 1.

McWeeney, T., Role of management and department heads in hospital occupational safety programs, *National Safety Council Transactions,* 18, 13, 1974.
Michigan University Health Service, Laboratory Safety, National Safety Council Doc. No. 71-2685, Ann Arbor, 1971.
Microelectrocution seen a growing patient peril, *Med. Trib.,* p. 1, 1971.
National electronic injury surveillance system, *Mod. Hosp.,* 118, 48, 1972.
National Fire Protection Association, Hospital Laboratories. National Safety Council Doc. No. 69-4122, 1969.
National Institute of Occupational Safety and Health, Health and Safety Guide for Hospitals, Publ. No. 78-150, National Institute of Occupational Safety and Health, Washington, D.C., 1978.
National Safety Council, Employee safety complacency is costly, in National Safety Council Hospital Safety Newsletter, National Safety Council, Chicago, 1965 1.
National Safety Council, Manual for Recording and Measuring Accidents in the Community, NSC Doc. No. 68-3156, National Safety Council, Chicago, 1968.
National Safety Council, Hospital safety identification systems, in National Safety Council Hospital Newsletter, National Safety Council, Chicago, 1976, 1.
National Safety Council, Implementation plan for a dynamic safety system, in National Safety Council Hospital Newsletter, National Safety Council, Chicago, 1976, 1.
National Safety Council, Accident Facts, National Safety Council, Chicago, 1977, 1.
Pennsylvania Department of Labor and Industry Report, Compensable Work Injuries in Pennsylvania, National Safety Council Doc. No. 67-7276, Pennsylvania Department of Labor and Industry, Scranton, 1967, 1.
Regan, W. A., Hospital deficient in investigating and recording accidents, *Hosp. Prog.,* 55, 28, 1974.
Rinder, L. J., Workshop on electrical hazards in hospitals, *IAEI News,* p. 36, 1968.
Rodstein, M., Safeguarding the elderly hospital patient, *Safety,* p. 2, 1968.
Ruck, D., Illnesses of Minnesota hospital staff puts new spotlight on ethylene oxide, *American Medical News,* p. 3, June 16, 1978.
Safetybriefs, *Natl. Saf. News,* 106, 12, 1972.
Sereda, P. J., Safety from fires and explosions in hospital operating rooms, *Canadian Building Digest,* August 1962.
Staff training finds hospital ready when fire hits, *Fire Eng.,* p. 40, 1968.
Stanley, P. E., Electrical hazards of medical instrumentation and their prevention, *National Safety Council Transactions,* 9, 13, 1968.
Stanley, P. E., Warns hospitals of the need for testing for shock hazards, *Hosp. Top.,* 48, 25, 1970.
Steere, N. V., Safety in the chemical laboratory, *J. Chem. Educ.,* 44, 3, 1974.
Stone, B., Patient safety program begun, *American Medical News,* p. 6, October 24, 1977.
Thomas, G. J., Safety from fires and explosions from anesthetics in hospitals, *J. Am. Osteopath. Assoc.,* p. 74, 1967.
Tiboni, E. A., Development and operation of accident control programs through health departments, in National Safety Council Doc. No. 67-7494, University of Michigan, Ann Arbor, 1967.
Trace amounts of anesthetics may imperil hospital workers, *Medical Tribune,* p. 3, November 10, 1971.
Turley, F. Y., Principles of accident control in hospitals, *Australian Safety News,* p. 6, 1976.
University of Minnesota, University of Minnesota employee and student accident experience in University of Minnesota Report, National Safety Council Doc. No. 67-7887, University of Minnesota, Minneapolis, 1967, 1.
U.S. Bureau of Labor Statistics, Work Injuries and Accident Causes in Hospitals, U.S. Bureau of Labor Statistics, Washington, D. C., 1968.
U.S. Bureau of Labor Statistics, Work Injuries and Work Rates in Hospitals, U.S. Bureau of Labor Statistics, Washington, D. C., 1968.
Accidents and the Nation's Health: Accidental Death Rates in the U.S., U.S. Department of Health, Education and Welfare, Washington, D.C., 1965, 1.
Packaged Disaster Hospital Custodian's Handbook, U.S. Department of Health, Education and Welfare, Washington, D.C., 1965, 1.
July start set for national system for injury reports from hospitals, in Food and Drug Administration Papers, U.S. Food and Drug Administration, Washington, D.C., 1971 35.
National electronic injury surveillance system, in Food and Drug Administration Papers, U.S. Food and Drug Administration, Washington, D.C., 1971 31.
Occupational safety and health act of 1969 hearings of November 18, 1969, U.S. House Committee on Education and Labor, Washington, D.C., 1970, 1179.
Verhalen, R. D., Keying product related accidents, *Trial,* p. 32, 1972.
Walter, C. W., Electrical hazards in hospitals and that green wire, *Fire J.,* p. 23, 1971.
Weilerstein, R., Health hazards of medical devices, *Calfiornia's Health,* p. 4, 1973.

What hospitals are doing to cut down accidents, *U.S. News and World Reports,* 80, 36, March 29, 1976.
Williams, B. R., Safety professional and the hospital: an appeal for action, *Professional Safety,* p. 34, November 1977.
Williams, H. L., Survey of mercury vapor hazards in hospitals, *J. Am. Ind. Hyg.,* 29, 186, 1968.

REFERENCES

1. **Latané, B. and Darley, J.**, Group inhibition of bystander intervention in emergencies, *J. Pers. Soc. Psychol.,* 10, 215, 1968.
2. **Rubinstein, J.**, *The Study of Psychology,* Dushkin Publishing Group, Guilford, Conn., 1975.
3. **Bryan, J. and Test, M.**, Models of helping: naturalistic studies in aiding behavior, *J. Pers. Soc. Psychol.,* 6, 400, 1967.
4. **Pablo, R. Y.**, Patient accidents in a long-term care facility, *Can. J. Public Health,* 68, 237, 1977.
5. American Hospital Association, Safety Guide for Health Care Institutions, Illinois: Chicago, National Safety Council, 1972.
6. California Division of Labor Statistics and Research, Work injuries in private hospitals, in Work Injuries in California Quarterly, California Division of Labor Statistics and Research, Sacramento, 1975a, 1.
7. California Division of Labor Statistics and Research, Work injuries in private hospitals, in Work Injuries in California Quarterly, California Division of Labor Statistics and Research, Sacramento, 1975b, 1.
8. **Theophane, M.**, Safety is everybody's business. *J. Am. Hosp. Assoc. (Hospitals),* 30, 44, 1956.
9. **Chaplin, J.**, *Dictionary of Psychology,* Dell Publishing Co., New York, 1968, 87.
10. **Worik, W.**, *Safety Education,* Prentice-Hall, Englewood, Cliffs, N.J., 1979, 30.
11. National Safety Council, Accident Facts, National Safety Council, Chicago, 1973, 23.
12. Ostrom, T., The emergence of attitude theory, in *Psychological Foundations of Attitudes,* Greenwald, A., Brock, T., and Ostrom, T., Eds., Academic Press, New York, 1968, 1.
13. **Newcomb, T.**, Persistence and regression of changed attitudes: long range studies, *J. Soc. Issues,* 19, 3, 1963.
14. **Litt, E.**, Civic education, community norms, and political indoctrination, *Am. Soc. Rev.,* 28, 69, 1963.
15. **Biondo, J. and MacDonald, A.**, Internal-external locus of control and response to influence attempts, *J. Pers.,* 39, 407, 1971.
16. **Zimbardo, P. and Ebbesen, E.**, *Influencing Attitudes and Changing Behavior,* Addison-Wesley, Reading, Mass., 1969.
17. **Allyn, J., and Festinger, L.**, The effectiveness of unanticipated persuasive communications, *J. Abnorm. Soc Psychol.,* 62, 35, 1961.
18. **Heyd, E. H. and Eader, H. C.**, Spelling out a pattern for safety, *J. Am. Hosp. Assoc. (Hospitals),* 30, 53, 1956.
19. **Surry, J.**, *Industrial Accident Research,* University of Toronto Press, Toronto, 1968.
20. **Fagin D., and Vita, M.**, Who, where, when, how: an analysis of 868 inpatient accidents, *J. Am. Hosp. Assoc. (Hospitals),* 39, 60, 1965.
21. **Weil, T. P. and Parrish, H. M.**, How did it happen, *J. Am. Hosp. Assoc. (Hospitals),* 32, 43, 1958.
22. **Williams, W. R.**, The patient's accident pattern, *J. Am. Hosp. Assoc. (Hospitals),* 22, 39, 1948.
23. Festinger, L., *A Theory of Cognitive Dissonance,* Row-Peterson Co., Evanston, Ill., 1957.
24. **Brehm, J.**, Attitudinal consequences of commitment to unpleasant behavior, *J. Abnorm. Soc. Psychol.,* 60, 379, 1960.
25. **Dweck, C.**, The Role of Expectations and Attributions in the Alleviation of Learned Helplessness in a Problem-Solving Situation, Ph.D. dissertation, Yale University, New Haven, 1972.
26. **Birch, H.**, The role of motivational factors in insightful problem-solving, *J. Comp. Psychol.,* 38, 295, 1945.
27. **Kling, J. and Riggs, L.**, *Experimental Psychology,* Holt, Rinehart & Winston, New York, 1971, 829.
28. **Selye, H.**, *The Stress of Life,* McGraw-Hill, New York, 1956.
29. **Weiss, J.**, Psychological factors in stress and disease, *Sci. Am.,* 226, 104, 1972.
30. **McQuade, W.**, What stress can do to you, *Fortune,* 85, 102, January 1972.
31. U.S. Department of Health, Education, and Welfare, Work in America: Report of a Special Task Force to the Secretary of Health, Education, and Welfare, MIT Press, Cambridge, 1973.

32. **Bankart, C.**, Heart Rate and Skin Conductance in Anticipation of Painful Electric Shock, Ph.D. thesis, Dartmouth College, Hanover, N.H., 1971.
33. **Ruff, G. and Korchin, S.**, Adaptive distress behavior, in *Psychological Stress*, Applye, M. and Trumbull, R., Eds., Appleton-Century-Crofts, New York, 1962, 205.
34. **Overmeier, J. and Seligman, M.**, Effects of inescapable shock upon subsequent escape and avoidance responding, *J. Comp. Physiol. Psychol.*, 63, 28, 1967.
35. **Ax, A.**, The physiological difference between fear and anger in humans, *Psychosom. Med.*, 15, 433, 1953.
36. **Lindsley, D.**, Emotion, in *Handbook of Experimental Psychology*, Stevens, S., Ed., John Wiley & Sons, New York, 1951, 473.
37. **Swets, J., Tanner, W., Birdsall, T.**, Decision processes in perception, *Psychol. Rev.*, 68, 301, 1961.
38. **Green, D. and Swets, J.**, *Signal Detection Theory and Psychophysics*, R. E. Krieger, Co., Huntington, N.Y., 1974.
39. **Kaufman, L.**, *Sight and Mind: An Introduction to Visual Perception*, Oxford University Press, New York, 1974, 63.
40. **Thorndike, R. and Yost, W.**, Statistics, measurement, and psychophysics, in *Foundations of Contemporary Psychology*, Meyer, M., Ed., Oxford University Press, New York, 1979, 92.
41. **Wallach, M., Kogan, N., and Bem, D.**, Diffusion of responsibility and level of risk taking in groups, *J. Abnorm. Soc. Psychol.*, 68, 263, 1964.
42. **Stoner, J.**, Risky and cautious shifts in group decision: the influence of widely held values, *J. Exp. Soc. Psychol.*, 4, 442, 1968.
43. **Clague, E.**, Work injuries to hospital employees, *J. Am. Hosp. Assoc. (Hospitals)*, 30, 37, 1956.
44. **Broadbent, D.**, *Perception and Communication*, Pergamon Press, London, 1958.
45. **Reynolds, A. and Flagg, P.**, *Cognitive Psychology*, Winthrop Publishing Co., Cambridge, 1977, Chap. 2.
46. State of New York Department of Labor, Characteristics and Costs of Work Injuries in New York State, 1966-1970, State of New York Department of Labor, Albany, 10, 160, 1970.
47. **Morris, J.**, Solving patient and visitor safety problems, *J. Am. Hosp. Assoc. (Hospitals)*, 30, 50, 1956.

THE HUMAN FACTORS OF HOSPITAL SAFETY

James L. Knight, Jr.* and Robert A. Howells

BACKGROUND AND CONCEPTUAL FRAMEWORKS

Definition of Human Factors

In the most elementary analysis, every accident involves two basic components — people and their environment. Accidents are produced by the unfavorable interaction of these two necessary ingredients. Though simple, this analysis emphasizes that safety can be enhanced by understanding and controlling either environmental or human factors. Indeed, it suggests that the most effective safety program will require attention to both domains since control of only one area of the person-environment diad will leave the other free to assume accident-predisposing characteristics. In considering this accident-interaction model, we must pay due concern to a version of Murphy's law: no matter how well the environment alone is designed and controlled, people will discover ways in which to have accidents. Clearly then, attention must be paid to the human elements of the accident phenomenon if continuing safety improvements are to be achieved. Indeed, when the immediate cause of an accident is identified, it is statistically far more likely to be categorized as behavioral, rather than mechanical failure or environmental misdesign.

Most of this book is explicitly devoted to consideration of the physical hospital environment. Recommendations and hazards associated with building features, equipment design, and operational procedures are presented in detail. However, implicit in even the most technical building code or hardware maintenance recommendations is a recognition of the human contribution to accident-producing interactions. Such codes and recommendations are fundamentally designed to eliminate hazards that untrained people would not normally recognize. Hence, they may be viewed as compensation for human perceptual and knowledge limitations which might otherwise lead to accidents.

In contrast, this section (along with its companion, Safety Considerations for Hospital Populations) departs from the mainline focus upon design or retrofit of the physical environment and deals explicitly with the human elements of hospital safety. The objectives of this section are to present and discuss some of the characteristics of human beings, their needs, expectations, limitations, abilities, and behaviors that have the greatest impact in person-environment interactions related to safety. While there is some necessary overlap between this section and its predecessor, the issues covered here are intended to be of a general nature; they are applicable to safety contexts beyond the hospital setting. The preceding section is concerned with the application of these general principles in the context of specific hospital subpopulations.

The term "human factors" has two distinct but interrelated meanings in the professional literature. First, this term refers to the psychological, emotional, and intellectual characteristics of people upon which human behavior, both safe and unsafe, is based. The manner in which people behave and respond within the hospital will depend upon their abilities to detect and recognize potential hazards and learn and remember appropriate remedies for hazardous features and situations that they encounter. Their behavior will also depend upon their levels of alertness, motivation, and emotional makeup. Thus, the first aspect of the term "human factors" can be taken as something akin to human nature.

* Currently at Bell Telephone Laboratories, Holmdel, New Jersey.

The second meaning of the term signifies a professional discipline comprising aspects of both psychology and engineering. This discipline concerns itself with the engineering of systems so as to make them compatible with their human users. Human factors in this engineering sense-of-the-term have traditionally focused upon the proper design of machines and tools which people must operate or use. As machines became larger and more complex, it became obvious that machine and man comprised a closely coupled system and that this machine-man system would operate only inefficiently — both slowly and with unacceptable levels of mistakes — unless the machine was designed to properly take account of limitations in human abilities.

While concern originally emphasized effectiveness of the Machine-man system, the focus of interest has increasingly shifted to the maximization of the comfort and safety of the human element in Man-machine systems. Luckily, it has turned out that the goals of increasing system effectiveness and improving the quality of the human users experiences with the system are entirely compatible goals. This point is especially worthy of note in connection with safety. Often safety programs are looked upon as impositions, sources of red tape, and hindrances to expeditious shortcut work methods. However, historically this has not been the case. An effective safety program can, and indeed usually does, lead to improvements in cost and efficiency of operation as well as the quality of life of those people living and working within the safer environment.

A trend that has developed in parallel to increasing concern for the design-for-human-welfare approach has been an expansion of the human factors engineer's responsibilities from the single machine or control panel to the entire environment in which the human must function. This expansion was motivated by the realization that a given piece of hardware could not be designed for optimal human use unless the environment in which that equipment would ultimately function was also controlled in dimensions such as lighting, available work space, and noise. As the engineer's sphere of concern thus expanded, it became clear that the concept of environment must encompass not only physical parameters, but also the social climate and organizational structures in which activity occurs. In the area of safety, it is now clear that such an overall systems approach is critical. This view is implicit in the contents of this handbook, which includes sections dealing with specific hardware and procedural details, human behavior and nature, and socioorganizational features of effective hospital safety programs.

This section embodies a similar structure. Several alternative yet complimentary models of viewing the accident-generating interaction between people and environment will be presented. These are intended to provide frameworks upon which subsequent material in this section and others can be organized. The section will then proceed to an overview of the human factors (in the human nature sense-of-the-term) of the individual as they relate to safety. A brief consideration of some social and organization human factors influences upon safety will then be presented. Finally, a discussion of the relation of the overall physical environment upon hospital accidents will be provided. The primary emphasis of this section, however, will rest in a consideration of the characteristics of the individual member of the hospital community.

Humans as the Cause of Accidents

While the logical arguments presented in the previous section support close scrutiny of the human element in accidents, statistical evidence provides even stronger justification. Deferring the conceptual definition of cause temporarily, accidents may be grouped into three general categories according to their proximal causes: human error, equipment failure or environmental inadequacies (e.g., poor lighting), and "acts of God" (e.g., an accident precipitated by a lightning bolt). In an analysis of 873 accidents at Mt. Carmel General Hospital in 1965, Fagin and Vita attributed human error or undue risk-taking (combining patient, visitor, and staff populations) with 95% of the accidents. Only 5% of the accidents observed during the study period were attributed to mechanical or environmental-design failures. The third category, which is all too often used as an excuse for the inadequacies of safety programs, was not represented at all in the Mt. Carmel data.

A similar pattern appears in the records of 1023 accident reports collected at Mt. Sanai Hospital.[1] This study revealed human behavior as the proximal accident cause in the vast majority of cases.

While such statistics support the importance of human actions in accident causation, they are somewhat arbitrary in classification as to cause. This categorization is reminiscent of a traditional debate between labor and management groups as to the causes of industrial accidents. The former group points to unsafe working conditions, while the latter lays the blame upon unsafe acts and failure to follow company rules and policies. In reality, the problem of cause is much more complex. It is generally accepted that accidents are due to a multitude of contributing factors, therefore it is somewhat unrealistic to single out a sole cause for any accident. While a broken ladder may be identified as the proximal cause of an accident, the failures of the ladder user to perceive the hazard and of maintenance and manufacturing inspectors to detect product flaws must be recognized as necessary ingredients in the occurrence of the accident. The point is that seldom, if ever, can the single cause of an accident be identified, and even less frequently, can an accident be described as having no component of human involvement in its genesis.

Preventability of Accidents: Humans as the Cure

Perhaps the biggest obstacle to overcome in a safety program is the implicit acceptance of the unavoidability of accidents. The intuitive concept of an accident is an event that occurs unexpectedly and fortuitously to an individual who just happens to be in the wrong spot at the wrong moment. While people are sometimes innocent victims of fate, statistics support the view that accidents are not random occurrences but appear with predictable frequencies related to specific situations. Additional statistical support for the contention that accidents are not simply the random slings and arrows of outrageous fortune are presented in a subsequent section dealing with the epidemiology of accidents. Furthermore, these statistics suggest that people are much less likely to be innocent victims than the agent which activates the final links in the accident chain. This latter statement is true even in the somewhat specialized context of hospital accidents where, for example, a patient may become the passive victim in an accident. Even most patient accidents are potentiated by the patient's actions, although often in conjunction with the activities of others as well.

Precisely because of the nonrandomness of accidents and because of the critical role of human actions in their occurrences, effective safety programs are possible. Thus, just as people are frequently the instigators of accidents, so can human actions become the remedy for safety problems.

The Special Nature of Hospital Accidents

There are several aspects of the hospital setting which make accidents occurring within it especially critical. The foremost issue concerns the obvious fact that the primary function of a hospital is to enhance the well-being of those whom it serves. Thus, the occurrence of hospital accidents is particularly distressing since these impact upon the central purposes of the institution. Consequently, hospital accidents can produce greater emotional trauma both to the victim (and in the case of patients, his sense of being adequately cared for) and the community at large. While a slip, fall, and broken bone are unfortunate events in any context, the impact of hearing that an individual received his injury at home or at the factory in which he works is far less dramatic than the emotional effect upon learning that this injury was received after the individual was admitted to a hospital for care.

An additional point to bear in mind is that accidents within hospitals involve patient injury far more often than staff or visitor harm. This is due to a number of factors, but it highlights another special feature of hospital accidents, namely that the population most frequently experiencing these incidents is physically under par and thus more susceptible to the consequences of accidents than would be a healthy population. Since minor accidents offer the potential for greater harm than they would outside the hospital setting, they warrant more concern and effort than they might otherwise receive.

Although accident precipitators are usually the victims of accidents they themselves cause, violations of this general rule are likely to be more frequently found in the hospital than in other settings. There is more opportunity for a patient to become the passive victim of another's errors simply because of the passive role assumed by patients in hospitals. It is generally unrealistic, for example, to expect the patient to be able to protect himself from medication errors or accidents that occur when he is unconscious or sedated. Thus, there is a certain heightened moral urgency about hospital accidents; outside the hospital, unsafe behavior is likely to be self rewarding (or unrewarding), while in the hospital this is less likely to be the case.

Finally, it is interesting to note that in the area of accidental injuries to staff, hospitals have a fair, but by no means excellent, safety record. While accident rates vary widely depending upon hospital size and staff position, an overall rate of 8.6 injuries per 1 million hr worked has been observed in hospitals.[2] Although this certainly compares favorably to the rate found in the logging industry (76.8), and general manufacturing (13.4), hospital performance is inferior to that of publicly owned colleges (7.4), synthetic fiber manufacturers (1.7), and even to the explosives manufacturing industry (3.6). Thus, there is room for both optimism and criticism in the safety ratings of hospitals. No matter how these figures are taken, however, they do suggest that significant improvements in safety can and should be achieved in an industry devoted to health.

Frameworks for Analyzing Human Factors in Accidents

Accidents are not randomly occurring events. An understanding of the processes that lead to accidents can be of help in guiding preventive and remedial action. In this section, several models of the accident process will be presented. These alternative viewpoints are helpful not only in understanding the interacting contributions of human and environmental factors in accidents, but also as means for directing and organizing the search for causes and corrections.

The models to be presented fall into two general categories — descriptive and predictive. Descriptive models primarily provide frameworks for organizing collected data so that occurrences which led to specific accidents can be adequately interrelated. Since they are more concerned with "what" happened than "why", to some extent they are necessary precursors to more sophisticated predictive models which offer explanations of "why" accidents occur and seek to verify these explanations by predicting characteristics of future accidents and accident patterns.

Chain-of-Events Model

One of the oldest and most traditional views of the accident process is that of a sequence of abnormal events that progressively leads to, and culminates in the accident itself. The description of an accident within this framework is reminiscent of the lady of nursery-story fame who died because she swallowed a horse to catch the cow she swallowed to catch the pig... and so forth in an effort to catch a primarily ingested fly whose consumption initiated the unfortunate chain of events.

According to the chain-of-events model, an accident can occur only if each link in the process is accomplished. If the chance (C) of any event (E) in the accident sequence is designated $C(E_1)$, then the chance of the entire sequence of events occurring is equal to $C(E_1) \times C(E_2) \times C(E_3) \ldots \times C(E_f)$, where E_f is the final step in the accident process.

One problem with this traditional approach is that it is seldom clear how far back in time the sequence of events should be traced. Eventually, of course, the causal links will become lost or unclear, as in the case of the lady who died from swallowing a horse; the cause of the first event, swallowing a fly, was cloaked in mystery.

This model also suggests that the sequence of events can be broken equally and effectively by removing links anywhere in the process chain. It is probably more reasonable to suppose that events occurring in the more distant past are less closely linked to the accident itself and are, therefore, less effective targets for preventive action in the future. Indeed, traditional users of this accident model have tended to concentrate only on events very close to the termination of the chain — that is, the accident itself. Increasingly, however, safety professionals have extended the chain of events further into the past by looking for such events as family arguments, job difficulties, or early developmental experiences that may have predisposed the individual to unsafe behavior later in the chain.

The chain-of-events model is essentially descriptive in nature. Thus, while it leads to an understanding, or at least a cataloging of, events surrounding a particular accident, it does not, in itself, provide any general theory or guideline for predicting future accidents. Nevertheless, this model can lead to second-generation predictive models through the careful analysis of a large number of accident chains. Such an analysis can reveal consistently occurring links and interrelations among links. Based upon such accumulated information, a predictive model may be constructed to allow the chain of events to be extended forward in time, rather than simply traced back through history.

Multicause Model

The main disadvantage of the chain-of-events model is that it does not adequately convey the well-recognized fact that any event in the accident process may depend upon not just one, but a multitude of antecedent factors to elicit its occurrence. It is now accepted that accidents seldom result from an inevitable, domino-like process that can be realistically traced along a single path. Far more frequently, accidents result from the unfortunate intersections of several event sequences developing in parallel. In this model, the single chain of events is replaced by a more complicated, tree-like structure in which many separate branches join together and eventually reach the trunk. A number of ways of representing these tree-like accident histories have been developed (e.g., multilinear sequencing) and these formal methods can be used to identify places where the accident-process tree can be most effectively attacked.

Even though a particular event tree might be unique (indeed, it may be unlikely to ever occur again), various branches or twigs may be recurrent elements in many accidents. Thus, while the multicause model is descriptive in nature, it can also, like the chain-of-events model, lead to more sophisticated predictive models.

As with the simple chain-of-events model, the multicause model requires some judgment as to how far into the past analysis of the accident process should proceed. In addition to this longitudinal problem, there must be concurrent latitudinal decisions regarding the causes convergent at each node in the accident process tree. Generally, if errors are to be made in accident investigations utilizing this model, it is preferable to gather too much information rather than too little. Much of the early research into the accident causes severely limited the information gathered and is, therefore, of little use today. This is unfortunate since such early data would be particularly useful in analysis of changing patterns of accident causes over long-time periods.

Epidemiologic Model

Like the two previous models, the epidemiological model is essentially descriptive rather than predictive. It is based upon analogy to the three-component disease model in which illness is viewed as an interaction among host, agent, and environment. By carefully accumulating and documenting the characteristics of these three factors in each instance of disease, the nature of their interaction is gradually illuminated. The classic example of these techniques is Snow's localization of a particular water supply as the source of a cholera outbreak by recording, among other data, the geographical location (i.e., environment) of numerous disease cases.

Gordon pointed out that these same epidemiologic techniques could be applied to accident research.[3] In this context, the accident victim is the host, the agent is the injury-producing material or object (e.g., the floor in the case of falls), and the environment comprises both the social and physical milieu in which the accident occurred. This approach can provide convenient direction for data collection, as well as a framework for data storage and organization. The best use of this approach is made when documentation concerning each of the three factors — host, agent, and environment — is complete. However, this can also present the danger of information overload.

Before concluding this brief discussion of the epidemiologic model, it is appropriate to present some representative hospital accident data structured according to this framework. These data are from an epidemiologic study at Mt. Sanai Hospital.

Host — Males are more frequent accident victims than females (45.6 vs. 19.1 accidents per 1000 admissions). Various medical conditions are not randomly represented among victims. Patients suffering neurologic, psychiatric, and orthopedic diseases are overrepresented in proportion to their percentage of the overall patient population. Patients suffering cardiovascular, neoplastic and obstetric diagnoses are underrepresented. In this particular study, "50% of the accident victims were found to be irrational, confused, senile, or had some other alteration of their mental-emotional status in comparison to 5% in the general hospital population."[1]

Agent — It is consistently observed that the floor is the primary agent of patient injury because the majority of accidents involve falls (80% falls vs. 10% all other agent categories combined). Furthermore, 46% of accidents involved falls from bed, thus implicating patient beds as the most common secondary injury agent in accidents. Wheelchairs, crutches, etc. were also frequent secondary agents. Knives, broken glass, razor blades, etc. were primary agents in 10% of accidents, while heat sources including matches, cigarettes, and hot water were primary agents in 5% of accidents.

Environment — The patient's bedside is the most frequent site of accidents accounting for 61% of the cases. Bathrooms and hallways are the next most frequent accident environments (both 11%). Accident rates have also been found to differ among hospital departments with the surgical ward involved in 39% of accidents, compared to 31%, 27%, and 3% for medical ward, children's ward, and clinic, respectively. Surprisingly, most accidents occur during the time when attendants are usually present. Accidents were almost twice as frequent during the day shift (46%) than during the evening or night shifts (both 27%).

Individual Differences Model

This view of accidents and safety focuses upon the psychological and physical characteristics of individuals involved in accidents. According to the various forms of this model, accidents can largely be attributed to, and predicted from, personal characteristics present in varying degree among individuals. Thus, this model differs from those previously described in that it is primarily predictive in intent rather than descriptive. Presumably, by identifying and giving special attention to individuals possessing accident-related characteristics, safety may be enhanced. The primary shortcoming of the individual difference approach tends to be its exclusive concern with personal characteristics out of environmental or situational context.

Research guided by the individual differences approach has attempted to identify a variety of safety-relevant personal characteristics. The most important of these will be discussed in a later section of this chapter. It suffices at present to note that these include age, job-related experience, physical health, risk-taking propensities, and some social adjustment/personality dimensions.

Modern application of this approach recognizes that personal characteristics change over time and that these features alone do not inevitably lead to accident involvement. Indeed, the connection between various personal traits and accident frequency is generally found to be rather weak. While these constraints seem natural and almost self-evident, it is important to note that their denial represents the foundation of the most universally accepted version of the individual differences model — accident proneness.

Accident-Proneness Model

It is important to deal with accident proneness as a separate model for two principal reasons (even though it is a representive individual differences model). First, belief in the validity of this model is particularly widespread and can result in the unfair stigmatizing of a few individuals who may serve as scapegoats for an inadequate safety program. Second, acceptance of this model inhibits more constructive accident-reduction efforts. This model is essentially tautological in that it identifies accident prones on the basis of accident involvement alone: Accident-prone individuals are those who have been in more than one previous accident. The level of explanation stops here. The intuition that underlies this model is that some people are simply "accident magnets" who will draw misfortune unto themselves no matter what steps are taken. Hence, beyond identifying and removing or isolating such individuals from the work or patient force, no additional safety efforts would be effective.

While the accident-proneness concept is rather vague and intuition-based today, the notion originated in the cautious statistical studies of Greenwood and Woods[4] and Newbold.[5] These researchers examined the distribution of accidents among groups of industrial workers. These distributions (how many workers have 1, 2,... or N accidents) were compared to distributions predicated upon a number of alternative statistical assumptions. One such assumption or hypothesis was that accidents are equally likely to befall any individual. This hypothesis is diametrically opposed to the unequal-liability assumption of accident proneness.

Statistical analysis revealed that although the equal-liability assumption provided an especially good first approximation to the distribution of individuals having 2 or fewer accidents (predicted number of workers = 640; observed = 622, a 3% error), it systematically underestimated the number of workers with 3 or more accidents (predicted = 8; observed = 26, a 31% error). Hence, although the equal-liability model provided a good approximation to the data in terms of absolute number of accidents, there were statistical grounds for rejecting this hypothesis. The researchers then tested several versions of the unequal-liability model and found improved fits to observed data patterns.

It is crucial to recognize that while individuals in these studies and indeed members of the hospital population appear to have unequal chances of being involved in accidents, the results of Greenwood and Woods[4] and Newbold do not suggest the source of the unequal liability. Before one could reasonably conclude that it rested in a personal characteristic of accident proneness, it must be demonstrated that individuals are equally exposed to accident risk. For example, it is certainly not reasonable to conclude that loggers are more accident prone than college professors simply on the basis that these groups differ considerably in accident frequencies. Clearly, the problem in supporting an accident-proneness position is to rule out a large number of equally, if not more probable explanations for the differences in accident liability which are revealed in statistical studies like those mentioned above. Furthermore, since accident proneness is assumed to be a personality characteristic of some sort, Surry points out that it is also necessary to rule out physical handicaps such as visual deficiency before assuming that a finding of unequal liability supports an accident-proneness interpretation.[6] Surry suggests that accident liability should refer to differences in likelihood of accident involvement due to all individual and risk-exposure differences, while accident proneness be reserved only for permanent, personality-related effects.

Much of the intuitive attractiveness of the accident-proneness concept rests on faulty use of probability laws. For example, a common bit of evidence cited in support of the accident-proneness model is an observation such as 5% of employees account for 80- or 90% of all accidents. A justifiable conclusion is that 5% of the work force is accident prone. In fact, this is not even support for the unequal-liability assumption, let alone hypotheses concerning the source of such unequal accident involvement. The fallacy can be seen most easily by extending the argument slightly. Suppose only one employee was involved in the single accident observed during a sampling period. Could one conclude that this individual was accident prone because he or she alone accounted for 100% of all accidents? Clearly, the answer is no, there were simply not enough accidents to ensure that all employees would experience accidents. The laws of probability which apply here do not require that every one sustain an equal number of accidents, only that every one have an equal chance.

Finally, it is appropriate to conclude this critique of the accident-proneness model by noting that if there is validity to the concept, its role in the accident problem is minimal. Even statistics such as those of Greenwood and Woods reveal only a very small percentage of accident repeaters (e.g., only 3% in the cited data).[4] If all of these were classified as accident prones and were somehow isolated from the work force, this would still leave 97% of the accident problem unsolved. Accident proneness is not an acceptable excuse for accidents.

Information-Processing Model

The information-processing model is a relatively recent approach to understanding the causes of accidents. This model posits an information-flow loop with people constantly receiving information from their environment, making decisions based upon their current perceptions and past experience, and carrying out responses in accordance with these decisions. Responses in turn, alter the environment and a new situation arises with which the human must deal. Accidents can result from failure at any point in this information-processing cycle.

A number of critical stages or information-processing functions have been identified. These include detection of information, recognition or identification of information, accessing appropriate material stored in memory, making decisions for action based upon identified information and past experience, carrying out responses, and finally, checking to determine that the desired changes in the environment have occurred. These abstract processes may be translated into the practical realm of safety as illustrated below.

After attempting to summon assistance and failing to receive aid, a patient may suffer a fall while attempting to get out of bed unassisted. The attendant who should have responded to the aid request may have been temporarily beyond the range of the assistance buzzer. Hence, a failure of information detection may have been responsible for this incident. On the other hand, the buzzer may have been misinterpreted as some other auditory signal — perhaps as a buzzer from another station. In this case, a recognition failure would have been to blame.

These two possibilities suggest that different remedies may be needed depending upon the type of information-flow failure responsible for an accident. A detection failure requires a more intense signal (or locating signal at several locations to distribute the information more effectively), while a recognition failure mandates the use of more distinctive signals (e.g., signals of different pitch for different stations).

Continuing along the information-flow path, an attendant might mistakenly "recollect" that another attendant was available to answer the aid request. Based on this memory error, an incorrect decision to delay responding may have resulted. Even if a decision to respond immediately was made, some other incident, perhaps an apparently more-pressing situation, may have distracted the attendant before the intended response was complete. Thus, a response failure caused by a competing distraction may have precipitated the accident described. Finally, being momentarily distracted and having forgotten the intended response, there may have been no follow-up signal to alert the attendant of the need for further action; i.e., the patient may have stopped signaling. In this case, a feedback failure could be assigned as the accident's cause since there was no environmental change to distinguish the effects of proper action from inaction. In both cases, the result would be the same — a silenced assistance buzzer. The remedy in this case would be a latching signal system (for example, a light that remained on until cleared by an attendant arriving at the patient's room).

It is evident that the information-processing model bases safe performance upon a set of fundamental, basic abilities which may be grouped into perceptual, decision, and response categories. Across individuals, differences in these abilities may be found as a function of age, for example. Specific changes in the environment may be required to compensate for these varying ability levels. Generallly, each of these basic abilities may be inadequate for safe performance for two reasons: (1) insufficient or inadequate information may be available as in the case of a weak auditory signal or dimly lighted stairway and (2) too much information may be presented for processing, thus overloading one or more stages. For example, it is quite difficult to follow two conversations simultaneously. Similarly, if a person is required to make several decisions in a short time period, errors are likely. Even in the response stages, problems of overload are present (balancing a food tray may be easy while walking but very difficult while running).

The information-handling capacities of the various basic-ability stages are thus of critical concern in the information-processing model. It appears that the capacities of individual stages may be quite sensitive to a variety of environmental factors. A primary human factors (in the engineering sense) goal is to design tasks to fall within the capacity ranges of all processing stages required in their performance.

PERSONAL HUMAN FACTORS

Personality Features Related to Safety

A belief long held in safety research is that accidents are related to certain personality characteristics. While this is undoubtedly true to some extent, the degree of relationship is controversial. In this section, a brief review of some of the findings in this area of safety research will be presented. Two points should be kept in mind. First, most, if not all of this work is concerned with identifying characteristics of the accident-causing individual. While the accident causer is frequently also the accident victim, this is not always so. The victim, especially in the hospital setting, may be the passive recipient of the consequences of an accident. This is likely to be the case, for example, in one of the most common hospital accidents — medication errors. While there may be some common characteristics among victims, the bond, if present, is undoubtedly very weak. Second, the relationships found between personality characteristics and accident involvement are generally weak even when statistically significant. It is unrealistic to assume that substantial improvements in accident rates could be achieved through such procedures as more intensive personality testing. Indeed, since the hospital has little control over the personality characteristics of patients or their visitors, concern with these features as important accident causes may be somewhat misplaced.

The notion that personality characteristics are related to accident frequency dates at least from the classic work of Tillman, a Canadian psychiatrist who extensively studied personality correlates of motor vehicle accidents.[7] His findings have been replicated in research with other accident types and are worth reviewing in the present context. Tillman interviewed low- and high-accident rate taxi drivers to obtain comparative personality profiles. The high-accident rate drivers were characterized by a higher incidence of family difficulties (divorce, alcoholism, etc.), childhood delinquency, and employment instability. The high-accident group also reported fewer hobbies and friends and were generally rated as emotionally immature and aggressive. Surprisingly, the high-accident group was generally in better health and exhibited fewer functional complaints than the low-accident group.

A more recent study by McGuire obtained results similar to Tillman and was a better controlled and more objective study.[8] McGuire also examined motor vehicle accidents and summarized his results: "When compared with the safe driver, the accident haver is less mature, less intellectual in his tastes and interests (although not necessarily less intelligent), has a lower aspirational level, expresses 'poor' attitudes toward the law and driving, is not as socially well adjusted and is the product of a less happy childhood." Similar findings by many other safety researchers support a relation between certain, usually negative, personality traits and accident frequency. Among other characteristics, people involved in accidents appear to exhibit less capacity for managing hostility, to be indifferent to the rights of others, to be excessively preoccupied with fantasy satisfaction, and to be generally less able to tolerate frustration.

Risk Taking

Somewhat more neutral (or even positively valued) personality traits have also been reported to characterize high-accident sample groups. Risk taking refers to the willingness of an individual to engage in an activity for which there is a perceived chance of failure and for which failure leads to a perceived harmful outcome. According to this definition, a danger need not be present. The only requirement is that the risk taker believe harm is possible. Risk-taking propensities seem to be related to a personality dimension characterized by the tendency to engage in exploratory behavior. While it is intuitive that both risk taking and explorativeness are related to safety, the existing evidence is unclear. Rockwell et al. tested a large sample of factory workers in a laboratory risk-taking study.[9] While a slight trend in the expected direction was found (i.e., high risk takers appeared to have a history of more frequent accidents), this trend was not statistically significant. On the other hand, a weak but statistically significant relationship was observed when risk taking was correlated with traffic violation history.

The concept of risk taking plays a central role in some theories of accident causation.[10] However, as Surry pointed out, the empirical relationships between risk taking and accidents are still in need of clarification.[6] An interesting finding is that risk-taking behavior is modifiable through training. In a study involving the training of truck drivers, Cohen found that trained drivers were less willing to accept risks than were drivers who did not undergo the training program.[11] In other studies not involving truck drivers, Cohen found that women consistently took less risks than men and that younger men exhibited a greater degree of risk taking than men over 30 years old.

Introversion/Extroversion

Another personality dimension of recent safety interest is introversion/extroversion. This personality characteristic is thought to be relatively stable. Generally, extroverts are characterized as socially outgoing while introverts avoid social interaction. The literature on the relationship between these personality types and accident rates is conflicting. Some reports show higher rates for extroverts while other studies reveal the opposite. Eysenck has suggested that extroverts exhibit involuntary rest pauses in brain activity, especially in repetitive, extended tasks.[12] Extroverts are more susceptible to accidents during these temporary mental lapses. Welford attempted to resolve the conflicting data on this issue by suggesting that extroverts tend to have higher accident rates in monotonous tasks while introverts exhibit higher rates in complex, demanding situations.[13] There is some support for this conjecture in the accident literature.

Relations to Accident Proneness

Before concluding this section on personality, the relationship between factors discussed here and accident proneness should be considered. While some of the criticisms leveled at the concept of accident proneness also apply to other personality dimensions, there are several important distinctions. First, the dimensions described in this section are defined on bases other than accident involvement itself. Hence, they avoid (at least with respect to accidents) the problem of circularity that plagues the accident-proneness concept. Furthermore, there is certainly no implication in the relationships noted to suggest that any of these personality attributes draw accidents to a particular individual. The accident-proneness concept, on the other hand, is frequently applied to innocent victims as well as accident causers.

Stress and Overload

The concepts of stress and overload were presented briefly in the discussion on the information-processing model of accidents. While susceptibility to these factors might be viewed as a personality feature, their implications go beyond emotional behavior and social interaction to include physical endurance, perceptual acuity, and decision-making performance. The effects of stress and overload are best discussed within the framework of the information-processing model. Humans have limited abilities to perform the basic functions necessary for daily activity. These limits may be significantly reduced under a variety of circumstances. At such times, the demands of everyday activities may exceed the limits of ability and one or more of the following consequences may result.

Consequences of Stress and Overload

The human under stress may begin to exhibit error-prone behavior. First, in an effort to meet all demands, a person may devote less than the necessary time to each of his tasks, thus partially completing each at the cost of low-quality performance. For example, a person under stress may shortcut those procedures specified for safe task performance. Second, when subjected to overload and stress, a person may begin to work at a slower rate or decide to selectively neglect some tasks altogether. Instead of speeding up and producing error-filled performance, a person may slow down and concentrate on only a subset of the tasks demanding his attention. Third, a person may react to overload with temporary physiological compensation. However, this transient mustering of physiological resources incurs a long-term debt that can lead to more severe overload and less adequate coping responses in the future.

There is considerable evidence suggesting that subjecting an individual to stressful situations increases the likelihood of accident involvement. Kerr suggested that an adjustment-stress theory of accidents could account for 45 to 50% of the variance in accident-frequency statistics.[14] One study of fatal accidents revealed 80% of the victims to have been subjected to some significant source of stress (e.g., severe interpersonal conflict) within the 24 hr preceding their accident.[15] Patients in a hospital are certainly under the load of significant stress, and hospital staff subjected to extended working hours without adequate rest are similarly afflicted. The degenerative effects of stress upon safe behavior may partially explain the finding that repeat accidents are most likely to occur within five days following injury in a hospital accident. This may reflect lingering physical and psychological stresses associated with the first accident. Stress in the present context is not limited to psychological events, but includes physical overload as well. This ranges from the overload of carrying too much weight, walking too far during the work day, or recovering from an operation.

Sources of Stress

Because of the close relation between stress, overload, and unsafe behavior, several sources of the two former items should be considered. Work loads in hospitals are frequently very high. Although these are often mandated by situational variables, emergencies, and budget requirements, their impact upon safety should be recognized. While work can induce stress by requiring excessive energy expenditures, its nonenergetic features such as monotony, eye strain, and boredom are more often to blame. The effects of these features upon safety are significant since they result in careless decisions, increased risk taking, increased irritability, and wandering attention.

An important aspect of work stress is fatigue caused by extended periods of sleeplessness. Studies of enforced sleeplessness show that one night of missed sleep produces no measurable physiological effect. However, there are effects upon mental efficiency; decisions take longer, learning becomes more difficult, vision begins to blur, and attention span reduces. After two sleepless days, these effects become more pronounced with failures of short-term memory and momentary hallucinations appearing. Effects of inadequate motivation are greatly compounded under conditions of sleeplessness or other fatigue-inducing stresses.

Stress in the Patient

While long working hours and lack of sleep are important sources of stress for the hospital staff, fear and anxiety are more significant for the patient. It is expected, of course, that a hospital stay will be accompanied by some apprehension and worry. This anxiety primarily interferes with decision making and judgment. High-anxiety levels interfere with manual skills requiring acute dexterity. Fear- and apprehension-induced stress also produce increased irritability and a reduced tolerance for safety regulations and procedures required in the hospital setting (e.g., those relating to ambulation). Although it must be recognized that a residual level of anxiety and heightened accident susceptibility will accompany hospital stays, there is much that can be done to mitigate this problem. Ronco pointed out a number of human-factors problems of the hospital environment that aggravate fear and apprehension.[16] They are associated with four problems: (1) the patient is cut off from his normal social supports, (2) the patient is deprived of the physical attributes of his accustomed environment, (3) the patient is deprived of information concerning his condition and procedures that he will experience, and (4) the patient is deprived of his autonomy.

Although reduction of physical freedom is often unavoidable due to lack of available space as well as regard for the patient's safety, the physical and psychological benefits of increased freedom should be considered. Aside from potential physically therapeutic effects, the ability to move around and explore one's environment promotes a sense of security by providing information about the nature of one's surroundings. Fear and anxiety are reduced in proportion to such familiarity. In addition to physical confinement, patients are subjected to psychological confinement as well. This results from both formal procedures and social conventions regarding the proper behavior patterns in the hospital setting. Formal procedures specify when, what, and how much a person may eat, when a patient must sleep, when visits with friends or relatives are permitted, etc. The patient finds himself under the complete control of the system. This counters entirely the conventions that apply outside the hospital. Consequently, control imposed by these policies is particularly frustrating and can lead to disregard for rules and procedures (including those designed to promote safety) whenever the opportunity to "strike back" at the system arises. The industrial psychology literature contains many instances of decreases in morale and increases in errors and hazardous behavior associated with excessive control.

Social conventions implicitly define the role the patient is expected to assume in the hospital, namely that of a passive recipient of manipulations and medications. The patient is not expected to question or otherwise interfere with the activities which occur around him or even those that involve him directly. This social convention has two undesirable consequences. First, it tends to isolate the patient and increase his sense of anxiety. Second, it deemphasizes the active role the patient could potentially play in improving hospital safety. Although the patient is not assigned any formal responsibilities for noting, reporting, or correcting hazards, neither should this behavior (within limits) be actively discouraged.

A number of simple improvements can often be made in the hospital environment, both physical and social/organizational, to reduce anxiety-related stress. Informing the patient as completely as possible concerning the nature of procedures to be performed should be considered. Information concerning hospital routines and physical arrangement is also beneficial. Such information should be conveyed by personal interaction as well as through printed material. In addition, some attention should be paid to the location and type of available bedside controls. Controls for lighting, summoning assistance, television or radio adjustments, etc. can enhance the patient's sense of control and thereby reduce the anxiety and frustration caused by his confinement. Additional steps such as allowing the patient some freedom to rearrange room furnitures should also be considered. Another factor that contributes to a patient's anxiety and fear is lack of familiar surroundings and social contacts that provide support and reassurance outside the hospital. Aside from minor personal articles, patients are typically not allowed to bring such familiar and psychologically stabilizing items as pictures, books, tables, or chairs into their rooms. While a balance must obviously be struck between the potential benefits of such freedom and the hazards associated with clutter and unsafe articles (e.g., electrical appliances), consideration of policy flexibility should be given.

As a final item, some mention should be given to the most obvious source of stress in the hospital — the patient's disease or health problem. While another section will consider some of the direct safety-related effects of disease, its relationship to accidents via stresses induced in its victims should be given its due consideration. Aside from direct decrement in physical and mental abilities, the patient's disease engenders apprehension and anxiety that can amplify the effects of other safety-related deficiencies. Under normal circumstances, an individual might be able to withstand the additional stresses imposed by physical and psychological confinement. These normally minor factors assume far greater impact when added to the stresses already accompanying the patient's physical condition.

Physical Limitations

Just as the limits of an individual's perceptual and decision-making abilities present safety implications, so too do a person's physical limits. While this may be obvious, there are several special considerations within the context of the hospital safety.

Patients in a hospital are frequently experiencing a rapid change in their physical capacities. Therefore, it is likely that they are somewhat unaware of the new limits imposed upon their behavior. Until patients have been able to adequately explore their new range of physical abilities, a danger exists that these limits will be exceeded. This initial unfamiliarity with one's new physical state may account for the finding that patients are most likely to become involved in an accident shortly after hospital admittance. One recommendation is to provide an adequately supervised opportunity for patients to explore the boundaries of their newly redefined abilities.[17]

A patient's inability to perform formerly simple tasks may become a significant source of frustration. This can lead to undue risk taking and intolerance for rules and delays that would otherwise be acceptable. Increased sensitivity to this problem of temporary physical limitation is warranted. This should be reflected in lowered bed heights, lights and phones that can be reached from a wheelchair, and windows and curtains that can be operated with minimal strength requirements. Physical limitations are especially critical in situations such as getting in and out of wheelchairs and when using crutches. Stairways also likewise present an obvious risk for temporarily incapacitated individuals. The recommendation for lowered bed heights is made on the basis of several safety surveys that revealed a high incidence of falls when getting into or out of bed.[1] Lowering beds at night has become a standard practice in some hospitals. The relationship between physical limitations and accident liability is suggested by statistics reporting accident frequency by patient category. A Mt. Sanai Hospital survey revealed the highest incidence of accidents among neurologic and orthopedic patients when statistics were corrected for the size of the population at risk.[1] This result is similar to that observed at the University of Illinois Research Hospitals where nearly half of the accident victims were localized among surgical-ward patients.

Finally, the patient population is unusual in its representation of chronic physical limitations. Because of this, long-term design decisions may be much more safety-effective than they would outside the hospital. These measures should include nonslip floor surfaces, installation of automatic door mechanisms, low-speed elevators, and frequent use of handrails.

Age

Age has been found to be consistently related to accident involvement both in and out of the hospital. Within this setting, the effect of age appears in the accident-frequency rates of patient, visitor, and staff populations, although it takes different forms for these groups.

Accident rates for hospital patients are often found to rise dramatically above age 60. Another peak is found for patients below age 15. Williams localized this youth peak at ages 5 to 14.[18] Weil and Parrish suggested that these peaks were partially due to different exposure rates.[1] However, after correcting their statistical analysis of 1036 accidents for risk exposure, they continued to find higher accident rates for patients below age 10 and in the 60 to 69 age range. The peak in accident rates among young patients is similar to a peak in industrial accidents observed among workers at about age 22. However, industrial-accident statistics show a consistent decline in accident rates with increasing age. This most likely represents the restricted age range encountered in industry as compared to the hospital.

A number of hypotheses have been advanced for the accident-rate age peaks encountered among hospital patients. Among these are the changes in physical ability that accompany old age. Also, the sensitivity to injury increases, thus enhancing the likelihood of an accident report. Among the young, explanations stress lack of knowledge of potential hazards, willingness to take higher risks even when hazards are recognized, higher activity levels, and personality characteristics of immaturity and lack of concern for rules and formal procedures. Indeed, a number of the personality traits which were previously discussed in relation to accident frequency are to some degree specific for age. The general physical awkwardness that accompanies the 5 to 15-yr range may also play a significant role.

Among hospital staff, as among industrial workers, there appears to be a reduced age effect compared to hospital patients. In a study of medication errors, Safren and Chapanis found a brief age effect consisting of a peak among the most youthful nurses.[19] However, this "age" effect was undoubtedly a manifestation of training and experience rather than the physiological result of aging.

This highlights one of the primary difficulties in attempting to interpret the apparent relation between age and accident frequency. Since young workers are generally less experienced than older workers, it is difficult to separate the effects of age from those of experience. In fact, experience seems to be a much more potent factor than age, producing about a 100-fold decrease in accident rate after 3 months job experience. However, a study by Van Zelst compared different age groups at comparable levels of experience and found some evidence for a decreasing accident rate as age increased to 60.[20] The effects of experience dropped quickly during the first three months of employment. Van Zelst attributed his findings to: (1) the relative immaturity of younger workers and (2) the tendency for employees unsuited for their jobs to leave during the early years of employment.

Another explanation for age effects is that it reflects a slowing of decision-making speed that is known to accompany aging.[13] There is also some deficit in short-term memory that may play a role in some accidents. However, it appears that these changes in cognitive abilities do not strongly influence accident rates until they become extreme. There is only weak evidence for any accident rate increases in the 30 to 60 yr span.

Basic Abilities

Safe behavior rests upon the adequate functioning of a number of basic abilities grouped generally into perceptual, memory/decision making, and response categories. Attention and alertness are two additional concepts which were not discussed previously. Although an individual may possess the necessary basic abilities for safe performance, he will not realize this potential if his level of alertness is low or his attention is diverted from the task at hand. In this section, the relationship of some of these basic abilities to safety will be discussed.

Perceptual Abilities

Perceptual abilities include the essential capacity to detect information in the surrounding environment and recognition which involves identifying and extracting meaning from the information detected. Detection depends strongly upon environmental factors such as illumination, noise, and the nature of competing distractions. It also depends upon features of the information signal itself such as distinctiveness, color, intensity, pitch, and duration. Finally, detection depends upon human factors such as visual acuity and experience. An experienced individual will know where and when to look for significant safety-related information in his surroundings. One function of warning labels is to direct attention to information that would otherwise be undetected. Several specific features of detection are important in the context of safety. Color information is particularly difficult to extract in dim illumination. Thus, color-coded labels, gas cylinders, controls, or cables should be utilized only under normal levels of illumination. Field-of-view and peripheral vision are also significant features in visual detection, particularly in relation to accidents involving collisions with objects. Normal field-of-view extends roughly 200° horizontally and 140° vertically.

Failures of detection are responsible for a significant number of accidents. If an individual cannot detect information needed to avoid a hazard, his accident liability is obviously increased. A number of human factors recommendations have been made to aid detection. For example, dome-shaped mirrors mounted above hallway intersections can provide a means for detecting on-coming traffic around corners. Similarly, the use of eye-level warning labels on glass doors is designed to improve detection of the hazard posed by the plate glass. Doors should be equipped with see-through panels so that the presence of individuals on the other side can be detected.

More sophisticated detection aids are also found within the hospital, such as on patient-monitoring equipment, fire-detection sensors, etc. These emergency-warning systems are designed to supplement human detection capabilities when events to be sensed are below human threshholds or when continuous vigilance is required. Such aids are effective only if their signals are detected. A number of guidelines have been developed for warning signals.

Auditory signals are generally preferable to visual indicators because the ears are less directive and the auditory signal can cover a larger area. However, visual signals mounted in distinctive locations or placed in several strategic positions can be effective. The best strategy, when possible, is to combine simultaneous auditory and visual signaling since the chance that both signals will be missed is small. This principle may have special significance in the hospital setting where sensory handicaps are commonly encountered. Intermittent (i.e., pulsed) or wailing signals usually attract more attention than steady signals. A pulse or wailing rate of 2 to 3 per second is most effective. Chimes or gongs are relatively ineffective alerting devices. Recommendations for sound intensities and frequencies can be found in several standard human engineering source books (e.g., Van Cott & Kincade[21]). One approach that should be considered to ensure adequate sound intensity over a wide area is placing multiple low-intensity sources at strategic locations. Another important principle in the use of alerting signals is that they should not be self-terminating. Warning signals should remain on until the action they demand is taken.

To be effective, warning signals must also be recognized. To facilitate recognition, the amount of information conveyed by the signal itself should be minimized whenever possible. There are limits to the information that humans can reliably extract from simple signals such as lights or tones. In pair-wise comparison, people can distinguish tones differing by only a hertz or two in frequency. However, absolute judgment (i.e., the ability to identify one of several tones presented in isolation) is far less effective. People begin to make errors when distinguishing among as few as five or six tones, even under optimal conditions. Under emergency stresses, recognition among as few as three or four signals may be unreliable.

Some ways of coding warning signals are more effective than others. Use of time-based or counting signals (e.g., a fast-pulsing tone indicates one situation, a slow-pulsing tone another; three chimes signify one condition, two chimes another) are particularly ineffective. Potential safety problems of color blindness are of traditional concern. Although this does not appear to be a major accident source, it should be considered. For example, color-coded warnings (green light means safe to enter, red light means danger) should be supplemented with other information (e.g., a "safe to enter" sign).

The detection and recognition of potential hazards represents a problem in vigilance.

Since the occurrence of hazards is relatively rare, rather long intervals may separate an individual's encounters with hazards. Vigilant performance is known to be sensitive to the interval separating successive signals (in this case, hazard-indicating information), with the likelihood of perceiving signals decreasing with increasing intervals. This perceptual deficit does not reflect a decrease in sensitivity to signals (i.e., hazards). However, after extended intervals without encountering a hazard, people become less willing to recognize a particular piece of information as representing a danger. In signal-detection-theory terms, decision bias, rather than sensitivity, is affected. This bias shift should be considered to ensure continued safety improvements. Since the intervals between hazard encounters will increase with the effectiveness of the safety program, sustained vigilance becomes more difficult. An individual will encounter hazards less frequently than the entire staff. Individuals are therefore more sensitive to vigilant decrements than would be expected on the basis of the actual number of hazards within the hospital. A potential remedy for this problem is to disseminate information concerning hazard-detection rates of the entire staff, thus providing a truer picture of hazard prevalence.

Another method for improving hazard detection is minimizing implicit reporting costs. The recognition process is complex even in the perception of a frayed electrical wire or drip of water onto the floor. According to one model of this process, people evaluate the likelihood of alternative "perceptions" in relation to some internal cost function. For example, perception of a hazard involves the implicit costs associated with additional follow-up action. The safety benefits of recognizing a hazard obviously outweigh these internal costs. However, when real hazards are exceptionally unlikely, even small implicit costs may deter proper perception. Thus, it is important that no subtle penalties be imposed for "crying wolf" in the reporting of potential hazards. These implicit cost effects may be even stronger in the case of patients or visitors who are unfamiliar with the hospital environment and thus run a greater risk of appearing foolish or overly concerned.

Detection and recognition of hazards can also be improved by training. Training should be directed toward the identification of specific hazards. Allowing personal examination of detected hazards is the most effective training procedure since it provides the most accurate hazard-matching template. The availability of such internal templates significantly enhances perceptual acuity. The use of pictures or sound recordings of actual hazards is also useful, though less effective than personal examination. Of course, verbal or written descriptions can be used. However, such descriptions are less effective in generating accurate pattern-matching templates.

Recognition of hazards is not the only role that perceptual processes play in accident prevention. Failures of perception can create accidents from otherwise commonplace occurrences. Misreading a drug label, physician's order sheet, nursing care card, or medicine ticket was the second most frequent (18%) cause of medication error in a study of this problem.[19]

Memory and Decision Making

Memory and decision making also play significant roles in safety. While no relationship between "having a bad memory" and accident frequency is apparent, memory failures are involved in a large number of accidents. Such situations may involve failure to recall proper procedure or to complete an interrupted activity. In the previously cited study of medication errors, 3% of the incidents occurred when a nurse administered only a partial drug dose (due to insufficient quantity available) and then later forgot to complete the dosage. Similarly, computation and decision-making processes affect accident-frequency statistics. For example, 6% of medication errors in the cited study were associated with calculational errors in computing doses, converting between measuring systems, etc.

Memory and decision-making processes are usually insensitive to deterioration from ongoing distractions since these can be filtered out rather effectively. However, decision making, in particular, will deteriorate quickly when an individual must divide his attention among two or more simultaneous tasks. This problem is especially severe if the competing tasks are similar to each other. For example, calculation of medication dosages will be degraded by a simultaneous task which demands counting. The duties of staff personnel should be examined for such potential conflicts. When detected, human engineering solutions may be available. For example, when simultaneous overlap of two numeric tasks is unavoidable, paper pads or a chalkboard could be provided for storage of intermediate results, thus reducing memory demands.

While a relationship between intelligence and accidents seems intuitive, the evidence for such a link is lacking when extreme cases are excluded (e.g., Farmer and Chambers[22] and Penn[23]). However, Biesheuval and White did report a relationship between intelligence and aircraft accidents.[24] It may be that this relationship only appears in situations involving rather high degrees of intellectual effort.

Training and Learning

The debate concerning the relative importance of innate and learned characteristics of human behavior has been long and tedious. However, it is clear that learning and training issues are central to the development of effective accident counter measures. We certainly cannot rely upon innate mechanisms to improve hospital safety. There are two aspects of learning to consider in relation to safety. First, it is necessary to learn when, where, to whom, and eventually why accidents occur. Descriptive models of the accident process promote this phase of safety learning. The second aspect of learning concerns the conveying of information about safe procedures and practices. This latter aspect essentially is one of training. How can safe-behavior practices be taught?

Learning-by-Doing

The most important principle of learning and training is that we learn those behaviors that we perform. If an individual is induced to perform a procedure or behave in a manner that enhances safety, that person will unavoidably learn something of that behavior and be more likely to repeat it under similar circumstances. Each time the behavior pattern is exercised, an increment in learning will occur. This principle dominates other issues such as motivation, reinforcement, the spacing of practice, etc. Although these other factors are powerful influences on learning, they are effective because they change the likelihood that a particular behavior will be performed; learning occurs when the action is carried out.

Two types of learning can be distinguished: (1) the acquisition and storage of basic information and (2) carrying out actions based upon this knowledge. The former provides a necessary foundation for the latter. One cannot solve a calculus problem until basic knowledge has been acquired to allow exercise of the activity. However, it is the performance of the action that leads to increased learning and proficiency.

Reinforcement and motivation assume significance through the following process. People are reticent to undertake action unless motivated to do so. This is not to say that a person will sit like a vegetable until externally motivated; humans have intrinsic motivations to instigate behaviors. However, reinforcement provides motivation to undertake a particular activity. Once the activity is underway, additional learning can commence. Reinforcement serves as a generator of motivation, motivation is a generator of action, and action is a generator of learning. Once performed, an activity becomes more likely in the future because it can be more easily motivated.

One implication of this learning theory is that safe behavior is best promoted by preventing unsafe activity during early exposure to the hospital environment. A patient may be tempted to risk a fall by getting out of bed unassisted. If this is done once, the unsafe-behavior pattern will be partially learned and will be more likely to reoccur. There is some controversy as to whether such learning can ever be "undone" entirely. Perhaps the best that can be achieved is to provide another safer behavior which can be learned better.

Thus, emphasis should be placed upon preventing initial performance of unsafe activity. This can be done by carefully instructing patients concerning dangers associated with particular activities and by providing instruction in alternative safer procedures. It is important that the alternative be as easy as possible, thus removing any "negative" motivation which may influence the patient's choice of future action. Returning to the example of the patient getting out of bed, a "practice" trial getting in and out of bed could begin the learning process. The alternative to such practice is to hope the patient will retain the verbally transmitted set of basic facts and that this will appropriately influence his motivational pattern the first time he decides to get out of bed.

The learning-by-doing concept is certainly not new. It provides justification for practice drills. Fire drills are probably much more disruptive of normal hospital activity than would be occasional administrations of paper-and-pencil tests concerning evacuation procedures. Most people would agree that a fire drill is a far more effective way of instilling and refreshing the correct procedures to be followed in a fire. Training-by-doing is almost always more effective than training-by-description and should be applied whenever possible in safety-education programs.

Learning-by-Watching

When learning-by-doing is not possible, the next best alternative is learning-by-watching. Seeing another individual behave in a particular fashion can be an effective training mechanism for the observed behavior. The reasons for this are not clear, but may reflect the possibility that basic knowledge of the activity details are more richly conveyed than with verbal, written, or pictorial description alone. Observing may produce some form of covert activity by the watcher (imagining oneself carrying out an action may be somewhat akin to actually performing the activity). Returning again to the patient getting out of bed, other patients in the room would be more likely to engage in this same activity having seen their roommate successfully perpetrate the unsafe practice. However, if the model patient's impetuosity resulted in an accident, his roommates would be dramatically less likely to undertake such behavior compared to someone who had not observed the incident.

The effectiveness of learning-by-watching is the basis for several phenomena. New arrivals in the hospital environment will behave more in accordance with the actions of those around him than with their words when these sources of information conflict. One reason why a peer group exerts such a strong influence on one's behavior patterns is that they represent the behavioral models most often observed. Similarly, the behavior of one's supervisor will be a significant influence since a person is likely to devote a substantial amount of attention in that direction.

Retention

Another important training issue concerns the durability of learning. Retention of procedures and motor activities seems more resistant to memory loss than rote learning of verbal material. However, even motor skills learned to an apparent peak of performance will deteriorate with time unless additional practice is given. Regression under stress will also affect safety-related training. Regression under stress describes the tendency to fall back upon simpler, earlier-learned behavior patterns under stress and overload. Under normal conditions, a nurse may follow routine procedures for drug administration exactly. But under stress-of-emergency situations, procedural steps and checks may be omitted, resulting in an accident. This reveals that the original learning was incomplete and training could have been profitably continued. While there are several reasons for regression under stress, the concern at present is how the effects of stress can be countered.

This training problem can be reduced by two methods. In the first, training occurs under conditions approaching, as realistically as possible, the actual conditions of stress that are later expected to occur. For example, fire drills are often more effective training devices when they are unannounced since the surprise of such tests mimics one stress-generating aspect of actual emergencies. The second approach employs overlearning. In this method, trainees are given continued practice with a skill even after having mastered it successfully.

Compatibility and Stereotyped Behavior

All patients, staff, and visitors enter the hospital with prior learning and behavioral predispositions. Frequently, it is possible to use such preexisting knowledge to promote safety. Unfortunately, the opposite often occurs. Through the years of experience, people acquire expectations concerning the way things should work. In the U.S., for example, most people have acquired an expectation for the way a switch should be moved to turn a light on or off. When displays, controls, and mechanisms violate such expectations, accident-generating errors frequently result. These stereotyped expectations in turn generate stimulus-response compatibility effects. In response to a given stimulus situation (e.g., a dark room) a particular response is selected (e.g., lifting the light switch) to accomplish a goal (e.g., lighting the room). When the required response matches the population stereotype, compatibility between stimulus and response is achieved. Compatibility facilitates performance while incompatibility creates interference. While such problems initially appear trivial, they are, in fact, a serious source of errors in complex systems (such as hospitals). These problems are compounded by regression under stress. Even though a person may learn a new response to replace a population stereotype, the preexisting expectation will very likely reappear in moments of emergency.

These problems produce specific hazards within the hospital. For example, people have expectations regarding the directions in which to turn a faucet to increase or decrease the water flow. If these conventions are violated, individuals run the substantial risk of scalding themselves when intending to turn off a hot water tap. Similarly, people have expectations regarding the way doors open (they don't swing into halls), the way controls should operate electrically actuated beds, the way switches should turn electrical equipment on and off, etc. Safety personnel should be alert to violations of population expectations; even if such incompatibilities don't directly contribute to an accident, they certainly reduce ease and convenience of system use. Many compatibility recommendations are embodied in building and equipment manufacturing standards. Nevertheless, it is easy to find obnoxious examples of incompatibility.

Motivation

In the previous section, motivation was described as a means of instigating action. In the present section, principles for generating motivation for safe behavior are discussed.

Motivation is generated principally through reinforcement. While the topic of reinforcement is rich in detail, only a few points will be emphasized here. First, positive reinforcement (i.e., reward) is much more effective than punishment in motivating a desired behavior. There are two reasons for this. Punishing incorrect or unsafe behavior, in itself, does not provide any information as to what constitutes correct behavior. Punishment increases the likelihood of future safe behavior only by reducing the likelihood that one particular example of unsafe behavior will not be selected for action again. In contrast, reward provides an incentive (i.e., motivation) for repeating the safe behavior and also implicitly indicates the nature of the desired activity. A second reason for punishment's relative ineffectiveness is that it generates a high level of stress. This stress inhibits learning the relationship between the punished action and its consequences.

Both reinforcement and punishment can be positive or negative. Negative reinforcement involves withholding punishment that would be delivered if safe procedures were not followed. Similarly, negative punishment involves withholding a reward that would otherwise be given. Although safe behavior is generally negatively reinforced (i.e., punishment is withheld), a general recommendation is to supplement this relatively weak motivator with a tangible reward such as formal recognition following a period of safety.

SOCIAL AND ORGANIZATIONAL FACTORS

The previous section concentrated on characteristics of the individual in isolation. The following section focuses upon the individual as a group member. Aspects of group behavior related to safety will be considered.

Since the classic Hawthorne Plant studies of the 1930s, it has been known that the socio-organizational climate of an institution can dramatically influence productivity and absenteeism. There is also evidence that a similar effect upon accident rates occurs. A study by Keenan et al. showed a high negative correlation between accident rates and social quality of the work environment.[25] Departments possessing comfortable social climates and characterized by a high degree of individual responsibility, good promotional opportunity, etc. were lowest in accident rate. The mechanisms whereby social factors influence accident rates is unclear. One possibility is that intercommunication is facilitated in friendly environments and group members are thus more likely to be cognizant of hazards. Another possibility is that work stress is reduced. It is not known whether such influences spill over to patient or visitor populations.

The most powerful influence upon the safety attitudes of a hospital staff member is likely to be the attitudes prevailing among his peers. These attitudes are likely to be communicated to patients as well. Two points should be stressed. First, since people are most influenced by their immediate peers, a successful safety program must involve a wide segment of the hospital population. It is definitely not sufficient to appoint a safety committee and delegate away all responsibility in the area of safety. A joint effort in this area is critical. Furthermore, a cooperative effort will tend to reduce potential friction caused by the imposition of rules by one group upon another.

The second point to recognize is that first impressions are the most important. When a visitor, patient, or staff member arrives at the hospital, a large measure of his attitudes concerning safety will be formed in the first few hours. Since this is the interval when the new arrival is most susceptible to persuasion, it is recommended that the importance of safety be actively promoted during this period. This can be done through printed material explaining potential hazards and safe practices or (more effectively) through personal discussions with new arrivals.

While an effective safety program must indeed instill the attitude that safety is everyone's concern, it must also provide clear channels of responsibility for action. For example, a general requirement to contact the safety committee to correct a problem is not sufficient. A more effective organizational structure would assign a specific individual to a specific area. Hazards noted in a particular region of the hospital would then be reported directly to the safety representative of that area. The name and office phone of each area representative should be prominently posted. Unless such clear personal links are established, diffusion of responsibility is likely, if not inevitable: while everyone may be aware of an area's hazards the problem will remain uncorrected.

Another organization obstacle which must be overcome concerns methods by which critical incidents and other hazards are reported. There is a natural reluctance to report incidents and conditions which might reflect on one's own performance or that of a colleague. This can represent a bottleneck in a critical-information flow. A number of possibilities for anonymous reporting schemes that do not involve revelation of identities could be devised. These certainly should be considered in an overall safety program.

HUMAN FACTORS ENGINEERING

The bulk of this chapter has been concerned with the ''human nature'' aspects of human factors. A few brief comments about the engineering and environmental modification aspect of the term is appropriate. Although there is a considerable body of engineering data regarding human behavior, capabilities, dimensions, and sensitivities, relatively little is known about the populations of greatest concern to hospitals, namely disabled individuals, the very young, and the very old. Even in the population of healthy middle-aged adults, the most commonly applied design-for-the-average procedures often lead to trouble. It has been reported that the chance of finding an individual who fits within the all-average tolerances for their age and sex is similar to that of finding two people with identical fingerprints. Hence, we all eventually encounter the rear-view mirror by which we can only see the roof of our own car, or the clutch pedal that is just out of comfortable reach. These problems are certainly magnified when similar principles are applied to the hospital patient population. At present, data are accumulating to allow proper human engineering to meet not only the safety needs, but also the convenience and comfort needs of these special populations.

SUMMARY

The key points stressed in this chapter include the following. In the vast majority of cases, people cause accidents by their own behavior. Accidents are not random and, just as people are the cause of accidents, so can people reduce accident frequencies. Because of the hospital's special role as health guardians, the impact of in-hospital accidents is particularly severe. Surprisingly, the record does not reveal an outstanding safety record for hospitals. Since accidents are interactions between people and their environment, both aspects of the problem must be simultaneously attacked for maximum safety-program effectiveness. Several ways of viewing and organizing the interrelationships among people, environment, and accidents were presented. Two central concepts were stress and basic information-processing abilities. Accident proneness was described as a counter-productive and discredited model. Perceptual problems were discussed in detail and some suggestions for improving hazard detection and recognition were presented. Also, the training and learning of safe behavior was discussed.

Some aspects of the social and organization environment were mentioned and the necessity for overall responsibility, rather than assignment of the burden of safety to a committee, was stressed. Finally, the dangers of design-for-average were stressed with regard to human engineering, particularly when the average was derived in a non-hospital population.

REFERENCES

1. **Weil, T. P. and Parrish, H. M.**, How did it happen?, *Hospitals*, 32, 43, 1958.
2. **Clague, E.**, Work injuries to hospital employees, *Hospitals*, 30, 37, 1956.
3. **Gordon, J. E.**, The epidemiology of accidents, *Am. J. Public Health*, 39, 504, 1949.
4. **Greenwood, M. and Woods, H. M.**, A Report of the Incidence of Industrial Accidents upon Individuals with Special Reference to Multiple Accidents, British Industrial Fatigue Research Board, No. 4, 1919.
5. **Newbold, E. M.**, A Contribution to the Study of the Human Factor in Causation of Accidents, British Industrial Health Research Board, No. 34, 1926.
6. **Surry, J.**, *Industrial Accident Research: A Human Engineering Appraisal*, University of Toronto Press, Toronto, 1968.
7. **Tillman, W. A. and Hobbs, G. E.**, The accident-prone automobile driver, *Am. J. Psychiatry*, 106, 321, 1949.
8. **McGuire, F. L.**, Personality factors in highway accidents, *Hum. Factors*, 18, 433, 1976.
9. **Rockwell, T. H., Galbraith, F. D., and Centre, D. H.**, Risk acceptance research in man-machine systems, Bulletin 187, Ohio State University, Columbus, 1961.
10. **Taylor, D. H.**, Accidents, risks, and models of explanation, *Hum. Factors*, 18, 371, 1976.
11. **Cohen, J.**, *Chance, Skill, and Luck*, Penguin Books, Baltimore, 1960.
12. **Eysenck, H.**, The personality of drivers and pedestrians, *Med. Sci. Law*, p. 416, 1962.
13. **Welford, A. T.**, On changes of performance with age, *Lancet*, 1, 335, 1962.
14. **Kerr, W.**, Complementary theories of safety psychology, *J. Appl. Psychol.*, 45, 3, 1957.
15. **Finch, J. R. and Smith, J. P.**, *Psychiatric and Legal Aspects of Automobile Fatalities*, Charles C Thomas, Springfield, Ill., 1970.
16. **Ronco, P. G.**, Human factors applied to hospital patient care, *Hum. Factors*, 14, 461, 1972.
17. **Morris, J.**, Solving patient and visitor safety problems, *Hospitals*, 30, 50, 1956.
18. **Williams, W. R.**, The patient's accident pattern, *Hospitals*, 22, 39, 1948.
19. **Safren, M. A. and Chapanis, A.**, A critical incident study of hospital medication errors, *Hospitals*, 34, 32, 1960.
20. **Van Zelst, R. H.**, The effect of age and experience upon accident rate, *J. Appl. Psychol.*, 38, 313, 1954.
21. **Van Cott, H. P. and Kinkade, R. G., Eds.**, *Human Engineering Guide to Equipment Design*, McGraw-Hill, New York, 1963.
22. **Farmer, E. and Chambers, E. G.**, A Psychological Study of Individual Differences in Accident Rates, British Industrial Fatigue Research Board, No. 38, 1926.
23. **Penn, R.**, An Investigation of Some Methodological Problems Concerned with Accidents, Department of Psychology, Carnegie Institute of Technology, Pittsburgh, 1955.
24. **Biesheuval, S., and White, M. E.**, The human factor in flying accidents, *S. Afr. Air Force J.*, 2, 25, 1949.
25. **Keenan, V., Kerr, W., and Serman, W.**, Psychological climate and accidents, *J. Appl. Psychol.*, 35, 108, 1951.

ORGANIZATION OF A HOSPITAL SAFETY PROGRAM

Allan J. McLean

BASIC ELEMENTS IN A HOSPITAL SAFETY PROGRAM

There are several principles common to the operation of any safety program whether it is in a hospital or other business. However, there are several specific areas that must be considered unique to a health care institution.

Appropriately, the first element is the most important. This is the necessary support and cooperation of top management. Without this support, a safety program can exist but not function, like a plant in just water; holding, but not growing. Effective management leadership consists of both financial and visible support. In many cases, the visible and active participation of the chief executive officer (CEO) and assistants is worth far more than money. Active, visible support will convince other staff that the safety program is important and should be considered. On the other hand, full funding and benign neglect from the administration will clearly tell everyone that the safety program is for show only, and will engender an attitude of disregard.

Policy Statement

A key element in an effective program, and the first sign of support from administration, is a policy statement. The policy statement is a simple statement of the responsibility and authority of the safety organization, including both a safety department (by whatever name it may have) and a safety committee. This policy statement should give an indication of who the organization reports to (hopefully the CEO and board of directors), the various functions and authorities the organization has (what it can do in the name of the CEO), and what departments and services are expected to be represented on the safety committee (regular members and consultants).

In addition to the policy statement, a policy and procedure manual, written safety program, or safety manual is needed. This manual should contain such items as the job description of the safety officer and assistants, descriptions of the safety inspection programs, accident reporting mechanisms, recordkeeping procedures, and training and inservice responsibilities. This is the source book for both the safety organization and others in the institution that have questions as to who and how various problems are handled.

Additionally, various departments and services should have their own safety manuals or safety sections in their policy and procedure manuals. Ideally, the program should hold each department or service responsible for the safety of its own employees visitors, and patients, with the safety office being used as a consultant and monitor for all of the programs.

Accident/Incident Investigation

Investigation

Accident/incident investigation and record-keeping will be covered first. It must be understood and accepted that the purpose of an accident or incident investigation is not to place blame. This is, perhaps, the most misunderstood principal in safety work. First, placement of blame will not undo the incident. In fact, it rarely ever minimizes the chance of similar future incidents. If its usual function is to attempt to punish the guilty it does little to advance safety. Worse, it actually inhibits the investigation because people are likely to give versions of the incident that protect themselves and friends, attempt to indict enemies, and muddy the water. Accident/incident investigation that identifies the parts of the two major elements of any incident and employs a policy that mandates that no punishing action will be taken against an employee (if the accident or incident was the only way to know that a violation had taken place) will better serve the purpose of locating the true causes and preventing future incidents. First, this attitude lends credibility to the concept that we are trying to help in order to prevent future incidents, not to find a scapegoat. Second, knowing that no punishment will come encourages people to come forth with accurate stories about what they saw. Incident reports should be designed to get information about both of the major elements in an incident, the personal side (i.e., who did or did not do what), and equally or more important, the physical or environmental conditions that allowed the incident to occur. Frequently, these are more important because there is often more that we can do to change conditions than we can do to change the actions of many employees. Also, changes in the working area affect everyone that comes into the area, not just one person.

Follow-Up

Following up an investigation is a three-phase program of using the results of the investigation. The first phase is to correct the immediate problem. This is the phase most usually done even when a safety program is minimal. Almost everyone will eliminate a hazard once it is pointed out so violently. However, the other two phases of information gathering and recordkeeping are often neglected. The second part of the process is analysis of the results in terms of trends and roots. This can be done with sophisticated computer processing, by mechanical systems, or by simple hand charting and analysis.

The process of charting, often called an awareness chart, is simply that of classifying all incidents (serious, first aid, and near misses) into appropriate categories, then tallying various incidents within each category against each department and service. This information suggests which departments require the most attention, which types of incidents and injuries require special attention, and whether various programs used to reduce injury are working as expected. The third phase is to translate the resulting information into figures usable with management. One way is to sample specific cases, develop an estimated cost per incident, and translate injury/accident data into direct cost figures.

Results

Because the language of management is cost and dollars, safety organizations that can translate at least a part of their data into cost figures are in a better position to justify requested changes, equipment, and physical modifications. Actual and estimated dollar cost figures, where applicable, are also usable in providing service and department heads with information about the safety operation of their responsibilities.

Within the process of awareness charting, an interesting phenomenon is noted. This is an offshoot of Pareto's law. We notice that specific accident types and specific departments and services occupy a large part of our attention. According to Pareto's law (roughly, 20% of all incidents represents 80% of our cost and time; the other 80% of the accidents requires the other 20% of our attention), we need to identify our "hot spots" and spend available resources (time, money, management attention) on these. If prevented or eliminated, these incidents will have an inordinant effect on the overall performance of the organization.

Analysis

The American National Standards Institute, in their Standard Z 16.2, Standard

I. Type of Injury

Cut or Laceration	Strain or Sprain	Amputation	Bruise
Fracture	Puncture Wound	Abrasion	Burn, Thermal
Needle Puncture	Back Injury	Bite	Burn, Chemical
			And Others......

II. Part of the Body Affected

Head and Neck		Extremeties		Body
Scalp	Ears	Forearm	Hips	Trunk
Face	Mouth	Upper Arm	Thigh	Chest
Neck	Teeth	Shoulder	Knees	Back
Skull		Wrist	Ankle	Abdomen
Eyes		Hand	Feet	Groin
				And Others......

III. Source of Injury

Needle	Glass	Razor Blade	Broken Dish
Spilled Liquid	Cart	Door or Doorway	Patient
Bed	Patient Care Equipment		Gas Cylinder
			And Others......

IV. Accident Type

Struck By	Struck Against	Caught Between
Carts	Table	Door and Frame
Equipment	Electrical Circuit	Cart and Wall
Person	Chemicals	Tool and Hammer
Falling Object	Sharps	
Strain and Overexertion		And Others......

V. Unsafe Condition

Unguarded	Defective tools	Hazardous arrangement or storage
Unsafe design	Poor Ventilation	Congested Area
Wrong Tool	Poor Housekeeping	And Others......

VI. Agency that Caused Accident

Equipment Type	Hot Water	Hot Foodstufs
Vehicle	Hypodermic Needle	Heavy Box or Patient
Chemical	Animal	And Others......

VI. Part of Agency that Caused Accident

Note part of item that caused Accident. (I.E. Protruding metal strip under cart)

VIII. Unsafe Act

Untrained	Operation at unsafe speed
Unsafe Position	Use of improper materials
Horseplay	Disobeyed instructions
	And Others......

FIGURE 1. Key factors in incident investigation.

Method of Recording Basic Facts Relating to the Nature and Occurrence of Work Injuries, list eight areas by which injuries and illnesses can be broken down. The eight categories are

1. Nature of injury; type of damage to the body or diagnosed illness
2. Part of body affected; inasmuch detail as required to identify and relate it to the injury or illness
3. Source of injury; item or object that actually caused the damage to the body or provided the vector for entry of disease
4. Accident type; can be broken into several types (see Figure 1) as required to effectively identify various problem areas
5. Hazardous conditions; part of environment within which the injury/illness was allowed to occur (e.g., wet floor, contaminated needle, patient with undiagnosed infection, etc.
6. Agency of the accident; specific thing that caused or allowed the accident to happen (in many cases, different from the source of injury, e.g., in the case of the painter painting from a scaffold, missing the handrail, and falling, the source of injury would be determined by the surface and objects the painter fell on, but the agency of the accident would be the scaffold)

7. Agency of the accident part; used when only part of the item noted in category six was involved (i.e., the agency of the accident part would be the missing guard-rail)
8. Unsafe acts; whether committed by the injured, or by another (includes such specifics as untrained, unsupervised, and widespread violation of the rules, as well as the specific acts of the injured party and fellow workers

The above-mentioned management oversights are as often an element in an accident as any act of the workers.

Severity

One last thought before we leave this area: consideration of injury/illness data and accident investigations is too often done on the basis of the actual severity of the incident. That is to say, even though the potential for a specific incident was serious injury and/or death, if the actual injury is minor, we tend to give thanks, and treat the incident as minor. The problem with this is that it ignores the warning inherent in the accident.

The treatment for this problem is called potential injury classification. The incident is considered and investigated at its potential severity, not the actual level. There are two advantages: first, we can investigate relatively free of the emotional overtones often present during the investigation of a serious injury, and second, we can often prevent the serious incident from occurring by catching it after a minor warning. All too often, we discover that after a serious injury several relatively minor incidents predated it, and had an effective investigation been made, the environment, training, or other factors could have been changed to eliminate the possibility, or significantly reduce the potential for that injury.

It is interesting to note that rarely does a serious injury occur during the first time exposure to an unsafe condition or action. Usually, it occurs after that act or condition has existed for many exposures. Thus, if we can identify and eliminate them before the serious incident occurs, we have no serious injury.

Training

The second phase of the three-legged stool on which a safety program needs to stand is training. This is the most underdeveloped area of most safety programs. Typically, a hospital safety program consists of a "new hire orientation" and inservice training about fire safety and body mechanics to nursing units and departments such as maintenance and food service.

Who

To be successful, training (and specific training at that) must be done for almost every employee. It is evident that such specialists as those in biomedical electronics must have and continue to receive training to stay effective in their field. It must also be recognized that housekeeping, maintenance, and dietetic personnel have as much impact upon the safety of the institution as the medical-related staff and often outnumber them. Two types of training are needed for almost all employees. First, there is general training by groups in areas such as fire, emergency services, body mechanics, and similar areas of general interest. In addition, a regular training program should be set up for each employee to train and refresh them in their present jobs. Also, both specific day to day jobs, with a medium-to-high-hazard content, and jobs that are done only periodically with particular hazards should be analyzed and trained on a schedule.

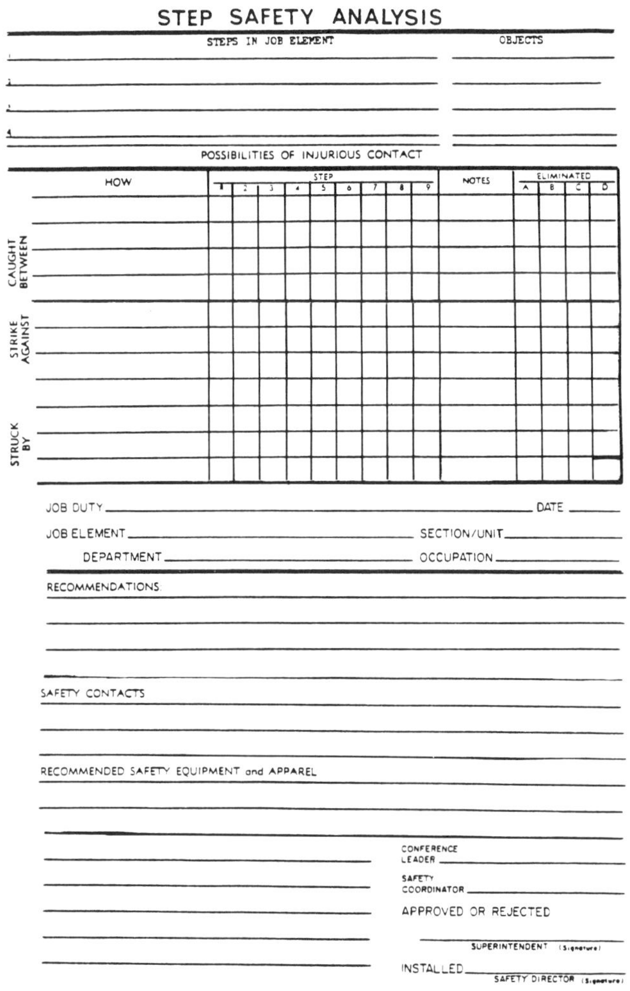

STEP SAFETY ANALYSIS

STEPS IN JOB ELEMENT | OBJECTS

POSSIBILITIES OF INJURIOUS CONTACT

HOW	STEP 1	2	3	4	5	6	7	8	9	NOTES	ELIMINATED A	B	C	D
CAUGHT BETWEEN														
STRIKE AGAINST														
STRUCK BY														

JOB DUTY ______ DATE ______

JOB ELEMENT ______ SECTION/UNIT ______

DEPARTMENT ______ OCCUPATION ______

RECOMMENDATIONS:

SAFETY CONTACTS

RECOMMENDED SAFETY EQUIPMENT and APPAREL

CONFERENCE LEADER ______

SAFETY COORDINATOR ______

APPROVED OR REJECTED

SUPERINTENDENT (Signature)

INSTALLED ______ SAFETY DIRECTOR (Signature)

FIGURE 2. Step safety analysis.

How

The mechanism for this training is known as "JIT-JSA" or job instruction training-job safety analysis. Developed by industry during and after WWII, this technique has proven successful in analyzing injury/illness potential and training millions of employees in hundreds of industries to do the job "right".

The first step is to look at a specific job and break it down into its steps. Usually, the skilled workers that are doing the job to be examined and their supervisor do the actual job breakdown and safety analysis, using forms such as those shown in Figures 2 and 3. This breakdown and analysis is then reviewed by the safety department and the head of the department or service affected, and compared to similar breakdowns made on other shifts by employees with similar jobs. The results of the best of all the analyses are combined to make a safe job procedure, and this procedure (see Figure 3) is then used as a training tool to train the worker in that specific job using the JIT method (see Figure 4). The JIT procedure is to: (1) prepare the work place to be sure it has the tools and materials needed to properly train the employee and (2) be sure the work place is in the condition the trainer wants it kept. Then, the actual training begins. First, put the employees at ease. Introduce them to the job and find out what

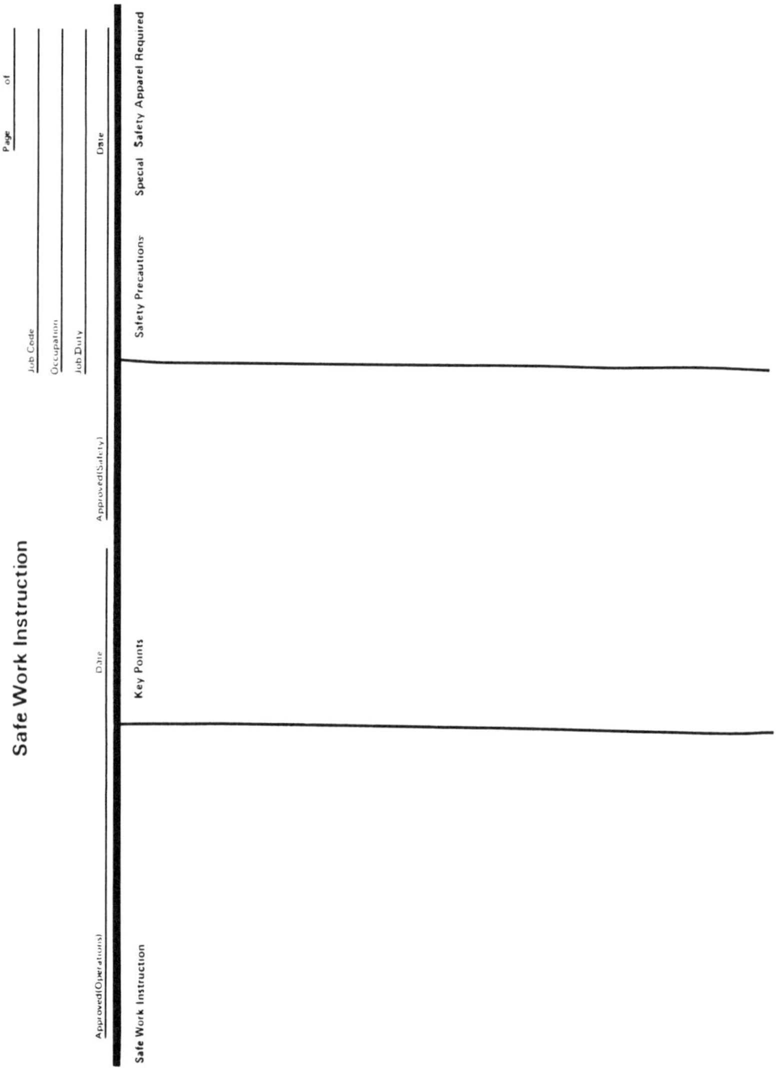

FIGURE 3. Safe work instruction.

Job Breakdown Sheet

Occupation ______ Task ______

Job Duty ______

Important Steps in the Job Step: a logical segment of the job when something happens to advance the work	Key Points • Will make or break the job • Injure the employee • A knack, trick, sound, feel, bit of special information.

FIGURE 4. Job breakdown sheet.

they know about it. It may be that the employees know already how to do the job, or think they do. After determining their level of knowledge on the subject, point out how important this particular job is to the department and the hospital as a whole.

Second, present the job step by step, demonstrating as you go. Be sure the employees understand each step before you go on to the next.

Third, have the employees do the job, telling you back what they are doing. Correct misunderstandings at this point, but do not press for speed. Accuracy is most important now; speed will develop with practice.

Fourth, put the employees on their own. Tell them how and from whom they can get help, and tell them you will check back with them from time to time. Then, check back later to be sure they are doing the job the way you trained them to, and compliment them on doing it right (or gently correct them if they make mistakes). Emphasize that you are counting on them to do the job right all the time. Also, you should record that they have had this training so you will not insult them by retraining them in a job they already know (unless, however, they are not doing it properly). Annual retraining of everyone, regardless of job skill level, reduces motivation to try to do the job well. Occasional rechecking, and recognition of the job skill level shows the employees that they are individuals, not nameless, faceless hoards, and provides some needed positive reinforcement and job feedback.

Proper and effective training and training records will do as much as anything you can do to provide and maintain a safe and secure working environment for all employees. The training and education of all employees is a crucial part of an effective hospital safety program. This training goes on all the time, whether you recognize it or not. If you do not provide formal training, employees will seek it out informally from their peers. Unfortunately, this training is often inaccurate and even counterproductive.

A differentiation between training and education is suggested by OSHA standards and definitions. Education, including inservice, is defined as information or intellectual activity; training is usually a physical skill, such as using a fire extinguisher. Both kinds of effort are required.

Orientation

To start with the first opportunity you have to reach an employee, at least on a formal basis, we need to consider new employee orientation. Each new employee that is hired should receive a short, specific program that tells them what you expect of them. Most new employees want to know where they fit into the organization, and how the organization will effect them. We can tell them both. Each and every employee needs to be told how they are involved in the safety program. This will include such basic items as how to report injuries and hazards to the safety officer, the proper response to a fire alarm or drill, and what specific hazards they will face in your institution, as well as how they can avoid them.

You should have this orientation done by a member of the safety staff or committee, so the employee will feel that at least they know someone that they can talk to if a problem arises. You must also emphasize that their supervisor will give them the specifics of the hazards at their jobs. (This is to alert them to ask for the information if it is not forthcoming and to reinforce the idea that the supervisor is responsible for safety in their own area).

In-service Education

Beyond the basic orientation, it is necessary to review much of this information on a regular basis. A yearly in-service session with a department or unit, stressing the basic response information and specific hazards and precautions unique to their area, is a useful tool. To be effective, it should be organized (perhaps with visual aids) and presented around the clock to all three shifts (and on the weekends) to ensure all or at least as many as possible are reached.

In addition, special purpose sessions can be used to cover a new problem or process, to reinforce a specific protocol, or to show the use of a specialist, e.g., a salesman or tech rep, a visitor from another hospital, insurance specialist, etc. (Where appropriate, you may wish to document this session on video or audio tape so that it can be used later).

Besides this general education, specific training should also be accomplished. This will usually include such areas as CPR, first aid, special fire brigade training, emergency response groups, chemical emergency training, and countless other subjects. You will not expect to train all of your employees this way, but supervisors, security, key maintenance, lab,. and service employees should be trained as to what to do in an emergency.

Specific skills training is also required. While the safety group is not usually directly involved in skills training, certain areas must be checked to be sure the training that is accomplished does conform to the necessary rules and practices.

Supervisor Responsibility

In most cases, the person responsible for the training is the supervisor. This is important for several reasons. One is that the supervisor is the ultimate source of authority of the safety rules for those employees. If their supervisor does not understand and believe the rules, the employees won't either.

An advantage of having the supervisor responsible for training is that the supervisor then knows what the employees have been trained in and how well they have used the training, which is useful for performance review techniques. The supervisor has a specific, step-by-step job description that makes it easier to do an objective job review.

The subject area of visual aids of training is too broad to be covered in this chapter, but a variety of visual training aids, from simple flip charts and chalkboards to video tape and slide/tape programs can be used to support and illustrate the training topics. It is important to note that films, video tape, and the like must not be used in a context that allows and encourages student questions and feedback; showing a group of employees a film is not effective training unless it is then related to their specific jobs and tasks.

As noted earlier, effective training records are very useful, even beyond their immediate and obvious value. Careful analysis of the records will allow you to discover areas where your training is incomplete, redundant, or old. The training record is also useful for documentation of compliance with various codes and regulations, performance review and discipline, and a valuable resource to employees that seek employment elsewhere, as it lists their skills and competencies.

Specific Topics

Back injury — There are several areas that almost all health care personnel need training in to avoid back injury. Back injury is one of the most widespread problems in all phases of health care. While sophisticated and effective technology is available in most areas of health care, the basics of patient movement and moving "things" is still a labor-intensive, body-using requirement. It is imperative that persons handling patients be trained and educated to assure the safety of the patient and the staff person doing the moving. Body mechanics (or some other term with less negative connotations) should be presented to nursing, patient assistant transportation, and any other persons that handle or come in contact with the patient (X-ray, patient interface lab personnel, etc.). In addition, similar techniques must be taught to housekeeping, food and dietary, environmental services, maintenance and engineering, as well as others that handle materials (such as receiving, central service, storeroom, building and grounds, etc).

Infection control — Another topic that needs wide coverage is infection control. In cooperation with the nurse epidemioligist or infection control committee, employees should be trained to recognize how their job affects and is affected by the potential to exposure contained in the medical facility. They must be taught how to minimize the exposure and what to do if they think they may have been exposed. The emphasis is to reduce panic and fear of the unknown.

Response training — Another area that should be defined is the expected response to emergencies, such as fire emergencies, weather, water loss, etc. This training usually takes the form of initial education and drills on a periodic basis to train and refresh actual skills, as well as the location of specific emergency items. One effective training method for such emergency skills is to provide a simple menomic such as R A C E (rescue alarm container extinguisher or escape); a simple set of instructions and frequent repetition are the keys to getting everyone involved in and knowing the program. It is particularly important to involve everyone in areas such as fire training because it is impossible to know who might discover a fire or suspected fire. Also, it is important to be sure that such training reaches all shifts (including the weekend and part-time employees), and if possible, to volunteers and medical staff. Effective training may be the most important part of an organized safety program. The safety director is only one person. If safety is to reach the whole facility effectively, everyone must be aware of and involved in the problems.

Inspection

The third leg of the safety program is safety inspection. This is a tool that, if well used, allows us to look into the future and predict and prevent future incidents before anyone is injured.

Standards

The first key item in an effective inspection program is standards. Unless people know exactly what is expected of them, they will perform to what they guess or deduce is the level of performance you expect. In fact, if you have not set standards, you yourself do not know if you are running your operation properly. There are two kinds of standards — internal and external. The external standards are set by various governmental, industry-wide, and voluntary groups including OSHA, NFPA, JCAH, AHA, etc. Also, federal, state, and local governmental groups, insurance companies, and local and national medical groups set standards for us. Your health care institution must look at all of these standards, and make choices of the level of risk and compliance you wish to maintain. Some standards are good enough as they are mandated or recommended. Other standards may not be strict enough for your conditions; you may want to impose more stringent internal standards because you cannot run an efficient operation with the mandated minimum. In addition, you may have to devise standards in areas where there are no outside guidelines.

Once you have decided upon your own internal standards, you must let everyone involved know about them. In fact, during the process of developing your own internal standards, it is useful to get input from the people that will have to live with the standards. This ensures that you have not developed standards that cannot be followed, contradict other standards, or are not strict enough. Often when involved, people working in an area will suggest much stricter standards than immediately obvious because they know about hidden or obscured problems others now working with the situation would overlook.

Check Lists

The second element is an effective memory aid for inspection most often in the form of a check list. The reason check lists are popular is that the user does not have to depend upon memory. An effective, properly designed check list has two elements (above others) worth mentioning (see Figures 5A and 5B).

One is the overall format, which includes double columns for the checkoff of items marked "OK", "Good", or some other work designation that indicates the conditions have been met and are within standards, and another for those marked "N/G", "Bad", or some other indication that the situation does not meet standards and corrective action is required. In addition there should be comment space on the page to allow for observed items not listed in the check list.

The second element for a successful check list is that the items or questions (if in that form) must be complete within themselves, to the greatest extent consistent with reasonable brevity in the check list. The user should not have to refer to external standards unless they do so out of curiosity. It is useful to note the origin of the standard so one can refer back, but the key parts of the standards or information must be there. Do not ask "Is the aisle wide enough?" as there can be many interpretations about how wide the aisle should be. Be arbitrary (if necessary); set a standard you can live with that allows a margin for safety and stick to it ("is the aisle 5 ft wide, marked, and clear of material?"). Even at the price of being arbitrary, you must assign specific concrete conditions to be inspected for so that the results will be consistent between different inspectors.

Response

In addition to creating a check list to implement inspection programs, you must

Date ____________

SAFETY COMMITTEE

	YES	NO
1. Does the committee have established goals and objectives?		
2. Are the following represented on the committee? Nursing, Maintenance, Security, Surgery, Employee Health Service, Office Personnel, Laboratory, Radiology, Food Service, Pharmacy		
3. Are other departments represented as needed?		
4. Does the committee meet monthly?		
5. Are employee incident reports reviewed at each meeting?		
6. Are recommendations made to prevent re-occurrence?		
7. Is there a mechanism established for follow-up to ensure recommendations are implemented?		
8. Are medication and procedure errors reviewed at each meeting?		
9. Are patient-visitor incidents reviewed at each meeting?		
10. Are recommendations made to prevent re-occurrence?		
11. Does the committee conduct regular safety surveys?		
12. Are survey reports reviewed at a safety committee meeting?		
13. Does the administrator or assistant administrator attend committee meetings?		
14. Are the minutes of the meeting sent to the administrator?		
15. Does the administrator comment on the work of the committee?		
16. Does the Safety Committee review the fire emergency plan at least once each year?		
17. Is there a representative of the safety committee on the following committees: Infection Control, Disaster		
18. Does the representative report to the safety committee on the work of the other committees?		

A

Date ____________

ADMINISTRATION

	YES	NO
1. Has a Safety Policy Statement been issued to all employees?		
2. Is there an active Safety Committee?		
3. Does the Administrator or Assistant Administrator attend Safety Committee meetings at least four times per year?		
4. Are there written regulations governing smoking within the hospital?		
5. Is there an up-to-date fire emergency plan?		
6. Are the fire alarm codes and emergency exit routes posted throughout the building?		
7. Is there an up-to-date external disaster plan?		
8. Are regular safety surveys made?		
9. Has the Administrator received copies of survey reports and made comments?		
10. Does the Administrator review incident reports?		
11. Are there procedures manual for every department?		
12. Is the Safety and Health Protection on the Job" poster placed in an area readily accessible to all employees?		
13. Is the poster clearly visible?		
14. Is the OSHA 100 Form, "Log of Occupational Injuries and Illness properly maintained, i.e.; entries made with six (6) days of all reportable injuries and illnesses?		
15. Is the OSHA Form 101, "Supplementary Record" or equivalent form being maintained?		
16. Has the OSHA Form 102, "Annual Summary" been posted prior to February 1st and left posted for 30 days?		
17. Are OSHA records being maintained for a period of five (5) years as required by law?		

B

FIGURE 5. (A) Safety check list — safety committee; (B) Safety check list — administration.

have an effective response system. There are three possible useful responses acceptable to a downcheck on a check list. To have no response is to fail to complete the feedback system and to destroy the effectiveness of the program. Seeing no response, those responsible for doing the inspection will soon no longer bother to conduct inspections. Seeing a response in the form of an item being repaired provides the feedback necessary to prove that the program is working and accomplishing something, thereby encouraging its use.

As noted, there must be a response through one of three modes of the response system. Most items will initiate a routine response, i.e., the item will be repaired in the normal length of time, usually a couple of days to a couple of weeks depending on the organization. If the item is regularly repaired within that time, the system is perceived as working. Some items, however, cannot wait. These are emergencies or "immediate" items. These usually indicate that a system or area cannot be used until the item is corrected. Some fire safety, electrical safety, and similar problems fall in this group. For these, you must have some method of getting immediate response. The other end of the spectrum is the item that will take weeks or months, even a year or more to correct. It may deal with major construction, or perhaps be covered in a program already underway, but in need of engineering, budget, construction, etc. In these cases, some form of feedback is still needed, usually in the form of a note or memo indicating what is being done and when it will be completed. This memo forms the feedback and tells the inspector that something is being done.

In addition to the above, there are several actions that will help a check list or inspection program succeed, including training of the inspectors, regular review of the check lists to be sure that they are still correct, and planning inspection schedules and routes.

Training of the inspectors is often overlooked, with the thought that anyone can see hazards. Unfortunately, this is not so. People working in an area often do not notice hazards they pass day to day. They may have seen them when they were new, but exposure has dulled their awareness. Effective training, including exposure to pictures of hazards, discussion of where and why, and practice trips with follow-up critique has been found effective. Inspectors must also have an understanding of their role in terms of authority and responsibility. Some organizations expect the inspector to simply observe and report, others give the inspector the authority to step in and correct, or even stop a job until conditions have been met. The inspectors must know their own limits and expectations.

Scheduling

To be effective, the inspections must be scheduled in a timely manner and cover the entire work place. Some inspections may be scheduled on daily, weekly, or longer periods. A rough rule of thumb for frequency is to figure how long it would take for a situation to turn sour, then inspect twice that frequently. Another guide is in standards (e.g., fire extinguishers should be inspected monthly, etc.). The other consideration is work hours available. It does no good to schedule an inspection daily if there is no work time to do it.

Inspection routes must also be covered. You must devise a method to ensure that each area is inspected. One method is geographic in nature; inspect one building or floor at a time, then move on to the next. Another method is to inspect by department or service. One way or another, you must be sure the entire institution is covered.

Record Keeping and Analysis

One of the most powerful tools of human knowledge is past experience. Without reference to past experience, we would still be living in caves, eating raw meat and roots. The experience in safety is no different.

Most progress in safety has been made by keeping accurate records of cause and effect of incidents, analyzing these records to determine causes, then developing methods to prevent or minimize risk.

Reporting

An effective incident reporting system has several elements. First is the incident or unusual occurrence report that should be filled out every time someone is injured or becomes ill from something related to their occupation, and each time a patient or visitor is injured in the institution. This report must be filled out either by the supervisor or the employee (or the person responsible for the area, in the case of patient/visitor), or by the treating agency (employee health, emergency room, or similar). Ideally, it is filled out by the supervisor, and checked and completed by the treating agency.

Collating

The second step is to collect and collate the information on the form. This information should include the type of injury, part of the body, location, time and date of the injury, and witnesses the human error involved, the environmental conditions that allowed the error to lead to injury, and the thing or things that contributed to the incident. Additional information that should be included, if possible, is when the injury was reported, the supervisor's name and phone (to expedite follow-up), age and date of hire of employee, employee's title and department, and other information useful to identifying cause and cure of the incident.

Tabulating

After collecting the data and reducing it to tabulation form, the third or analysis phase takes place. Here, we are trying to tie related facts together in order to find a pattern. Often, additional information will be needed that may be gathered by incident investigation and interview. The fourth part is the evaluation and correction of the conditions causing the incident, and the training and education of those whose inadequate training may have contributed to the incident.

It is important to note at this point that training alone will not solve most problems. In most cases, there are environmental factors that also contribute to the injury. It is important not to stop with personnel factors, but to dig in and find all the causes. All too often the incident is capped with a notation that it was "so and so's fault", with insufficient attention to conditions that, if changed, could prevent that and other like incidents, (bedrails for patient falls are a good example).

The incident investigation itself should also be discussed. With the resources available to most safety staffs, it is not practical to thoroughly investigate all incidents, therefore, a selection must be made. It is important that the selection be made not on the basis of the severity of the actual injury, but upon the potential severity of the injury. In other words, if the injury received was minor, but only through luck, and the potential was severe injury or injury to several people, that incident must be looked into. The same goes for minor incidents that are often repeated (e.g., a broken plate causing lacerations in a dietary service).

Documentation

The second use for effective reporting and recording of incidents is documentation. This documentation has two sides, the required records you need to comply with to show recognition of standards and regulations and litigation if needed, and the records that allow you to check and chart your progress. The first set, those required of you, include OSHA, JCAH, state and local fire, insurance, and other regulations. Accurate and clear records are valuable not only for the immediate results, but because they show "good faith" efforts to comply with and meet requirements. Records that allow you to evaluate your own performance may include areas not usually noted. For instance, an increase in the total number of incidents reported is not only not bad, but actually good. Most institutions receive only a small percentage of the incidents actually occurring; and increase may mean that the word is getting around and more people are reporting previously ignored incidents.

A great deal of useful information is contained in the American National Standards Institute (ANSI) Standard Z 16.2 "work accident reporting and analysis" if you translate the industrial consideration into those appropriate for a health care institution.

Medical and First Aid Systems

An often overlooked area of safety responsibility is the area of first aid and medical services. It may seem unusual to suggest that first aid is an important element in a hospital or health care institution, but consider the following. Almost all employees work in areas more than a couple of minutes from emergency facilities. Many employees are exposed to the same hazards any light industry has each day (maintenance, electrical, lab, food service, housekeeping, etc). Many nurses have little or no first aid training. All of the above indicates that seriously injured employees may wait several minutes until emergency-trained personnel reaches them (and remember, a person can bleed to death in 90 sec, and suffer brain damage 3 to 6 min after breathing stops).

It is important to train a wide cadre of employees in first aid and CPR. At the least, supervisors, security personnel, fire brigade, and others should be trained. Ideally, all employees should receive instructions. Reality, hopefully, lies somewhere in between.

The Employee Health Service (EHS), by whatever name it may be called, is a key element in a good safety program; close cooperation will be to everyones benefit. Some of the areas that cooperation is useful in is in mandating pre-employment exams (with emphasis on being sure the potential employee is fit for the proposed job) and establishing baselines for employees that will be in jobs where, for instance, they must handle toxic chemicals, or heavy lifting is needed.

Another area where cooperation is needed is in scheduling employees for regular checks where they do handle toxic, carcinogenic, or other dangerous materials.

The EHS can also be a great assistance in follow-up of accident/incident situations, in monitoring, helping monitor work places and workers, biosurveillance of toxic carcinogenic, bio-hazardous areas, and in similar responsibilities.

Another area where safety and personnel must closely work together is in placement of handicapped employees. Because of federal laws and because they are usually superior employees when fitted to the job, there is wider hiring of personnel with some type of physical or other handicap. It is important to look carefully at the work environment, access, and other facilities to be sure they are compatible with the situation.

The EHS is a key element in this process, both in identifying the potential employee and in advising what modifications may be useful. In reference to this, it is useful, and in some areas critical, to establish specific standards for physical fitness for some jobs. You may wish to specify certain screening tests (in conjunction with and through EHS) for those that will have to lift heavy loads, stand for long periods, or have some specific agility.

Another consideration that EHS may enter into (if they have or can tap the expertise) is emergency reaction to specific situations, such as chemical spills, weather extremes, and other emergency conditions.

Maintenance of Interest

Safety Committee

One area that receives constant attention (and with good reason) is finding ways to catch and maintain the interest and involvement of all the employees. Employee involvement is widely recognized as critical to the real and long-range success of any safety program. No safety staff can be everywhere and see everything at once. Therefore, it is necessary that as many employees as possible be involved. One of the most effective methods of involvement of key employees is a safety committee or task force. This activity includes a wider group of people, therefore, they in turn can impact still further.

Saftey Newsletters

Another technique is the employee newsletter(s). This vehicle can reach all employees, even into their homes. If the newsletter is published on a regular basis and includes articles of interest to all, it can be an effective tool for reminding people that you exist. A real effort should be made to get feedback from the readers so that it continues to contain information they want and use. Contests, puzzles, word games, even letters from the readers all help to maintain interest and enthusiasm.

Other people-reachers are displays and posters. Often, a display that involves the viewer (with a quiz or "which of these things") will get people talking and arouse questions. Posters, particularly those made by people in your institution, are also a real vote-getter. A poster contest may be an effective way to kick a campaign off or hammer home a slogan or phrase.

Feedback

One element that is necessary in all these media is the requirement that a feedback channel be built in some way. Feedback is the most important element in a communication system. Without feedback, you do not know whether the message has gotten through. The assumption that, after you hang a poster or put up a display (or for that matter, show a film, give an inservice, or talk to your boss) you have gotten through is risky. Experience shows that rarely does an idea get through the first time. You have to repeat it, change it, restate it, and answer questions before it gets into people's minds. All of this is impossible without feedback.

Feedback systems may be as simple as talking to the audience after a film and asking them what they think it means to their job. It may be a questionnaire, a contest, or a quiz. Whatever you use, consider how to get feedback before you decide on the media you choose to get the message across.

Performance Feedback

A modern technique that is adaptable to the field of safety is that of performance feedback. This technique, which is to tell people how they are doing compared to a specific standard, uses the natural desire of most people to do their job well. It simply is finding a way to measure the effectiveness and assigning it a number or ranking. Most people want to do better and will try to do so. One safety-related use is in housekeeping; rank various areas as to their housekeeping. Be sure the criteria you use are known, and publish the scores. Good areas will work to stay on top, and other areas will try to get higher. It is important that you use only positive reinforcement. Do not punish or ridicule the bottom; they will get the message.

This kind of positive reinforcement is also useful for contests and awards, and is based on intrinsic vs. extrinsic value. Consider for a moment the amount of time and effort someone will put into winning a trophy. Common sense will suggest they could go to a sporting store and order the same trophy for far less effort and cost. Why then do people value those inexpensive reminders of achievement? It is because they earn them. They have value because of what they represent, not what they are. They have extrinsic value. In contests, we often choose expensive prizes. Unfortunately, when that prize is used up, the reminder is gone. The trophy or certificate stays on the wall or mantle for a long time.

Effective public recognition of good employee performance, both job skill-related, and safety-related, will pay dividends in production, safety, and attitudes.

Safety is not a straightforward mechanical engineering exercise; the intangible human factors often play a much larger part in the bottom-line outcome of a program than all the equipment details you may discover.

SPECIAL PROBLEMS IN HOSPITAL SAFETY

There are a number of specific considerations within the area of hospital and health care safety that require special consideration. These are not always unique to the health care area, but are of specific concern.

Fire Prevention and Reaction

Foremost among these is the area of fire prevention and effective fire emergency responses. Fires have always been visible; they are understandable to the public, and have known and frightening results. Fire protection/response in a hospital has been regulated for many years. Hospital fire protection is usually based on a concept of compartmentalization and containment, and upon the needs to train all employees in an effective response. Continued drills to ingrain the response and polish the system are not only good practice, but required by local fire protection agencies, insurance carriers, and hospital accrediting bodies.

The fire response system is covered in detail in another chapter, but one aspect will be reinforced here — the need for comprehensive training and practice. Effective drills are more than simple repetition; they require analysis and change of procedure when problems are identified. Drills should be as realistic as possible without endangering the patients. Using empty rooms and providing real victims may make the employees responding more aware of the problems and dangers of bad handling practices. Where possible, efforts should be made to allow employees to actually handle fire extinguishers, use self-contained breathing apparatus, move "real victims" (actual people in order to get the weight and response), and follow through on the drill (i.e., to do more than go through the motions and then drop it).

In addition to the requirements of the drill, other fire prevention activities must be worked into employees' daily schedules, e.g., inservice education about basic prevention, fire inspections (part of housekeeping), specific hazard awareness, and special instruction on special problems, such as flammable-liquids storage and disposal. Training must be done by both the safety department and the various working areas to ensure that everyone is covered.

Lab Safety

Lab safety is an area often neglected in a health care safety program, although it has recently come under much closer scrutiny by accrediting authorities. Key areas to be considered here include fire safety, flammable-liquid storage, fire blankets, self-contained breathing apparatus, and eyewash and emergency showers. Chemical and biohazard storage and disposal are also of importance.

Current standards require that flammable liquids (with flash points less than 140°F) be stored in metal and in small quantities. If a lab or other area needs to have more than a total of 5 gal, the flammables must be kept in a properly designed flammable-liquids cabinet (as defined by NFPA 30), except when in use. If chemicals must be in glass for purity reasons, they must be in small-sized bottles (less than a gallon). Venting flammable-liquids cabinets is considered good practice (they should be vented from the bottom, as most flammable liquids have vapors that are heavier than air).

Fire Blankets

Current lab standards also require that clinical labs have fire blankets installed. The fire blanket is a versatile fire fighting and personal protection tool, but is often misunderstood. If a person's clothing catches on fire, he should not run for a fire blanket. First, running fans the flame, and second, the products of combustion rise into the breathing zone. A person with clothes on fire should lie down and roll onto the flame. This will smother the flame. However, if another person is nearby, he should use the blanket to help smother the flame and treat for shock, if necessary. The fire blanket is also an effective tool for escape. Cover yourself with the blanket if you must make your way out of a burning area. The blanket will protect flame impingement and to some extent provide protection from radiant heat.

A fire blanket can also be used to contain and extinguish a small flammable-liquid fire or smother a small area fire (such as a wastebasket), or piece of electrical equipment.

Self-Contained Breathing Apparatus (SCBA)

A self-contained breathing apparatus is suggested for all lab areas, and training in its use should be extended to provide 24 hr coverage. This equipment will be used in a fire situation to assure trained personnel that all people are out of the fire scene. It will also be used to fight the fire, and is needed in case of a chemical spill or emergency. Many common chemicals produce vapor or smoke that is hazardous in large quantities, (although many of these seem to permit working, they have delayed effects). Ideally, two kinds of SCBA equipment would be available. The 5-min escape packs are ideal in lab locations, as they allow anyone (even those with glasses and facial hair) to wear them, and escape from chemical vapor or products of combustion. The 30-min backpack type should be used if emergency work is to be done in the danger area. This apparatus requires training and periodic refreshing, and the equipment should only be used by fully trained personnel.

Eyewash and Shower

Emergency eyewash and shower facilities should be available to anyone working with corrosive materials. Even mild acids and hydroxides can do serious and permanent damage if not washed off immediately.

Squeeze-type bottle eyewashes are not recommended except in the most unusual conditions. Portable units should be able to deliver at least 1 gal/min for at least 15 min. Ideally, the hose type, connected to allow water temperature control, should be within 25 to 30 ft of areas where employees may handle corrosives or irritants. A quick test is to close your eyes, spin around three times, and go to the eyewash. You should be able to get there in 15 sec. (The spin is to simulate the disorientation caused by pain and surprise.) Emergency showers, the type where one handle is pulled to turn them on (or a step-on platform is used), and another is used to turn the water off, are recommended in most labs where areas must be kept clear. In small labs, the shower might be placed at the door in the hallway. Again, it should be where it can be found by someone who is disoriented and whose eyes are closed. Many institutions plumb in showers where there are no drains; in the event of emergency, simply vacuum the area after the incident.

Chemical Storage

Chemical storage is often overlooked in day-to-day operations in labs. Chemical storage shelves become overloaded, bottles get pushed to the back of the shelf, and infrequently used materials, often large bottles get put on high shelves. Acids and corrosives are stored on top shelves or on the floor, and reactive materials are stored in proximity to each other.

Chemical storage areas should be purged at least yearly, and no longer-used chemicals, outdated materials, and improperly labeled materials should be properly disposed of. Chemical labels should be reviewed and checked for hazard information, date opened, expiration date, if appropriate, and concentration and mixture information.

Flammables (140°F and lower) should be in metal containers or a flammable-liquid cabinet. Using a hood to store flammables is poor practice because (1) it does not protect the flammables in case of fire, and (2) the flammables block the hood for its designed purpose.

Because bottles may be broken, acids and corrosives should be stored in plastic trays designed to contain the contents, and transferred in rubber or plastic buckets to reduce in-route accidents.

Large amounts of strong chemicals should be stored just above floor level, but not on the floor where they may be bumped and broken. Smaller bottles that are stored on shelves must be kept back from the edge, and a lip or restrainer should be at the shelf edge. Care should also be taken that incompatible chemicals are not stored together.

Sharp Waste Disposal

One of the unique problems found in a health care environment is the abundance of needles and other sharp objects, most of which are expected to be used once and then disposed of. The disposal of so many dangerous objects (dangerous because of their potential to cut, as well as infection which may be on or in them) leads to EPA standards requiring that they be handled differently than ordinary trash.

The list of objects in this category leads off with hypodermic needles, both on syringes and i.v. sets, and on blood-drawing equipment. These are used in patient care areas, exam and treatment rooms, offices, labs, and even in mobile equipment. The key to effective control of these wastes is to have disposal sites immediately available as near the point of use as possible. Two major types of disposals are widely used.

The most common method uses a needle-cutting device to destroy the hypodermic needle, as well as to eliminate the puncture hazard. The syringe is then destroyed and disposed of separately, or simply put into a disposal box and compacted. The hazards remaining are the possible puncture from the cut off needles.

The second system is more secure and requires slightly more space and workers. The used syringes are simply tossed whole into heavy walled containers. These containers are picked up by trained personnel and ground in a special sharps grinder. The final material is a granular mix of glass, plastic, and metal, disinfected, and ready to put into landfill. This system is most useful where a large institution is serviced or a service area is shared, as a large quantity of used sharps are necessary to justify the expense. Disposable lab glass and plastic may also be handled in this way.

The overall problem of lab disposables has two sides: infection control (both cross infection and quality control) and the problem of safe disposal of the used material. The best way would be to accumulate the used glass, culture medium, and specimens in autoclaveable bags, autoclave the entire mass, and then dispose into landfill. While this method renders the contents harmless, it requires autoclave space and time. Many smaller labs handle this by having someone do the autoclaving in the central service or laundry area on the off shift. If this is done, particular attention must be paid to the storage and handling of the material prior to sterilization, and to careful routing so as not to mix contaminated material with clean supplies.

Another answer to lab waste is to chemically disinfect the waste during and after it is ground or mashed, and then landfill. This is a rather messy method, and requires special care on the part of the people controlling the destruction and separation of liquids and solids.

The whole area of disposal of sharps is regulated by the Environmental Protection Agency (EPA). Careful attention to their requirements will reduce problems.

Chemical Waste Disposal

One of the increasing problems for health care institutions is the proper disposal of wastes. The EPA defines all hospital, lab, and similar wastes as "special" wastes, and requires that they be effectively neutralized before disposal. Waste can be subdivided into several groups: pathological, including tissue samples and specimens and certain lab wastes; chemical, including materials that are reactive, corrosive, flammable, toxic, and carcinogenic; and sharps, which in themselves offer a puncture/laceration danger and an infection problem because of their use and contamination.

Chemical waste requires some special training as to the hazards and the correct identification and categorization of them. The technicians in the lab also need to be trained as to the hazards of the chemicals they use. It is not safe to assume that a competent lab tech knows those hazards. Most technical people are taught what a chemical or process can do for them, not what it can do *to* them. A well-supported policy of chemical storage purging and order limiting is necessary, as is safe storage within the lab area. Insufficient space, a problem endemic to all labs, is not just reason to jam chemicals together regardless of their potential interaction. Sooner or later in any lab, bottles will be broken, and according to Murphy, at the worst possible time. (Murphy obviously worked in lab safety.)

Pathological

Safe disposal of pathological waste is best done in a pathological waste incinerator which burns the material, burns the smoke, and then scrubs the resulting effluent. Suitable storage must be available for the waste between burning (usually a freezer), and protocols must be observed to be sure that all wastes are in bags which will retain all liquids. Double bagging, with absorbing material in the outer bag, is often used. The personnel that will burn the material must be trained and made aware of the hazards involved and have suitable personal protective equipment in case a bag ruptures. They must also be trained to safely clean up after such a spill.

If your institution does not produce a large enough amount of pathological waste, an effective alternate may be used to make arrangements with a nearby larger hospital to handle yours. This would require both a freezer to store the material and insulated transporting equipment. However, it is very important to be sure that any outside firm handling your waste disposal is licensed by local, state, public health authorities, and by state and federal environmental protection agencies. Wastes that are improperly handled by "gypsies" or hospital personnel may come back to haunt you later. If you have disposed of (or allowed someone else to) regulated chemicals improperly, your institutuion is held liable for both punitive fines and the extraordinary costs of cleaning up the mess when the improper handling is discovered. There are hundreds of illegal dumps across the country that are now being discovered, opened up, and by means of labels, the original generators identified.

Your protection is the company that you hire. If the company handles hazardous materials for disposal, it must be licensed by the EPA, and you should see evidence of this license. The company should also be able to tell you exactly how the materials you entrust to its care will be transported, categorized, and finally disposed of. Many better disposal contractors, as a part of their service, provide a certificate of disposal that specifies where the waste was finally disposed of.

Pest Control

Strange as it may seem to a visitor, most health care institutions have pest management problems not because of poor conditions, but because of the basic situation. The facility has people in it 24 hr/day, 365 days/yr and food is handled around the clock, throughout the building. The personnel often have no time to eat in a central area, so food is consumed in nonpatient areas also. Finally, constant cleaning and mopping provides moisture for the infestation even in a carefully kept institution. Common areas for problems are in and around the central kitchen and its related storage. Another common problem is the receiving area because incoming material brings insect and even rodent infestations with them.

The best method of prevention is housekeeping. Heavy infestations are most common in areas with poor housekeeping, such as long-term patient rooms, storerooms (particularly storerooms used covertly for eating rooms), and areas with hard-to-move fixed equipment which is infrequently cleaned behind. Other areas include infrequently visited places such as elevator wells, sump pump pits, pipe and electrical chases, the underside and backside of sinks, dish and lab washers, and counters.

Common pests include roaches and rodents. Roaches prefer dark, damp areas with cracks and crevices, access to wet cardboard and paper, and areas not often disturbed. They will thrive in two out of three, and survive even with only one of the above conditions. The best defense is good housekeeping, but this alone may not be enough. You must seal cracks and crevices in suspect areas with a good grade caulking, plaster, or cement. Frequent turnover of material in boxes and storage of boxes on metal racks off of floors and away from walls not only keeps them dryer, but makes it harder for the insects to move around.

Rodents (particularly mice) like many of the same things people like, e.g., packaged foods, warmth, and peace and quiet. In addition, mice can gain entry through holes no larger than a pencil or pen. They also gnaw well. In fact, they must gnaw in order to survive. Since their teeth grow constantly, they must gnaw in order to keep them short enough to close their mouth. They can get through wood, plaster, and cement. The best way to stop them is with metal sheeting or metal mesh imbedded in plaster or cement.

It is important in a health care setting not to indiscriminately spray insecticide, and to spread bait around to control these pests. It is best to get trained, licensed exterminators who are familiar with the FDA and EPA regulations as to which materials can be safely used around areas where food is prepared and patients stay. The ideal approach is to have a consultant/specialist prepare an effective program and then monitor the service of the exterminator. Therefore, you have an independent outsider to ensure that the exterminator is following proper protocols.

Air Quality and Environmental Considerations

There is a renewed interest in the health of those that work in health care institutions, and much of this interest concerns lab and operating room workers.

Both because of the recent tightening of regulations affecting the amounts of contaminants in the air and the related studies being done on the long-term health problems of hospital workers by governement (NLOSH) and labor unions, the quality of breathing air in labs needs to be examined.

The Occupational Safety and Health Administration publishes maximum allowable concentrations (MACs), time weighted averages (TWAs), and short time exposure limits (STELs) which indicate the amounts allowed in the work place over a normal work exposure of 8 hr. These limits are set for most of the common lab chemicals we use and are under consideration for operating room exposure to waste anesthesia gases.

Air Samples

There are inexpensive tools available to do rough sampling to determine whether you are over the limit or within range. Colormetric tubes are glass tubes with specific reactive chemicals that stain when exposed to specific amounts of air contaminants. They are used with simple hand pumps and can determine, within 25%, the amount of a specific contaminant at a specific point in time and place.

For more sophisticated testing, charcoal-filled tubes are used to absorb the contaminants, then they are desorbed in an environmental lab and equipment such as gas chromatography is used to accurately determine the amounts of chemicals present. Usually, if a contaminant of greater than acceptable limits is found in an area with colormetric tubes, further sampling with charcoal tubes is recommended, along with the expertise of a trained industrial hygiene technician. Other equipment which may be used includes IR gas analyzers used for ethlene oxide (a sterilizer gas) and anesthetic gases, and organic vapor analyzers to detect hydrocarbons, chlorinated solvents, alcohols, ethers, and other airborne chemical vapors.

Hoods

Another area which needs some consideration is air movement both in lab areas and chemical and biological hoods.

Air circulation and air supply/exhaust need to be checked to ensure that enough air moves through the lab, reducing chemical levels to those considered safe. Also, the chemical fume hoods and biological hoods used to protect workers from higher concentrations of dangerous materials need to be checked frequently to ensure proper function. Hood airflow switches are a good precaution to be sure air is flowing, but they are not enough because they do not respond to partial air movement.

At least 100 to 125 ft/min of air is the generally accepted minimum, but is higher for specific materials and situations. A velometer is needed to measure the speed of the air; from the speed and area the air passes through, the amount in cubic feet per minute can be calculated.

Noise

Most health care institutions do not have dangerous (as defined by OSHA) levels of noise, but noise on a patient floor or in audiometric testing areas can be a problem. A sound level meter is used to measure levels of noise in units known as Db usually on the A scale, the scale closest to normal hearing.

Gas Detector

The last air testing tool is often known as the "electronic nose" or flammable gas detector. This instrument uses an electronic sensor to detect even small (about 50 ppm or 0.005%) amounts of flammable gas. This is useful for detecting and tracing gas leaks, flammable-liquid spills, and with some models, using freon as a tracing gas to check air ducts, etc. It is also useful in reassuring people that the smell they think is gas is not flammable.

THE SAFETY PROFESSIONAL AS A CONSULTANT

The job of safety director is a relatively new one in the health care setting. As a result, not only do newly appointed personnel not always know what is expected, but the administration often does not know how to use them best. First, some basic thoughts.

Staff vs. Line

The safety director is staff, not line. In the classic military and management theory, there are two classes of those at the top: the line personnel that have direct authority/responsibility in the chain of command, and the staff people that are expert in some specific area, but do not have a direct chain of command job. This means that staff people do not have the authority/responsibility to direct work, tell people what to do, etc. This means that their job is to advise, recommend, and suggest, not to tell. The traditional approach is to send a memo or letter to the person that does have the responsibility, and if that does not have the desired impact, to the boss, and on up until they reach the top person that they report to. Then, they should wait. If the top people do not wish to act, the staffer has still done the expected job, i.e., to inform the boss. The final responsibility is the boss.

In practice, this is often somewhat modified. The boss may delegate some of the authority/accountability to a staff member who will then act in the boss' name (this, among other things, should be in the statement of authority required by the Joint Commission on Accreditation of Hospitals).

Thus, the safety professional may have some direct authority/accountability to direct that specific jobs be done and specific procedures be followed. It is important to understand just what the chief executive and associates want you to do. Some of this must be committed to paper in order to define the basic job and satisfy the accrediting authorities, but much more is a verbal or tacit understanding. The delegated authority/accountability usually increases as time goes on and the CEO gains trust of the safety director/staff and begins to trust their judgment.

It is important, however, as a safety staff person to remember where you fit into the scheme of things. Your responsibility is not to effect change, but to keep your boss informed and point out relevant problems and solutions. In short, to keep them from being "caught with egg on their face". However, if your boss wants to ignore your recommendation, even after you have given him all the information, remember that this is his decision, and do not give up, simply go on to other problems.

Maze Brilliance

The term "maze brilliance" is used to describe the training a mouse or rat gets in psychological circles. When first exposed to a maze, they go thither and yon, finding dead ends and traps, finally stumbling through the maze to the food. As successive trials unfold, some rats get through them more and more quickly as they learn shortcuts and avoid traps and dead ends. So it is with the safety job. First, you may stumble, get caught in political traps, and chase up blind alleys, but as time goes on, you should be able to identify areas where you have impact and can do some good. Spending your time there, learning where to concentrate your time and available resources, is probably the best way to serve both your institution and yourself.

Consultancy

One of the best and fastest ways to get started and to impact the various problems you face is to think like a consultant.

You know what a consultant is: the outsider you hire when you cannot solve your own problems. You bring them in because they know a lot more about a specific area than you do. Also, they often get a lot of money and operate with a specific frame of mind.

The key, the thing that gets consultants hired again, is that a good consultant offers answers. Any hospital has a host of people that can point out problems: inspectors, surveyors, governmental officials, insurance people, and even hospital employees. The trick is to offer answers to these problems; specific answers, with alternatives ranging from the cheapest through the logical approach, to the top-of-the-line-with-all-accessories approach. They also list their advantages and costs (all costs: people, money, space, and time).

It has been suggested that most bad management decisions come about because the manager does not have enough information upon which to base an effective decision. Most managers do not have the time and expertise to research and design answers to safety problems. This kind of expertise requires a knowledge of codes, regulations, and laws, a background in science, psychology, some engineering, and a current working knowledge of what is happening in the field. (It also helps to have friends that know more about specific areas.) In short, this is the job of the safety staff professional, to help develop solutions, not just find the problem.

It should be understood, however, that if safety professionals do not look for problems, then they are not doing their jobs. It is not nice to find out about problems "by accident". You must do more, however, and be the source to develop or help institute the solution.

A second key concept a good consultant uses is to work as far down the line of command as possible. The best person to solve a problem is the person directly responsible for it. If you start too low, you waste time, and if you start too high, you waste the time of high management (the most precious resource). You must learn to define the level at which the problem starts and work one level above this. If you have a housekeeping problem, it is useless to start with the worker. If the problem is isolated in one area, talk to the immediate supervisor. If it covers several areas, talk to the manager, and if it is everywhere, talk to the environmental director. There are several reasons why this approach works. First, that specific person is closest to the problem and is the one that must solve it in the end anyway. Second, it offers that person the respect of being responsible and important, and third, it wastes as little of the time of upper management as possible. If the effort at this level fails, move up one level and try again. Remember, however, if the boss does not want to do anything, learn that part of the maze and profit by it next time.

Cost vs. Price

When you assess the costs of accidents, remember to assess the nonaccountable costs: supervisory time, rooms not usable, materials wasted, etc. It is estimated that the nonaccountable costs are usually at least four times the accountable costs (workers' compensation, medical, insurance).

Good consultants (i.e., those that get hired again) (1) have answers to the problems they or others point out, (2) offer alternatives, along with their advantages and costs, (3) start as low on the chain of command as possible, and (4) are available to answer questions as necessary about the specifics of their specialty. You may not always know the answer to a question, but should always have a source for an answer. Do not be afraid to say "I do not know yet, but I will find out and get back to you."

Good consultants also belong to professional organizations. Participation in national organizations such as the National Safety Council, National Fire Protection Association, National Safety Management Society, and others offer almost unlimited access to the expert knowledge available.

The yearly National Safety Congress offers programs both directly for health care industry and other industry groups having some impact or similar problems. Bi-yearly meetings of NFPA allow members to comment and vote on proposed standards, as well as comment on what standards are needed.

Other sources of information include some of the many seminars, classes, and courses offered by the above organizations (and groups such as JCAH) aimed at providing both answers to specific problems and contact with the best professionals in the safety field. Constant education and reading in the field is necessary both because of the rapidly changing nature of the regulations that affect the industry and the new developments that are created to solve those problems.

REFERENCES

1. Accident Prevention Manual for Industrial Operations, National Safety Council, Chicago, 1974.
2. Guide for Safety in the Chemical Laboratory, Manufacturing Chemists Association, Van Nostrand Reinhold, New York, 1972.
3. Regulations of the Occupational Safety and Health Administration, Department of Labor, 29 C F R Part 1910, latest edition.
4. Accreditation Manual for Hospitals, Joint Commission on Accreditation of Hospitals, Chicago, 1979.
5. **McLean, W. T.,** *Safety Training and Employee Record Cards,* McLean Association, Chesterton, Ind., unpublished.

Specific Safety Practices

BIOLOGIC SAFETY: SANITATION AND INFECTION CONTROL

William C. Beck

INTRODUCTION

The physical safety within the health care institution is usually regulated and monitored by a safety committee. Biologic safety falls under the purview of the infection control committee, a requirement of the Joint Commission on Hospital Accreditation (JCAH). Each hospital and each extended care facility must have an infection control committee with specified responsibilities. This committee is charged with the creation and implementation of policies to ensure a biologically safe environment.[1] This is necessary because between 3 and 6% of all of the patients who enter our acute care hospitals today acquire infections while residents of the facility.[2] The number of the institutional staff and patient visitors who develop infections as a result of hospital exposure is unknown. Some probably also become carriers and compound the problem.

Hospital-acquired infections have been recognized for centuries. Before Pasteur related infection to bacteria and Lister devised methods for the control of microorganisms, almost all surgical wounds became infected. A century and a half ago, before Semmelweis and Oliver Wendell Holmes recognized that organisms could be transferred by the attendant's hands, more than one of each ten women delivering their babies in a hospital died of infection. Our present infection rate, by such a comparison, is greatly improved, but is still far too high.

Separate hospitals (or "pest homes") for the isolation of patients with communicable diseases have disappeared. Even the tuberculosis sanitoria — their last vestige — are waning. Each innovation in medical infection control, such as antibiotics, seems to bring us closer to the disappearance of hospital-acquired (now dignified by a new term — nosocomial) infection, but still fall short. Although the percentage is small, the total number of nosocomial infections is still large. In 1967, of the 31,600,000 admissions to hospitals in the U.S., 2,101,037 (6.5%) were said to have acquired an infection in the hospital. The costs of 1,400,000 postoperative wound infections alone in 1967 was estimated to be $9.8 billion.[3] This did not even include the costs of pain, discomfort, and even death, to say nothing of the loss of the patient's output due to disability or premature death. Also not included was the loss of attendant time and the added costs of isolation practices (e.g., the use of disposables) and treatment of isolated dishes, drugs, and silverware (Figure 1).

The mortality rate of hospital-acquired infection is not inconsiderable. Dixon reports that 1% of affected patients die as a direct result of infection.[4] This may also be related to malpractice suits. See Table 1.

Careful planning, universal vigilance, and continued monitoring can and does minimize the hazard. However, the very nature of the health care institution's occupants creates a milieu that is predisposed to the dissemination of infection and also to acquiring them. The hospital houses patients who bring infectious illnesses. It also houses patients who by their disease or by their therapy are rendered incapable of resisting this microbial invasion that would be harmless to a normal person. The extended-care facility is occupied by persons of advanced age who are deficient in their biological resistance mechanisms. The pediatric section houses infants too young to have acquired immunity.

Particularly susceptible are patients with burns, cancer, or anemia. So also are pa-

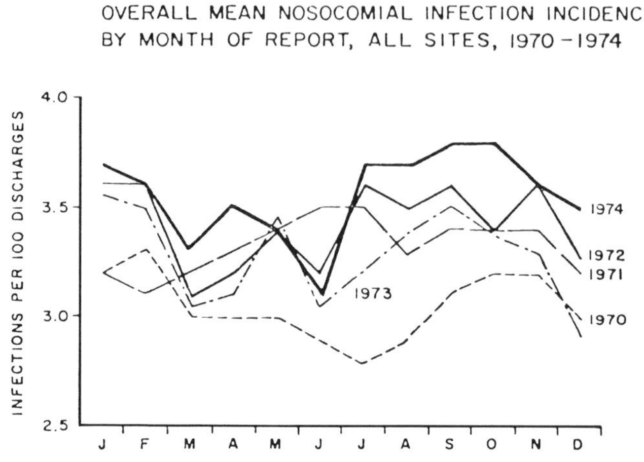

FIGURE 1. The incidence of hospital-acquired infections by year. (From U.S. Department of Health, Education and Welfare, National Nosocomial Infections Study, Center for Disease Control, Atlanta, 1977.)

tients being treated by radiation or chemotherapy. Some patients may have their immune processes therapeutically depressed, e.g., the recipients of organ transplants or implants of foreign bodies such as prosthetic joints, heart valves, or eye lenses.

The skin is one of man's greatest organs of infection resistance. When it is broken by the surgeon's knife or by an injury, a new portal for the entry of infection is created; 3 to 5% of surgical wounds succumb. When a normally sterile cavity such as a urinary bladder or vein is opened to a foreign body (e.g., a catheter), infection is a very frequent complication.

Carelessness on the part of any person involved can initiate a dangerous and costly train of events. To alert all of the hospital's personnel is one of the most important and potentially helpful goals of both the safety and infections committees. The understanding of their responsibility and their cooperation can have a significant benefit. For this continuing educational process, all hospital employees, whether or not they have an intimate patient contact, must have knowledge and understanding of safety procedures. This is not a responsibility borne only by the professionals, the physicians, nurses, dentists, and technicians. It is also a constant challenge for the maintenance, dietary, housekeeping, and engineering personnel. It is also a problem for the patient and his visitor. All must learn to respect the rules, understand their meaning, and meticulously exercise the controls.

BASIC PRINCIPLES

The Environment

To understand the reasons for the procedures of sanitation and infection control, all persons working in the hospital must be aware of the problems. Living microorganisms are universally distributed. In every gram of earth, in every drop of water, and in every cubic foot of air, there are a large number of microorganisms. However, these microbes (bacteria, viruses, fungi, and protazoa) are not equally nor evenly distributed. In the outside air, in the sea, and even in agricultural soil, the contaminants are not "people" germs and thus are generally and usually not harmful to man. In people enclosures such as homes or hospitals, there are people bacteria that cause most of our problems.* See Figure 2.

* Exceptions to this are frequent. For example, earth soil contains the bacteria that cause lockjaw (Tetanus).

Table 1

NOSOCOMIAL INFECTION RATES[a] BY SERVICE AND CATEGORY OF HOSPITAL, 1976

	Medicine	Surgery	Obstetrics	Gynecology	Pediatrics	Newborn Nursery	All Services
Community	2.4	3.8	1.6	2.4	0.9	0.9	2.6
Community teaching	4.0	5.2	1.3	3.2	0.4	1.1	3.6
Federal	4.5	5.9	2.0	4.9	0.6	0.3	4.8
Municipal or county	7.2	7.1	3.8	5.4	3.0	3.1	5.5
University	4.8	5.8	2.0	2.6	1.5	3.0	4.4
All hospitals	3.7	5.0	1.9	3.0	1.1	1.6	3.6

[a] Rate per 100 patient discharges (%).

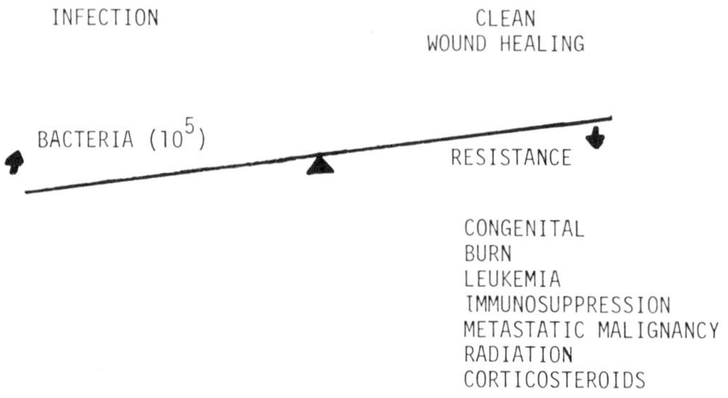

FIGURE 2. Infection or clean wound healing is the product of the bacterial challenge and the elements involved in resistance. A bacterial load larger than 10^5 is usually required to create an infection in the normal patient. Some of the elements which reduce resistance are listed in this diagram.

The quantity of the bacterial load is also a factor, particularly in patients of reduced immunity, such as those with burns, cancer, or under treatment. The "bioload" or "bioburden" of a surface on a potential source is the type and number of microbes on it at a given time. It may vary greatly from time to time, however, unless a specific process of sterilization or removal of organisms takes place, some are always present or contamination is always present.[5]

At one time, bacteria were classified as pathogens (capable of producing disease) or nonpathogens (harmless). However, we no longer assume that there are any nonpathogens. Under special circumstances, it is probable that any or all bacteria can produce an infection. As yet, not all have been incriminated. However, more and more of the apparently harmless ones are producing infections. For example, there is an organism (*Serratia marcesens*) that when growing on an agar plate produces brilliant red colonies that are easily recognized. At one time, this was considered to be an entirely harmless organism. In order to observe contamination from his breath, this author gargled with a solution of this organism and spread plates throughout the hospital to observe where my breath settled and contaminated the air. After hearing of the first fatality (in a hospital 1000 mi distant) from this organism, I cultured myself from scalp and throat, to toenails to be certain I did not still continue to harbor them. This organism has been added to the growing list of the dangerous.

Ecologic Transport

Bacteria have no wings or feet so they cannot swim, walk, or fly. However, they can ride a mote of dust or a droplet in the breath. A touch from hand or finger to sheet or pillow can cause their transport from place to place. They move from human to human in the handshake or finger touch, to food, or to any surface. They move from human to inanimate objects and back again through contact. They also move from human to air in the droplet of cough, sneezing, talking, or shedding from our body surface (Figure 3).

A droplet may evaporate leaving a bacterial cluster to float — like smoke — in the air, either gradually settling upon a horizontal surface or inhaled by another. From any surface, the bacteria or its dust-mote-carrier may again be entrained by wind, sweeping, or shaking. People or any warm, moist surface such as animals, soils, or

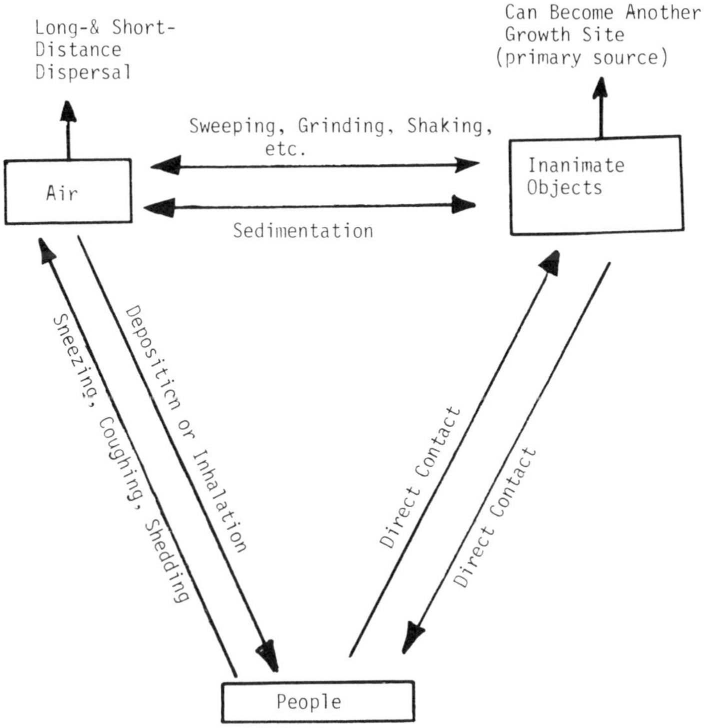

FIGURE 3. The source of most infections is people. However, the infectious agents may reach other people through either the air or inanimate objects.

stagnant water may be the breeding place and source of the bacteria. They may be carried from the source by flies, rodents, or mosquitoes.

A patient may become contaminated by direct contact and spread this organism to a physician who examines him. The physician may in turn carry it to another patient when his supposedly immaculate white coat touches the second patient's bed. The methods of spread exceed our imagination. Fortunately, however, the quantity and power of the bacterium to cause trouble when removed from its natural habitat usually diminishes. An exception is epidemics.

Immunity and Resistance

Physical Protection

Man from birth possesses a natural resistance to the invasion of microorganisms. The most efficient of these is the skin, the largest organ of the body. Although it is at almost all times covered with bacteria that live contentedly upon this warm, moist surface, it protects the tissues beneath it. The hairs in our noses and ears protect the internal surfaces from bacterial ingress, just as the hairs of the eyelids and eyebrows protect our eyes from flying particles. Secretions such as tears rid our eyes of contamination. The celiated (hairy) cells of our respiratory tract and their moving mucus tend to entrap and rid us of bacteria reaching these areas by inhaled air.

Immunology

Furthermore, we possess an efficient system, or group of systems, designed to protect us from the bacteria that have passed the external defenses. There are immunities passed to us from our mothers before birth and those we have acquired. Some of these are responses to challengers such as the disease itself, while others are artificially induced by vaccines, killed microorganisms designed to induce immunity.

Our white blood cells are defenders that are not specific and usually succeed in engulfing invaders and neutralizing them by ingesting and digesting them. These immune processes of the normal human are at their weakest in the first weeks of life and advanced age. For this reason, the child is most susceptible and the old person's life is usually terminated by bacterial victory. Certain disease states also result in a reduction of these immune processes, e.g., extensive cancer.

The immune process is what causes the rejection of incompatible organ transplants. In fact, organ transplants were not really possible, except between twins, until methods were found to suppress the immune process. The advanced cancer patient accepts skin grafts without the power to reject them as would the normal patient; this shows his loss of immunologic protection. For this reason, most cancer patients actually die of infection.

Patients into whom relatively large foreign bodies are implanted are at special risk. Many years ago it was demonstrated that the challenging number of microorganisms sufficient to produce an infection can be exponentially reduced by simultaneously introducing a foreign body.[6] Apparently, there is also a propensity for such foreign bodies to harbor and permit the elaboration of unusual infectious agents such as yeasts or the serratia marcessens previously discussed. One factor rarely given consideration is that an infection complicating a surgical implant will usually necessitate removal of the implant so that the operation itself is rendered a failure. Furthermore, these infections, for some reason yet unfathomed, may be delayed in their clinical manifestations, often up to a year or even two.

The implantation of such foreign yet generally compatible materials is, without question, one of the growing areas of surgical endeavor. Both small and very large artificial joints are being introduced to replace worn-out arthritic joints, from the small finger joints to the huge hip joint. New heart valves are being implanted to replace defective or diseased ones. Almost all of the body's blood vessels are being replaced or bypassed, often with artificial materials. Plastic eye lenses are replacing those removed for cataracts. Each year, new implantables are being created from artificial hearts to pacemakers, and other nerve stimulators. To have these life and limb savers and essential surgical procedures spoiled by an infection is a terrible blow; not only is the operation a failure, but the infection adds cost, discomfort, and even death.

Inflammation and Infection

Any tissue insult, whether it be by trauma or by microorganisms, calls forth a body response. It is characterized by the slowing of the blood stream in the area of injury so that more blood is present. The clinical evidence of this is a reddish hue to the skin and increased local heat. While this is taking place, fluid leaves the blood vessel carrying white blood cells into the tissues. This causes a swelling of the area. Finally, the swelling and surge of arterial blood trying to get into the area results in a throbbing pain. The sum of these activities manifested by redness, increased temperature, swelling, and pain is descriptively called inflammation.

Successful inflammation will resolve the effects of the injury, initiate any needed reparative process, and destroy and remove any foreign body or bacterial invader. Unsuccessful inflammation is called infection. This means that the bacteria have (at least in that area and for the time being) won and will remain viable while inflammatory products such as the white blood cells die. The admixture of dead white blood cells in a liquid medium containing live dangerous microorganisms is called pus. Dead protein matter, warm and moist, is ideal for bacterial growth, and successive generations are created in rapid succession. Thus, it is important to give the pus a way out and remove it as soon as possible. We must also treat it with great caution, for it is alive with dangerous organisms.

Moreover, collections of pus (called abscesses) are difficult to treat biochemically, as antibiotic medications have difficulty in reaching them. The only way antibiotics can affect microbes is if they can reach them. The blood stream is the only method by which an antibiotic can reach an abscess without surgical invasion (by needle or by incision). Therefore, abscesses containing bacteria are relatively inaccessible to blood-borne antibiotics.

SANITATION

The residence of hospital-based microorganisms is on the personnel working and residing in the hospital and in the soil accumulating within the hospital. Control, therefore, devolves into personal hygiene and the maintenance of a clean environment. Since most of the problem microorganisms that concern us are people ones, personal hygiene cannot be stressed too much. All employees of the hospital, whether or not they have immediate patient contact, contribute to the microbial milieu of the institution because all are constantly shedding superficial skin and exhaling mouth droplets into the air. Bacteria contained in these are often a hazard to the resistance-deprived patient.

Personal hygiene means washing. Repeated handwashing will remove huge numbers of dangerous bacteria, particularly when carried out with a germicidal soap. Showering before coming to work is also an important component of personal hygiene. If it is done before coming to the hospital, the natural skin oils will be replaced and will limit the scurf (shed skin cells such as dandruff) discharged into the environment. We tend to shed more immediately after the shower. Wearing clean uniforms or clothes is also helpful, as well as esthetic, in the institutional atmosphere.

Care of all hair is particularly important as it is constantly shed. Modern fashion enhances this. Hair is heavily contaminated with bacteria. Therefore, cleanliness, neatness, and containment in areas of concern are imperative.

The value of repeated handwashing cannot be sufficiently emphasized. Finger contact probably disseminates more problem microorganisms than any other mode of spread.

Soil Removal

Soiling in the hospital is a very complicated problem. The institution — even the small one — is a complex of buildings, rooms, and corridors all of which present a variety of surfaces that must be regularly cleaned. The usual mechanism is by covering the surface with a detergent-disinfectant and then removing it. The detergent-disinfectant is chosen not only for the type of soilage, but also for the quality of the water used for dilution of the concentrates. The type of surface that must be cleaned will also govern the materials and methods to be used. Some may be injured by strong solutions or even by water.

It would be impossible in the scope of this treatise to detail the schedules, the exact materials to be used, and the practices to be followed in the housekeeping of the hospital. The housekeeping executive has been educated on how to choose them. He is also guided by many special textbooks on the subject.[7] However, certain general guidelines can be given, particularly to assist a nonhousekeeper's understanding of the activity.

Zones of Cleaning

Sound cleaning practices differ with the environment in which they are employed.

In hallways, waiting rooms, and storage areas, it would appear that the cleaning problem would not differ materially from similar institutional structures such as hotels, office buildings, schools, etc. However, they do. The populations differ. In the hospital, there are sick and even dying patients disseminating unusual and virulent microorganisms towards patients with reduced powers of resistance. This holds true for the ancillary hospital zones including food service areas, interstitial floors (if present), and service closets.

The housekeeping of isolation rooms, critical care areas, and surgical and obstetric suites is the most critical in the hospital. They need to be accurately defined and identified. The cleaning plan of each area needs to be the joint effort of the supervisor of that area and the housekeeping executive, with review and approval of the infection-control committee.

A variety of suggested plans for this activity have been reported in the literature. For certain areas, such as the operating room, a standard has been created by the Association of Operating Room Nurses (AORN) which details the techniques.[8]

Cleaning Materials

Soil consists of a wide variety of ingredients, some soluble in water, some organic, and others inorganic. There is no single material that will universally facilitate its removal. Furthermore, all cleaning methods should remove soil, not redistribute it. Brushes and brooms have no place in the hospital. Any brushing or sweeping action must be accompanied by an aspirating method such as a vacuum system.

Wherever possible, wet systems are employed because they are the simplest to remove and dispose. Helping soil get into an aqueous solution or suspension involves emulsification or saponification. Surfaction reduces the surface tension of water to increase its ability to penetrate soils. Dispersion helps to break up clumps of soil into tiny particles and peptization breaks up proteins.

Most water contains magnesium and calcium ions in varying degrees that cause hardness. This precipitates soap, causing it to form a distressing, hard-to-remove scum. For this reason, organic chelating agents or inorganic sequestrating agents are often added to soften the water. They precipitate an insoluble magnesium and calcium.

New cleaning agents are being created constantly and the available choices are large. Many are added to hot water, itself a surfactant. Biodegradability is particularly sought for in hospital cleaning materials because large amounts are used. It is imperative that the cleaning agents, usually supplied as concentrates to be mixed with water, are accurately diluted. Many are supplied with measuring devices. However, the supervisory personnel must be vigilant in reviewing this. Many are haphazardly mixed, either endangering by over-concentration or spoiling results by over-dilution.

The character of the soilage in the hospital poses special problems for the housekeeper. Often blood, feces, urine, pus, or even tissue creates special problems. They are compounded if they dry. Immediate soaking with cold water can be very helpful and should be carried out by all personnel.

Disinfection in Cleaning

The admixture of antimicrobial agents with the cleaning detergents for surfaces is almost universally adopted. The regulation of the antimicrobials is a charge of the Federal Environmental Protection Agency as auhorized by the many amendments to the Insecticide, Fungicide, and Rodenticide Act of 1964. All disinfectants are included in this act and must carry labels that identify the material and give adequate directions for their use.

The person choosing the disinfectant for use in the hospital is faced with a large number recommended by persuasive salesmen, who provide them at a wide spectrum of cost. The yardsticks that are employed include the phenol coefficient and the more widely accepted Association of Official Agricultural Chemicals (A.O.A.C.) use-dilution test.[9] The latter is the more valuable, but still is not entirely valid in revealing what the actual results will be in the hospital with the local water source and local cleaning conditions. For most purchasing agents it will, however, provide the simplest method of comparison. Another microbiological criterion that should be observed is the effect of the germicide upon the organism *Pseudomonas aeruginosa*, as this is difficult to kill and is ubiquitous in the hospital environment, as well as dangerous. Similarly, the Gardner Straight Line Washability Test and Detergent Capacity Tests will help in evaluation.[7d]

A comparison evaluation of the relative effect of the germicide on the flora of the hospital is really beyond the capability of most of the clinical laboratories. However, the opinion of the microbiologist and of the infection-control personnel should be obtained. It should be discussed with the employees, using their opinions on the odor, skin irritation, rinsability, and other physical phenomena as guides. All other criteria being equal, cost will prevail, estimating this on the basis of its dilution factor.

Housekeeping Techniques

Most of the expenditure for housekeeping is for labor.[10] In 1970, Mallison estimated the cost to be $2 per patient day. In the Robert Packer Hospital (340 beds) in 1977, it amounted to $5.70 per patient day. This amounts to $180/ft^2$ of cleaned space. This excludes areas cleaned by department personnel. Salaries account for 90% of this amount. Cleaning by housekeeping includes care of the floors, walls, and other surfaces.

As most contamination of the fixed environment occurs by the settling of particles, the horizontal surfaces are the ones that should be of greatest concern and should occupy the most time and effort. Vertical surfaces should be cleaned whenever they become visibly soiled by splashes and spots, and stains should be promptly cared for. However, floors and other horizontal surfaces need routine care.

Litsky and Litsky have clearly demonstrated that dusting should be done only with chemically treated single-use cloths.[11] It has also been demonstrated that oily surfaces entrap microorganisms and prevent their dissemination through subsequent entrainment, and that commercially treated cloths are not imperative.

Floor cleaning has repeatedly been shown to be of great value. It is, of course, dependent upon the surface. Carpeting is being widely employed; if used, it should be chosen with great care. Carpeting entraps microorganisms and actually removes soil from shoe soles and wheels. However, it must be efficiently and frequently cleaned by agitating vacuum cleaners that have good filtration at the exit portal.

For the cleaning of hard flooring, the most efficient method is flooding with a detergent-disinfectant and its subsequent removal by a wet vacuum with exit filtration. In areas of special concern, such as surgical suites, this is the method of choice and should be done daily.

Double-bucket mopping with a clean mophead is the second choice. Litsky believes it should be sterile and presents biological evidence for this.[12] Here the disinfectant-detergent is contained in one bucket and rinse solution in another. The mop is always rinsed prior to dipping into the detergent-disinfectant. This system minimizes reapplication of contamination and extends the useful action of the disinfectant-detergent. A third bucket may be added for wringing out the mop before immersion into the rinse bucket. Mopheads must be clean, and this is best done by laundering and thorough drying, not by soaking. Steam sterilization gives added assurance.

In isolation facilities, all mopheads and rinse waters are treated with other contaminated materials. Most of these have hard floors suitable for this treatment. The frequency of floor treatment should be decided consistent with the cleaning of other horizontal surfaces.

All forms of brushing and sweeping are contraindicated in health care facilities. A possible exception is the scrubbing machine often employed in corridors. This may be particularly useful in areas of (and at times of) exceptional soiling or special hazard. This has been recommended particularly for the food preparation areas.[9]

It has been suggested that some of the techniques of floor care should be adopted from industrial clean rooms. These include the use of "tacky mats", "mud rugs", and shallow containers of liquid germicides. The tacky mat has not achieved a significant place even in the entrances of surgical suites because of its great expense and the danger of tripping. The traffic of the surgical suite is much greater than that of the industrial room. The shallow pools of germicides also have resisted popularity. The use of entrance rugs (such as those often employed on muddy days) with a napped surface on a rubber base do clean shoes and wheeled carriages or gurneys if they are themselves kept clean by repeated vacuuming. These are used in industry to clean even truck tires. They are useful in the hospital and are inexpensive and easy to maintain.

AIR HYGIENE

Air Contamination

Historically, the passage of disease was thought by Semmelweiss and Homes to be by hand contact. However, Lister, at first, believed that airborne contamination was the source of surgical infection, and he attempted to destroy this source by the use of a carbolic acid spray.

There is no doubt that some infection is spread via the air by particulate matter-carrying microorganisms. As the air in the hospital is constantly in motion, the vertical settling of these particles onto horizontal surfaces is usually not direct. If there is any consistent directionality to the airflow, their spread is usually downwind from the source. Today, there is usually a turbulent flow in air-conditioned hospitals. The undirectional flow, called laminar, rarely exists even in planned, specially designed rooms.

The source of the air contaminants is invariably from human room occupants and may be from shed particles, exhaled moist droplets, or the entrainment of settled particles. The shedding of particulate matter from the body surface has been carefully studied in industrial clean rooms.[14] (See Figure 4) It has also been studied in surgical operating rooms, therefore, special clothing with air-exhaust systems are worn in some operating rooms to achieve ultra asepsis.[15]

Droplets emanating from the nose and mouth are also sources of air contamination. The droplets have actually been photographed and counted. They are obviously at peak during talking, sneezing, or coughing.[16] The droplets procede for a meter or more propelled by the exhalation, and then evaporate, leaving a clump of microorganisms and dry secretion to float in the air like smoke. The settling of these particles 10 to 20 μm in size may take several hours. Masks designed to protect the air from this source are designed to entrap the droplets and thus retain the contaminants. They are not bacterial filters, but rather droplet filters.

The entrainment of particles by cleaning operations has already been discussed, and filters for the outflow of vacuum cleaners recommended. The dissemination of lint and other particulate matter in such activities as bedmaking, draping of surgical fields, and from laundry chutes probably is of even greater importance. For this reason, fomites must be handled with great care and immediate containment.

Air Flow and Air Quality

Containment of the sources is the essential part of air hygiene. On the other hand,

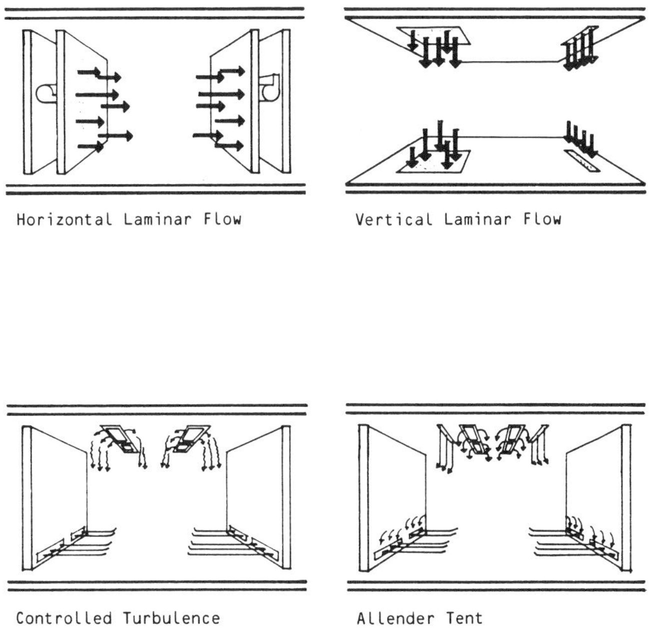

FIGURE 4. Illustrated here are methods of distributing filtered "clean" air in ultra-clean operating rooms. All have found limited use for procedures requiring ultra asepsis.

management of the air flow is also of significance. The recirculation of ambient air is an acceptable technique. Recirculating warmed or cooled air through filtration cleaning will certainly conserve energy. This is permitted even in surgical theaters.

The design of the filter banks is dependent upon the quality of the air to be cleaned, as well as the requirements for the final air to enter the room. Rough prefilters are useful to preserve the final filters. The final filters probably never need to be of the ultra high efficiency particulate (HEPA) type employed so widely in industrial clean rooms. High efficiency filters, 90% effective, will probably remove all of the biological hazards even in sensitive areas such as operating and recovery rooms. For less sensitive areas, the final filter quality need be of medium efficiency only (60 to 90%). They should be placed as close as possible to the site of delivery.

Filters must be certified as to their quality and their mounting. They must be tested in place to be sure that they secure in the air stream within their confines and that leaks do not occur around the frame. The pressure differences on both sides of the filter can be very useful to monitor filter function and to indicate when the filters need replacement.

The directionality of the airflow from room to room is described in the Federal Hill-Burton Code.[30] It is described by requiring positive or negative pressure with relationship to other rooms. This is theoretically ascertained by measuring the cubic meters (or feet) of air delivered into the room in comparison with that leaving into an adjacent space. This is correct under laboratory conditions and assuming that the temperatures are equal, doors are shut, etc.

The exchange of air through open portal is not simple. There is a two-way airflow if temperatures are equal on both sides (Figure 5).[17] Therefore, concerned clinical engineers should be able to test airflows and know its directions.[18] It can be done by smoke tests or by simply hanging toilet tissue on the door jam.

In certain places, the airflow either into or out of the room can be very significant

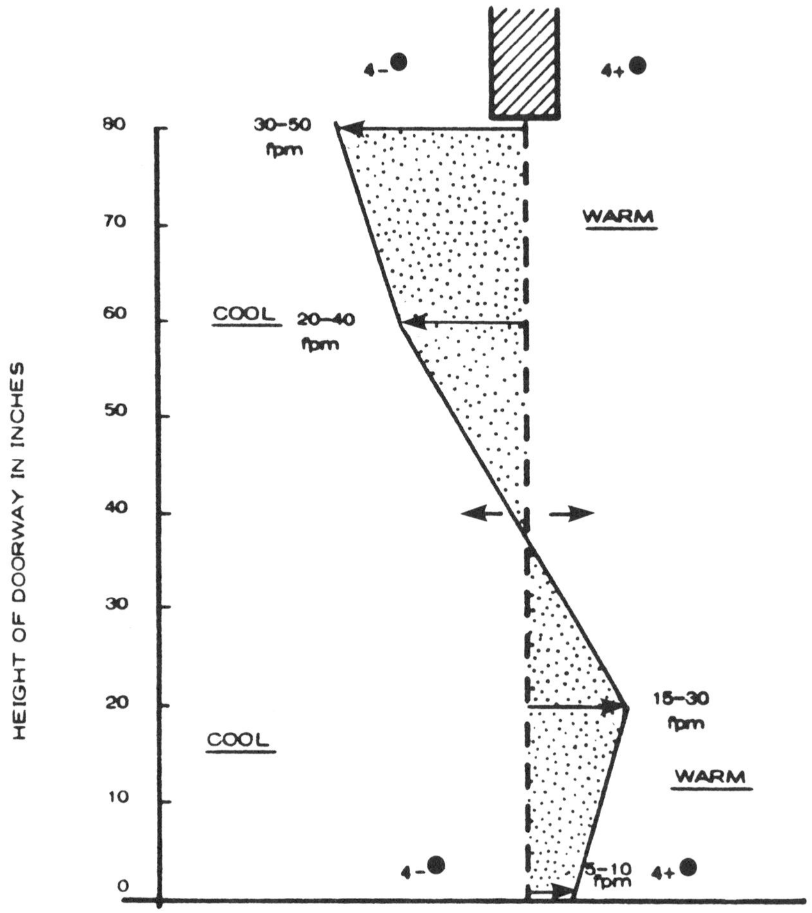

FIGURE 5. This diagram illustrates the exchange of air through an open door. It is assumed that the chamber of one side of the door is 4° warmer than that on the other. It is to be noted that there is a difference in direction of flow in the upper and lower sides of the portal with the flow to the warm side in the lower half and towards the cool side in the upper.

and removal may be as important as delivery. Pressurized exhaust and scavenging systems may be considered. Airflows within rooms of special infection potential, such as surgical operating rooms or immunity deprived patient quarters, have been outfitted with a variety of unidirectional flow systems often called laminar airflow. No hard evidence has been produced to show that these ever reduce infection. This has been enunciated by the Committee on the Operating Room Environment of the American College of Surgeons.[19] However, laminar airflow systems are being employed in a variety of designs and configurations.[20] Their evaluation is extremely difficult because the statistical basis is very hard to design. A huge number of cases of a single operation must be reviewed because the basic infection rate is so low.[21]

Air Changes

In addition to the directionality of the airflow and its cleansing by filtration, the air exchange rate is of importance. This does not mean the entire replacement of the air within the exchange zone by an entirely new air (unless a total, true laminarity has been established, which is probably impossible except in one completely empty of fur-

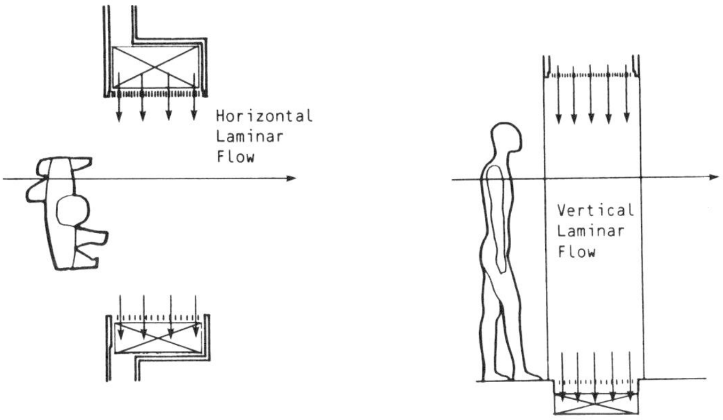

FIGURE 6. Laminar airflow can be used as a door. This can be done by (A) horizontal flow or (B) by vertical flow.

niture, etc.). However, it will provide dilution. By definition (Federal Standard 209B), laminar airflow requires a flow rate of 100 ft/min.[22] For turbulent systems, the Federal Code requires a specific number of air changes per hour.[23] This is figured by ascertaining the size of the room in cubic feet, the size of the air delivery grille, and the average rate of airflow over the grille.

An operating room 20 × 20 × 10 ft contains 4000 cubic feet. Two 4 × 2-ft entrance grilles have 16 ft^2. If air is introduced at an average of 100 ft/min, this would produce 96,000 ft^3/hr. Dividing 96,000 by 4000 would result in 24 air changes per hour. Air changes, however, must be validated by controlling the entrances to a room. This may be accomplished by air portals. See Figure 6.

Where air contamination is a problem, the biologic cleanliness has been defined and classified.[24] The classification is by the number of viable particles per cubic foot of air and is accomplished by a volumetric sampling device that aspirates a known volume of air and impinges it against an agar plate within a certain time. The plate is then incubated and the colonies are counted. A variety of instruments are available for this purpose, including single-use ones that will even sort out the particle size. Merely exposing open Petri dishes acting as settling plates is a simpler system, but does not permit an accurate definition since the rate of settling differs for particles of different sizes.

ISOLATION

The technique of isolation is accepted as an important part of infection control.

Local Isolation

In recent years, isolation of parts of the body has been practiced with success. When a body part, particularly a surgical wound, is draining large amounts of contaminated material or large numbers of microorganisms, it can be sealed off by surrounding it with a plastic. The plastic is securely fixed to the surrounding skin. The secretions may be removed by aspiration into a closed system, or into dressings that can be handled through an opening into the plastic, without contamination of the air or the environment.[25]

Total Isolation

There are two types of total patient isolation — positive and reverse. The most usual

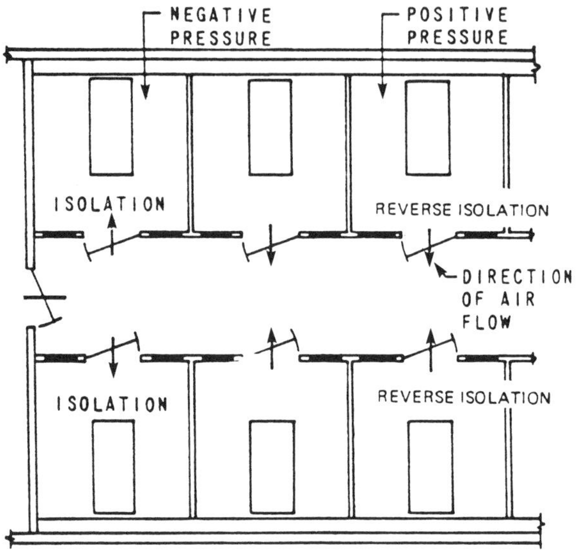

FIGURE 7. Isolation facilities require special air management. The difference between positive and reverse isolation air directions is illustrated here.

positive isolation — the infected patient — is isolated to prevent the spread of infection to other patients or hospital personnel. The patient is put into specially designed quarters that prevent the outward spread of contaminants by air, contact, or fomites. See Figure 4.

The second type is called reverse isolation. Here, a highly susceptible patient is protected from infection by the hospital environment. Such patients are protected from the inward spread of hospital air and contact with harmful bacteria. Examples of such patients could be patients with extensive burns, those with extensive malignant disease being treated with radiation or chemotherapy, and those under immunosuppression receiving organ transplants.

Reverse isolation is carried out in some institutions in environments surrounding only their beds so that they may even be treated in open wards.[26] In other situations, large quarters are assigned to these patients and they are managed in practically germ-free units.[27] While in actual use, these techniques are still considered experimental and their results are being studied. See Figure 7.

All of the isolation techniques associated with special problems for the hospital personnel are expensive to build and maintain, and impose psychological restrictions for the patient. There is a variety of types and degrees of isolation. These include strict, total isolation, enteric isolation, respiratory isolation, and precautionary isolation for skin and wounds, etc. The Public Health Service produces Isolation Techniques for Use in Hospitals (Public Health Service Publication 71-8043), and colored cards for display for each of the isolation techniques. (See Table 2.) Other references are given in the bibliography.[28]

Isolation rooms or areas are usually provided in the adult hospital, in pediatric sections, and often in recovery and critical care units. These usually have an anteroom separating the isolation facility from general hallways. These can act as airlocks and can be used for gowning and handwashing. Special containers are provided to discard the single-use items employed in patient care, e.g., gowns, masks, gloves, etc. The prominently displayed, colored cards described above should be read by all persons

Table 2
INFECTIOUS DISEASES GROUPED ACCORDING TO DEGREE OF RECOMMENDED ISOLATION

Private room	Mask	Gown	Gloves	Excreta and excreta-soiled articles	Blood	Secreta and secreta-soiled articles	
Strict Isolation							
x	x	x	x	x	x	x	Smallpox
x	x	x	x			x	Anthrax, inhalation; plague, pneumonic; vaccinia, generalized and progressive, and eczema vaccinatum
x	x	ⓧ	ⓧ			x	Burn, skin, or wound infection, major, with *Staphylococcus aureus* or group A streptococcus that is not covered by a dressing or that has copious purulent drainage
x	x	ⓧ	ⓧ		x	x	Lassa fever, Marburg virus disease
x	x	ⓧ	ⓧ			x	Pneumonia — *Staphylococcus aureus*, group A streptococcus
x	x	ⓧ				x	Diphtheria (pharyngeal or cutaneous)
x	x*	x	x			x	Varicella (chickenpox); Herpes zoster, disseminated
x		ⓧ		x	x	x	Congenital rubella syndrome; disseminated neonatal *Herpesvirus hominis* (herpes simplex)
x			ⓧ			x	Rabies
Respiratory Isolation							
x	x*					x	Tuberculosis, pulmonary (including tuberculosis of the respiratory tract), suspected or sputum-positive (smear)

Table 2 (continued)
INFECTIOUS DISEASES GROUPED ACCORDING TO DEGREE OF RECOMMENDED ISOLATION

Private room	Mask	Gown	Gloves	Excreta and excreta-soiled articles	Blood	Secreta and secreta-soiled articles	
				Respiratory Isolation			
x	x						Meningococcal meningitis; Meningococcemia
x	x*					x	Measles (rubeola); mumps: Rubella (German measles); pertussis (whooping cough)
				Enteric Precautions			
D		ⓧ	ⓧ	x			Cholera; enterocolitis, staphylococcal; gastroenteritis — enteropathogenic or enterotoxic *Escherichia coli, Salmonella* species, *Shigella* species, *Yersinia enterocolitica;* typhoid fever
D		ⓧ	ⓧ	x		x	Diarrhea, acute illness with suspected infectious etiology
D				x	x	x	Hepatitis, viral, types A, B, or unspecified
				Wound and Skin Precautions			
D			ⓧ			x	Gas gangrene (due to *Clostridium perfringens*)
D	x*	x	x			x	Herpes zoster, localized
D	ⓧ	ⓧ	ⓧ			x	Burn, skin, or wound infections, limited, including infections with *Staphylococcus aureus* or group A streptococcus, that are covered by and the discharge ade-

Table 2 (continued)
INFECTIOUS DISEASES GROUPED ACCORDING TO DEGREE OF RECOMMENDED ISOLATION

Private room	Mask	Gown	Gloves	Excreta and excreta-soiled articles	Blood	Secreta and secreta-soiled articles	
Wound and Skin Precautions							
							quately contained by a dressing; plague, bubonic
D		x	x			x	Burn, skin, or wound infections, major (except *S. aureus* and group A streptococcus that are not covered by a dressing or that have copious purulent drainage; melioidosis, extrapulmonary with draining sinuses

Note: X — recommended at all times; ⓧ — with direct contact; X * — for susceptibles; and D — desirable, but optional.

From U.S. Department of Health, Education and Welfare, Isolation Techniques for Use in Hospitals, Publ. No. (CDC) 76-8314, U.S. Department of Health, Education and Welfare, Washington, D.C., 1975.

entering and leaving the isolation area, in compliance with the requirements of the particular case. This is especially true for personnel not normally in contact with such patients. Engineers, technicians, and maintenance staff can comply with the precautions when their presence is required in the isolation facility. This is important not only for protection of the patient, but also for the hospital employee.

Maintenance and inspection of all the engineering of isolation facilities should be a special administrative concern. Since they are isolated from the general hospital systems, air systems in these areas are often neglected. Housekeeping personnel need to be particularly alert to the hazards in these rooms. At one time, when air systems were treated by fogging or closing them for a period of time, their special demands were obvious. This is not emphasized by present methods.

WATER HYGIENE

The water supply of the health care facility must meet the high standards of governmental regulatory agencies, and is monitored to assure that these standards are maintained. The biologic and chemical qualities are reviewed in a large variety of standard publications describing routine testing.[28] The physical qualities of clarity and colorless appearance, along with the tasteless and odorless consistency are self-evident. Their radiologic characteristics require special investigative methods. The standards of the U.S. Public Health Service[30], and the values recommended for ideal water by Beam[31] are worthy of review and should be available in the hospital's engineering file.

Purity

Special demands for water purity will be made by laboratories, pharmacies, and dialysis sites. Therapeutic bathing and washing tanks may also require higher standards for water cleanliness, particularly if they are used in the care of patients with extensive burns. If any of these departments require water supplies, special sources and controls will have to be arranged. In addition, arrangements will have to be made for their treatment, storage, and distribution.

Quantity

The amount of water used by a hospital varies from 150 to 350 gal per bed per day. The higher figure is for a hospital maintaining its own laundry service. In extended-care facilities, the quantity is usually estimated at 150 to 200 gal per bed per day. The peak use time is usually during the morning hours from 9 to 12, when Searcy and Furman have found that the use may approximate 600 gal per bed per hour.[32]

When the water supply of a hospital is derived from a municipal water system, the hospital authorities should assure themselves of its adequacy both in amount and quality. For the former, it is important to know that the supply will be adequate and of sufficient pressure during times of maximum demand. The adequacy of distribution systems, as well as emergency alternate systems, should be available from local or state utility and health departments. Also, knowledge of the number and types of tests conducted by the utility should be an administrative concern.

Testing

Testing carried out within the health care facility and its frequency will be dependent upon the size of the hospital and the facilities available in it. However, arrangements can also be made with independent laboratories for this service. Tests should include samples from the point of entrance to the hospital, as well as from several delivery points.

While the source of water should be from municipal sources whenever possible, an auxiliary source (preferably from ground water) may be useful, particularly for fire fighting and lawn requirements. Such sources must be independently tested for coliform organisms to assure that it is uncontaminated.

Distribution Systems

The original distribution systems within the hospital will have been designed and approved by knowledgeable and responsive people. Repeated samplings with a consistent absence of coliform bacteria, as well as good chemical formulation assures that the water system is well designed and functioning. If there are fluctuations, frequent testing is indicated. However, in every hospital there are repeated invasions of the system by additional and often innovational equipment. The engineering staff will have a special responsibility to review the equipment and its installation to be certain that effective contamination-control principles are maintained.

A thorough knowledge of the type of water distribution system is essential whether it is an upfeed system with booster pumps or a downfeed system with a storage tank above the facility. The dangers of invasion of either systems for repairs or introduction of new equipment will have to include a review of the safety systems of each. This would include the shunting that might occur between drinking-water systems and the general systems or protection devices in air vents, etc.

Plumbing cross connections that may occur between various water supplies present a special hazard with retrograde flow of contaminated liquids into the water supply. This is particularly possible if there is an insufficient pressure in the delivery system. Cross-connections between systems may be innocuous, such as certain kitchen appliances or dangerous ones such as bedpan washers, washer sterilizers in the sterile supply areas, and hoses on sinks in housekeeping areas.

Aspirators have a great potential for cross contamination. They may be used in a variety of places, however, their use in connection with the water distribution system has been condemned. Operating rooms, autopsy rooms, and some special care facilities are their more common sites. For these, special isolated pump systems should be used. They also should be protected by bottle traps.

Processing tanks in photography and X-ray may be sources of cross connections. Water stills in various locations, as well as a huge variety of pieces of equipment, may be connected to water supply systems in the health care facility. Any equipment used in the hospital that will have any water supply connection should be reviewed by the clinical engineering service for safety. Where back siphonage occurs, effective air gap or nonpressure vacuum breakers must be present.

Where there are a large number of potential cross-contamination possibilities, an area may have a system installed to provide this area with a break from the general hospital system. When this is done, the nonpotable nature of the water should be appropriately labeled by painting the pipes yellow or banding them and putting signs at the outlets. This may also be accomplished by the use of a barometric loop as described by Michaelson and DeRoos.[33]

Ice

Ice can also be the cause of contamination, even though it may be produced from a sanitary water source. Most of the ice used in our health care institutions is manufactured by a variety of machines that produce cubes, chips, or flakes. The machines not only supply the ice to be used on demand, but also store it for use. Accurate information for the requirements can be ascertained only by observation of the amount of use because it will vary with the climatic conditions of the geographic location, the season of the year, and the presence or absence of atmospheric cooling. In general, however, the need has been estimated at roughly 6 lb per bed per day and 4 lb per meal for the cafeteria in central food service. It is, of course, used for purposes other than food, such as ice bags, etc.

Distribution

When ice must be delivered to parts of the hospital in containers, it may be handled by several persons and be touched by several hands. This creates an opportunity for contamination, particularly when it is handled by nonprofessional personnel. The cold moisture will preserve the microorganisms. Thus, many food and drink products may become contaminated. Furthermore, ice chests may be employed as a temporary storage for specimens. Thus, they are ample sources for cross contamination. Koren reports a study in which 88% of all the commercial ice used in an institution was contaminated with Escherichia coli.[34]

The cleanliness of the ice makers, flakers, and shavers can be maintained only by a careful inspection and cleaning routine. Twice weekly, complete emptying and draining has been recommended along with the discard of all contained ice.[34] The exposed surfaces should be cleaned inside and out with a disinfectant-detergent and then sanitized with a second sponge. Once each month, the machine should be defrosted and then similarly cleaned. If a scoop is used, it should be kept in a cool clorox solution and not in the ice chest. This solution should be changed daily.

LAUNDRY HYGIENE

Laundry Collection

In the patient-resident quarters of the hospital, bedmaking can be a significant source of air contamination.[35] This is also true for the filling of laundry bags and the transport of dirty laundry in halls and chutes. However, it is almost impossible to avoid some of this except by the exercise of care, and the limiting of the shaking, pounding, and stuffing of soiled linen. Clouds of contaminated lint pass through rooms, halls, and stairwells.

The use of lint-free single-use sheets and linens are prohibitively costly. They also pose a problem in disposal. Gravity chutes for vertical transport can be a chimney for dispersion of contaminants in multistoried buildings. The use of plastic bags may help but these can break in the chutes. Water-soluble bags may be useful in the transport of linens from contamination and isolation quarters, but wet linens should never be placed in them.

Exhaust fans and cleaning sprinkler heads have been suggested for laundry chutes, but they do run counter to some fire safety regulations.

Cart collection of soiled laundry (preferably in stainless steel carts) is an expensive but relatively safe method of soiled laundry collection. These carts can be steam cleaned. This system is particularly feasible when stainless steel cart facilities are used for other delivery systems of supply, and sterilizing systems are at hand for their care.

Laundry Processing

In many laundries, the linens arriving from isolation areas are handled separately. They are pretreated for decontamination before going through the regular laundry cycles.

To process soiled linens from the nonisolation areas, many laundries empty the bags and perform a presort so that like linens can be washed together, and the handling of clean linen is minimized. When this is done, it is particularly important that the air pressure within this room be less than neighboring hallways and that airflows will all be from the corridor into the room. Exhaust of air from these rooms needs to be carefully planned and the exhaust air may be rough filtered.

The laundering process is usually carried out with multiple sudsing stages at relatively high temperatures from 150° to 170°F for about 30 min. The general methods are described in U.S. Public Health Service Publication 930-D-24 on hospital laundry. Cold methods have been suggested that might be economically advantageous, but so far they have not found acceptance and there is no laboratory proof of their efficacy in decontamination.

Clean Linen

The mangle and folding machines are particularly valuable in destroying gram-negative organisms and providing relatively sterile linens. These must be sorted, and possibly packaged for distribution, in clean carts.

Personnel working in this section of the laundry should observe the same meticulous hygiene, attire, and, hair restraint as food handlers. Handwashing practices and skin care are of paramount importance.

Clean linen can be tested. Wetzler and Quan have recommended that the laundry product be free of known pathogens and be limited to $6 \times 10^3/\text{in.}^2$ of micrococcus species and bacillus spores.[36]

Table 3
ACCEPTABLE TEMPERATURES FOR MAINTAINING VARIOUS FOOD PRODUCTS

Food	Temperature
All perishable foods	45—50°
Fruits (except bananas), vegetables, and most other perishable products	34—45°
Dairy products	38—46°
Meat and fowl	33—38°
Fish and shellfish	23—30°
Frozen foods	0—minus 20°

FOOD HYGIENE

The safety problems of food are an important part of the health care safety program because the patients, particularly the very young, aged, and debilitated, are highly susceptible to gastrointestinal microbial infection. Foodborne diseases are discovered largely when they cause outbreaks of clusters of cases with symptoms referable to the gastrointestinal tract, such as vomiting, abdominal pain, and diarrhea. In the acute-care hospital, however, such symptoms may also be attributed to the primary illness for which the patient was hospitalized and thus go unrecognized, or recognized only when additional patients are affected.

Gastrointestinal infection is, moreover, the result not only of the ingestion of a certain dosage of microorganisms, but also of their virulence and their elaboration in the contaminated food. If several persons eat the same contaminated food, not all will exhibit symptoms; some may be resistant. In the hospital, only a very few patients may show symptoms. Thus, the contagion will be disguised.

For these reasons, food hygiene in the hospital must be meticulous and continuous vigilance must be observed. Food service managers bear a heavy responsibility to observe all of the prescribed measures and to continually inspect and correct deficiencies. Some guidance will be given by certain standards of the National Sanitation Foundation[37], the American Hospital Association[38], and the Public Health Service (Table 3).[39]

Personal Hygiene

All food service workers in the health care institution should be impressed with the responsibility they bear for the well being of the patients. This implies a high degree of personal cleanliness and the reporting of any skin disease (acute or chronic), and open sores or cuts promptly to supervisory persons. It also means the wearing of clean, fresh garments.

Hand Care

Handwashing facilities should be easily available to food service personnel. They should be exclusively for handwashing; the sinks should not be used for food processing. Hands should be washed whenever the food area is entered, after handling any soiled or contaminated article, after visiting the toilet, after coughing or sneezing into the hand, and after smoking. The wearing of loose-fitting plastic gloves is valuable for persons actually handling food, setting up trays, etc. Fingernails should be neatly trimmed and jewelry is best avoided.

Hair Restraint

Hair is constantly being sloughed. It is highly contaminated with microorganisms. This is true of scalp hair, facial hair, and all orifice hair that protects the eyes, ears, and nose. Scalp hair restraints such as caps or hairnets are only a partial restraint; they do apparently discourage playing with or rearranging hair while at work, so they are of value. Since most of these motions are habits and are not premeditated, the cap or net serves as a useful reminder.

Facilities

The facilities available to the food service personnel provide the milieu for good hygienic practices. Adequate toilet, washing, and lounge facilities will be of great assistance in the maintenance of good practice. It is, however, imperative that these do not degenerate into breeding places for problems, therefore, their inspection and maintenance should be a part of the service manager's or administrative's inspection and control. All reminders of responsibilities, such as the use of foot-control sinks and adequate signs, are of help.

Food Choice

Repeatedly, certain foods have been demonstrated to be potentially hazardous.[40] The hospital dieticians are aware of these and will avoid their use when making menus. However, unclean utensils, improper refrigeration and storage, and lack of maintenance of proper temperatures are probably the causes of most difficulty. The American Hospital Association's Manual (1966) provides guidances for these systems.

SOLID WASTE MANAGEMENT

As landfill areas become increasingly scarce and the disposal of waste assumes a major role in all of our lives, consideration of hospital waste disposal will become increasingly important. Hospital wastes are often attractive to scavengers. Needles and syringes may find unfortunate use and provide embarrassment to the hospital. Moreover, these wastes pose an infection hazard not easily recognized at the time of their disposal.

The collection, handling, processing, and disposal of waste are becoming of increasing importance, particularly in these days of energy conservation. A certain percentage of waste is biodegradable. Another might be valuable for recycling. A third segment might actually be employed as an energy source, while an obviously infectious fourth segment must be subjected to special decontamination and disposition. Another consideration is the injury of hospital personnel in the disposition of these wastes. Needles that are not broken and are hastily discarded into trash bags will penetrate them and injure housekeeping persons. This can become a very real problem for safety committees.

Amounts

The volume of solid waste in the hospital and other health care facilities has been growing tremendously in recent years, particularly since the widespread acceptance of single-use items. Packaging methods designed for the preservation of disposable and preprepared materials are voluminous. In the Robert Packer Hospital (340 beds), about 15 lb of solid waste is created by each patient per day. Thus, it is possible to multiply this figure (the average for each hospital) by the patient days to arrive at the figure of solid waste that must be handled. The 15 lb in our hospital consist of those materials compacted and sent to landfill. This is in addition to the amounts that are incinerated.

Sources

Every section of the institution contributes to the solid wastes. Iglar studied the sources of waste for a doctoral thesis at the University of Minnesota in 1970.[42] He found that half of the waste came from the kitchens and dietary facilities. Nursing stations contributed 20% while surgery and obstetrics contributed about 8.5%. The laboratory contributed just over 2% while X-ray, storerooms, and administrative offices contributed about 1.5% each. Small amounts came from other sources (each under 1%), while 8% was mixed or unknown in origin.

Receiving and Containing

Solid wastes are usually collected in 3-mil plastic refuse bags placed within supporting containers. Wastes should be separated so that they are ready for ultimate disposition. Those that are highly infectious, such as growth plates (Petri dishes, etc.) in microbiology should be stored in containers that can be accessible to steam in an autoclave. The use of open plastic bags for this purpose has been questioned. The Center for Disease Control (CDC) has recommended that the open loaded bag be laid on its side. Others have recommended filling the bag only half full, while others recommend tying the bag loosely. Probably the best way is to experiment using spore strips. Adding water to the content may also be done. Sterility of the spore strip is proof of the efficacy of the method.

Plastic bags containing wastes that may putrefy should be tied and transported to the incinerator in appropriate carts. The tops of the containers should be closed. Bags of 0.0015 to 0.0030 guage should be used for the average waste. Heavier bags should be used for wet and heavy wastes, while lighter bags may be used for dry light-weight materials. For dangerous materials, double bagging is recommended.

Glass and metal should be separated from other wastes. Syringes and needles pose a special problem and the latter are a major hazard to housekeeping when they pick the bag from the container. The only prevention is education of the professionals. For this purpose, whenever a needle is seen to protrude from a receptacle, it should be grasped by a hemostat, removed, and retained in a test tube. These should be presented at safety committee meetings and shown to the department head in the area of their source.

Disposables often come in special styrofoam containers. These make excellent coffins for their disposal and should be so used. Gravity chutes and pulp-waste systems are not widely employed.

Transportation

Wastes are transported to the site of their disposal in suitable carts. Two exit centers are usually present for the disposition — one for the incinerator and one for the compactor. The residues should be stored in watertight containers with firm closure, outside of the building.

Incinerators are governed by local and federal legislation that determine the permitted particulates and toxic chemicals that they may discharge.[42] As the act does not include biologic limitations, the hospital assumes liability. Incinerators should be particularly adapted for hospital use because pathology wastes have a high moisture content and will probably require one or several auxiliary burners. The design and function of the hospital incinerator is complex, and its management is usually assigned to a single person who is knowledgeable on this subject. This person needs to be familiar with the function and operation of the incinerator as well as its hazards. Fire protection is described in a special NFPA publication.[43]

Hospital wastes have been studied as possible sources of energy production. Falick found that the heat value of hospital wastes had risen from 2500 to 6500 Btu/lb from 1955 to 1965.[40] He estimated that they would rise to 14,000 by 1975. Thus, our 340 bed hospital's waste might produce 158.2 million Btu/month. Actually, however, oil will produce 140,000 Btu/gal so that the energy potentials from the hospital's solid waste are not great.

Incineration, while probably the biologically safest disposal method for hospital waste, is not infallible. Viable microorganisms have been recovered from stack emissions. Barbeito and Gremillion have shown that firebrick temperatures of 385° for a 26.5-sec retention of the content was necessary to sterilize stack gases.[45]

ASEPSIS

The techniques of asepsis become a ritual to those concerned professionals who carry out sterile procedures. It is, as Walter states, "rooted in a philosophy of total patient care".[46] It is basically taught to the physician, the surgeon, and the nurse who are charged with not only setting an example, but also guiding the nonprofessionals to avoid their being inept and thoughtless, thus breaching the technique.

Asepsis is a plan to keep a sterile area sterile. This is, of course, of primary concern in a surgical operating room. But the techniques hold true throughout the hospital, even for the introduction of a hypodermic needle.

Asepsis for Nonmedical Personnel

A sterile area is defined for every procedure. All items used within this area must be sterile. Sterile items to be used in this sterile field must be maintained in a sterile fashion. When a package that contains sterile material is opened, the entire inside cover is considered sterile. Special opening techniques are used to assure this.

The pattern of movement of nonsterile personnel in the area is controlled so that there is no opportunity to touch and contaminate. All persons in the room where a sterile field exists should be attired in the manner prescribed for it. It may be a special scrub suit in an operating suite or street clothes in a patient room. Caps or masks may be required in certain zones. A nonsterile person should never touch or reach over sterile equipment. A nonsterile person should always approach a sterile area facing it and never pass between two sterile areas. Nonsterile liquid should never be poured in a room containing a sterile unprotected zone.[47]

The application of the principles of asepsis depends entirely upon individuals and their conscience. Integrity and honesty concerning possible breaches of asepsis should be immediately reported. Embarrassment is of no importance when so much is at stake.

Asepsis in the General Hospital

In the patient quarters of the hospital, it is anticipated that all of the patient's aseptic skin sites will be sealed by dressings or other similar barriers. Therefore, with the exception of personal cleanliness and hygiene, visitors or other persons need have relatively little concern. There are so many potential sources of contaminants in the hospital that care must be exercised in going from one patient to another. Between visits to each patient, handwashing or its acceptable substitute (an alcohol foam) is a rule.[48]

Asepsis in Critical Care

These sections of the hospital usually house patients who have a special sensitivity to infection. Hands should be carefully washed and thoroughly dried on entering each unit and again on leaving it. Nothing should be touched except those elements that are necessary to accomplish the mission. If at all possible, the patient, his bed, and bedding should not be touched. Handwashing facilities (or their substitute) between patients is required.[48] Special housekeeping plans are written and known by assigned housekeeping personnel.

Asepsis in Surgical and Obstetric Suites

Usually these suites are zoned, and special clothing or overclothing must be worn in certain areas. Jumpsuits, bootcovers, caps, and face masks are supplied. The supervisory personnel will usually be very cooperative in explaining the rules in the particular suite and how the accouterments are to be worn.[49]

STERILIZATION, DISINFECTION, AND DECONTAMINATION

Sterility is classically defined as the complete absence of all living matter, including all microbial life. This state is attained by the process of sterilization. The process of killing microorganisms follows a law that states that the filling of living cells proceeds at a uniform rate and that the death rate is a straight line when plotted on a lagarithmic scale. Thus, the same percentage of living bacteria die in each given unit of time. If 10% of a population of bacteria die each minute, at the end of 10 min almost all — but not all — will be killed.

Theoretically, there will always be a residue of living bacteria; an absolutely sterile state is never quite reached. The rate of killing is determined by the power of the killing agent or mechanism and the resistance of the microorganism. Instead of referring to a death-rate constant, it is more common to refer to a D-value. This is defined as the time value for a one-log (90%) reduction in living cells at any given temperature for a given species of microorganism. Knowing this value and the number of microorganisms in the sample to be sterilized, one can calculate the time and temperature required to be assured of there being only a remote chance (e.g., one in ten) of the survival of a single living organism. See Table 4 and Figure 8.

It should be mentioned that an alternative method, the Z-value, has also been devised. This is the increase in degrees Centigrade that is required to bring about a one-log (90%) change in the D-value.

While sterilization represents the concept of the killing of all microorganisms, lesser states are also recognized. It has already been mentioned that there is a specie differentiation in the ability to resist sterilization methods. Certain microorganisms have the capability of acquiring a mantle or capsule by which they protect themselves from lethal situations. This formation is called a spore form, and is particularly resistant. However, this capability is present only in microorganisms called spore-formers.

In general, microorganisms fall into three definable classes from the standpoint of the sterilization process. The most difficult to destroy are the spores. An intermediate group is typified by the tubercle bacillus, which is not quite as resistant as the spore, yet defies some chemicals. The least resistant are the so-called vegetative organisms. This last group contains most of those that are an infectious threat once they by-pass the body's normal defenses such as the skin or mucous membranes that line the internal body surfaces. See Figure 9.

Unfortunately, this simple classification is no longer applicable to our infection potentials. Medical progress now employs modalities (such as immunosuppression) created by drugs, ionizing radiation, or the implantation of large foreign bodies (e.g., artificial joints, heart valves, pacemakers, eye lenses, etc.) in which microrganisms never before known to cause infection, may now be causative of severe or fatal disease.

At one time, we were able to speak of disinfection as the killing of microbial forms potentially pathogenic to humans. This term will have to be redefined because there are *probably* no microbial forms entirely without such a potential.

Table 4
THE TYPE OF DISINFECTION OR STERILIZATION FOR HEAT SENSITIVE OBJECTS

	Disinfection				Sterilization	
	Will not come in contact with skin or tissue		Will come in contact with skin or mucous membrane		Will enter tissue or vascular system	
Object	Procedure	Min	Procedure	Min	Procedure	Hr
Smooth, hard-surfaced objects	A	≥10	A	≥30	C	18
	D	≥10	C	≥30	K	mfr rec
	E	≥10	F	≥30	L	12
	G	≥10	H	≥30	M	10
	I	≥10	J[a]	≥30	P	mfr rec
			L	≥30		
			M	≥30		
			N	≥30		
Rubber tubing and catheters			F	≥30	K	mfr rec
			H	≥30	P	mfr rec
			M	≥30		
			N	≥30		
Polyethylene tubing and catheters[b,c,d]			A	≥30	C	18
			F	≥30	K	mfr rec
			H	≥30	L	12
			M	≥30	M	10
			N	≥30	P	mfr rec
Lensed instruments			L	≥30	K	mfr rec
			M	≥30	L	12
					M	12
Thermometers (oral and rectal)[c]			B	≥30	C	18
			M	≥30	K	mfr rec
					L	12
					M	10
Hinged instruments					K	mfr rec
					L	12
					M	10
					P	mfr rec

Note: A = ethyl or isopropyl alcohol (70—90%); B = ethyl alcohol (70—90%); C = formaldehyde — (8%) alcohol (70%) solution; D = quaternary ammonium germicidal detergent solution (2% aq. solution of concentrate); E = iodophor germicidal detergent (100 ppm available iodine); F = iodophor (500 ppm available iodine); G = phenolic germicidal detergent solution (1% aq. solution of concentrate); H = phenolic solutions (3% aq. solution of concentrate); I = sodium hypochlorite (100 ppm available chlorine); J = sodium hypochlorite (1000 ppm available chlorine); K = ethylene oxide gas (for time, see manufacturer's recommendations); L = aqueous formalin (40% formaldehyde); M = alkalinized glutaraldehyde (2% aq.); N = wet pasteurization at 75°C after detergent cleaning; and P = heat sterilization (see manufacturer's recommendations).

[a] Not recommended for metal instruments.
[b] Be certain tubing is completely filled for disinfection.
[c] Instruments or catheters that enter tissue or the vascular system should be sterilized.
[d] Investigate thermostability when indicated.
[e] Thermometers must be thoroughly wiped (preferably with soap and water) before disinfection or sterilization. Alcohol-iodine solutions will remove markings on poor-grade thermometers. Do not mix rectal and oral thermometers at any stage of handling or processing.

From U.S. Department of Health, Education and Welfare, Isolation Techniques for Use in Hospitals, Publ. No. (CDC) 76-8314, U.S. Department of Health, Education and Welfare, Washington, D.C., 1975.

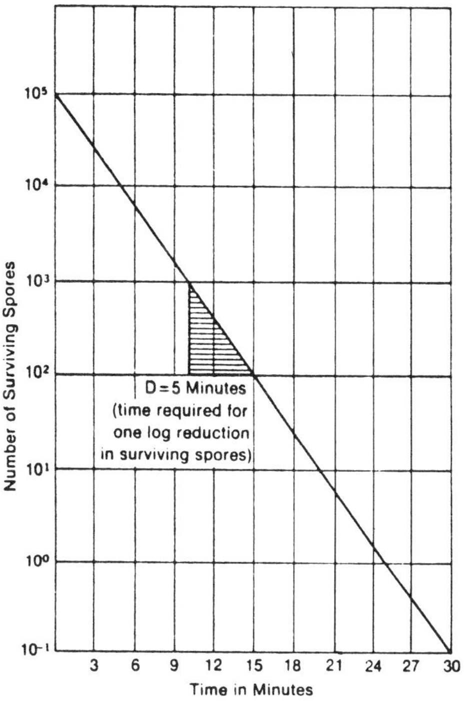

FIGURE 8. The D-time is the time in minutes required to achieve a 1-log reduction in spores. This means that in the D-minutes, 90% of the organisms in the sample will have been destroyed.

The word antiseptic is employed to describe the reduction of microorganisms on surfaces such as the skin of the surgeon's hand or the patient's surgical field, by the application of antiseptic drugs (e.g., alcohols or iodine or chlorine compounds).

Disinfectants are chemicals that will destroy vegetative organisms and possibly the tubercle bacillus, but will not kill spores. These will be discussed in some detail.

Sterilization Methods

Sterilization can be achieved by either physical or chemical means, or by combinations of these. The physical methods include (1) flame, (2) dry heat, (3) wet heat interpreted as saturated steam under pressure, and (4) ionizing radiation. Chemical sterilants include gaseous agents such as ethylene oxide, and the lesser used formaldehyde and beta-propalactone. Some liquids can also produce sterility in proper concentration and in sufficient time. We have recently worked with a combination physical and chemical method that seems promising, but is yet experimental. This is the combination of ultrasonics and chemicals using chlorine compounds.[50] (see Table 4).

Other methods have been suggested for special purposes, e.g., ultraviolet light for air sterilization and boiling water or oil. These will be discussed later, but actually should not be considered as sterilizers.

Basic to all sterilization methods are the following concepts that must be carefully observed.

1. Objects to be sterilized must be bare of any soil. Soil is an effective insulator and will defy penetration by heat, steam, or liquid. Thus, objects for sterilization must be meticulously clean.

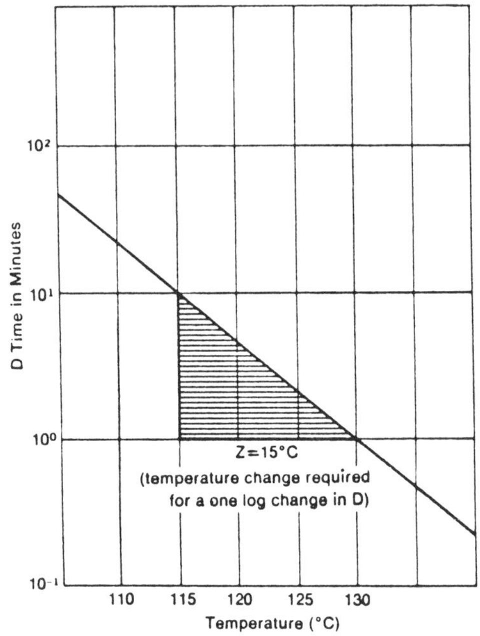

FIGURE 9. The Z-time is the number of degrees centigrade required for a one log reduction in minutes for any specific bacterium.

2. The steam, if this is used, must be saturated and pure. Saturation means that it will be at the density and pressure necessary to release heat. Purity means that there will be no air pockets to prevent contact. For ethylene oxide, the temperature and relative humidity are important.
3. The sterilant must be able to come into contact with all surfaces to be rendered sterile. This means that all instruments (particularly if they have box lockjoints) must be open. Whatever wrappings are used must be penetratable by the sterilant. Oils, greases, and powders may vitiate the sterilizing process.
4. Monitoring capabilities for both the physical and chemical process must be used in accordance with the plan required by the Joint Commission on Hospital accreditation.[51]
5. A cycle for drying and/or aeration must be a part of the sterilizing process.
6. Accurate records of each sterilizing cycle must be maintained to permit backchecking for the assurance of sterility. This includes the marking of each lot. These records must be on file for a time required by state regulations.
7. All sterilized items in the hospital must be dated for the time when they are no longer considered sterile.[52]

Steam Sterilization

The steam sterilizer (autoclave) is the instrument of choice for all hospital sterilization whenever the object to be sterilized can withstand the heat of the process. Some cannot, however, such as lensed instruments, certain catheters, and some rubber and plastic materials. Procedures for steam sterilization follow.

Wrapping materials for steam sterilization should be based upon a standard of double (2 layers each) 140-thread-count muslin (4 layers). If other materials such as two-way crepe paper, nonwoven fabric, or paper-plastic combinations are used, their relative penetratability in comparison to this muslin must be ascertained. Plastic dust covers are recommended if shelf storage exceeds 3 days.

Steam for the sterilizers is usually centrally generated and piped to the point of use at high pressure (60 to 80 lb/in.^{2}). This must be reduced to the pressure required by the sterilization temperature of the particular unit. For the high-temperature 270°F (132°C) rapid sterilization cycle, the pressure requirement will be 27 to 28 lb/in.^{2} For the lower temperature 250°F (121°C), the pressure requirement will be 16 to 18 lb/in.^{2} A trap is usually inserted close to the sterilizer to avoid excessively wet steam.

Steam sterilizers are generally of two types, a gravity downward displacement type or a high-temperature prevacuum type. In both, the aim is to secure a complete contact of all surfaces with the temperature for sterilization. The greatest enemy to overcome is the entrapment of air so that the steam is withheld from contact. In the gravity displacement autoclave, the steam is forced under pressure into the rear of the chamber and the air is forced out through a port at the lower front. The steam, being lighter, rises to the top and displaces the air past a thermostatically controlled check valve into the air discharge line. At this point, which is the coolest part of the system, the temperature is taken and recorded onto a calibrated time chart. Obviously, the loading geometry of the chamber is important, and all air must have an unimpeded opportunity to flow out and down, just as water would flow following a gravity course. The timing of sterilization is begun when the discharge temperature has reached the appropriate level.

In a prevacuum autoclave, the evacuation of air by a vacuum pump can be achieved by drawing a vacuum to an absolute pressure of 25 mm of mercury. This will secure a much more rapid removal of air, which is followed by the introduction of the steam. Dangers in this system are caused by compaction of air within a load (small load effect) or by air leaks. A malfunctioning of the vacuum pump is also possible, as is the malfunction of the control switch that may cut off evacuation too soon. These faults are simple to recognize by the Bowie-Dick test that will be described later under test procedures.

Failure of sterilization can take place because of equipment malfunction or improper loading into the equipment. This is discovered by observation of the sterility tests that are applied to the equipment. The multiplicity of the testing methods affirms not only the importance in which the sterilization process is held, but also the shortcomings of the test methods. Without exception, all concerned insist upon precision of the sterile quality of the product from the sterilizer. The user, however, is prone to blame the malfunction of the equipment while the maintenance personnel lean towards a suspicion that the test is inaccurate. Since both need to be satisfied, suspect loads must be withheld from use by recall or nonissuance until all are satisfied that they are safe to use. This requires a somewhat complicated system of records mandated by Joint Commission on the Accreditation of Hospitals.[47]

Unloading of the sterilizer is also very important, as contents must be thoroughly cooled. If the load is still warm and is placed upon a cool surface, condensation will take place and the wrapper will become wet. Probst has demonstrated that a wet wrapper permits bacterial transfer and must be considered contaminated and reprocessed.[53] Dust covers should only be applied to cool packages.

The distribution of sterile supplies is frequently done in covered, enclosed stainless steel carts. More and more, they are used as individual case carts for surgical procedures. Prior to reuse, carts must be decontaminated and dried. Packages contained in them should be inspected for integrity and labeling before issuance.

Care and preventive maintenance should be written and carried out by the sterilizing personnel with the cooperation of the engineering and maintenance department. The manufacturers offer service contracts that are useful. The manufacturers also supply instructions for daily inspection and cleaning. A weekly inspection and cleaning, including all of the accessories, is usually also prescribed.

It is recommended that the time/temperature recorders and the pressure guages be recalibrated at least semi-annually, recording the dates of this service. The steam traps should be checked and replaced as needed. For maintenance records of each sterilizer, a log should be kept giving the sterilizer serial number, the date of service, character of the service, and list of parts replaced, as well as the signatures of the person carrying out the work. The log should also include any notations on malfunction or failures of sterility tests.

Dry Heat Sterilization

This method has very limited application, usually to laboratory equipment. It does not erode ground-glass surfaces as steam does. It is also used for anhydrous powders and greases. Ovens with circulating hot air are the most frequently used, and temperatures of 160°C (320°F) for 2 hr is the most frequently used cycle. However, 170°C (340°F) for 1 hr or 121°C (250°F) for 6 hr in a forced air circulating-type oven has also been used.

The moisture contained in spore cultures and dryness of the air (relative humidity) have also been shown to be factors in dry heat sterilization. The circulation of the air in the chamber must not be impeded by improper loading.

Mixed Physical and Chemical Sterilization

With the concern expressed over gaseous chemical sterilization methods by government, there is an active search in progress for other monitorable sterilization techniques. One such technique that appears to offer some promise is the combination of ultrasound cleaning with liquid chemical sterilization.[50] In the future, this may be particularly useful for decontamination.

Gas Chemical Sterilization — Ethylene Oxide

Originally used as a fumigant for spices, ethylene oxide is now widely used in hospitals and industry. In hospitals, it is found to be particularly valuable for the sterilization of items that cannot withstand the high temperatures of steam sterilization, and its use should be limited to this function.

Ethylene oxide is a colorless, pleasant-smelling, highly penetrating gas. It is also highly toxic, mutagenic, possibly carcinogenic, flammable, and, in its pure state, explosive. Thus, it can be dangerous unless properly controlled, used, and disposed of. This has concerned the environmental protection agencies who have made efforts to control its use, and impose stringent safety measures.[54] Because of its unique properties and its unquestioned value, the substance is not banned, but is strictly controlled.

Ethylene oxide is now being used almost exclusively in gasclaves, and mixtures with freon or carbon dioxide. Usually, 450 mg/ℓ of ethylene oxide is used in a 5- or 6-hr cycle.

The temperature of the gas is important and optimum at 66°C (130°F). Higher temperatures do not help much and may damage the materials to be sterilized. The effectivensss of the gas is greatest with a relative humidity at 30 to 40%. The available water before treatment may be as important as the humidity.

Ethylene oxide exerts its lethal effect upon microorganisms very slowly. The gas must be in solution at the cell membrane. Spores are more resistant than vegetative organisms, and the tubercle bacillus and some viruses are particularly resistant. The gas is highly soluble in water and penetrates many substances with ease. Desicated materials are relatively impenetrable, as are certain plastics. The latter includes laminate polyethylene films, linear-type nylon, mylar, aluminum laminates, etc. Some wrapping materials are lightly penetrable such as paper, cloth, nonlaminated polyethylene film, etc.

Materials once sterilized by radiation must not, as a general rule, be subsequently sterilized by ethylene oxide. Apparently, the radiation weakens the bond with chlorine ions. Then, when they are exposed to ethylene oxide, they form the toxic compound ethylene chlorhydrin.

Ethylene oxide is a toxic material. After all, it is being used as a lethal agent. Toxicity occurs both in its liquid gaseous state, as well as when it is a residue within certain materials. It may produce burns and eye irritation and can be toxic if inhaled. The number of parts per million are determinable concentrations and are limited by regulation.

At the end of the sterilizing cycle, the gas is usually removed from the chamber by evacuation at a negative pressure of approximately 25 in. of mercury. To return to atmospheric pressure, filtered air is then introduced. A second cycle is used for further evacuation of gas. At the end of the cycle, a waterwash may be used to clear the equipment of any residual gas because ethylene oxide is soluble in water. Drain pipes to remove this water, by code, usually cannot be connected to floor drains. For this reason, a gap is left between the sterilizer and floor drains. This has been reported to be a source of release of the ethylene oxide into the ambience where it can exert toxic effects.

Ethylene oxide reacts with many chemical groups. Residual ethylene glycols and chlorohydorines can pose problems, and their permissible quantities are being determined by a proposed Association for the Advancement of Medical Instrumentation (AAMI) standard.[55] There is much conflict on this subject at the present time. The toxicity of residual ethylene oxide on human tissues is of great importance. The rate of dissipation of the ethylene oxide from exposed material is dependent upon the nature of the material and the condition of the surroundings of the materials after removal from the unit. Solid surface items of glass, and metal of simple construction will discharge the gas rapidly. On the other hand, tubing may have to be stored in open, well-ventilated storage for 7 days. Aerators may speed up the process and if functioning properly, heat and circulate HEPA filtered air (114 to 130°F) or 40 to 54°C) in 24 hr, removing all of the ethylene oxide. Usually, the manufacturers will disclaim responsibility, however, so that many users employ both aerator exposure and shelf life for implanted prosthetic materials.

Testing for Sterilization

Obviously, it is not possible to check each item in each sterilized load for satisfactory technique. Therefore, reliance is upon mechanical, chemical, and biological monitors. The mechanical ones are installed as a part of the sterilizer and provide a graphic display of the warm-up time, sterilization time, temperature, and cooling time. Added pressure guages show that the conditions of sterility have been achieved. Far better would be thermistors placed within the packs such as have been used by Litsky in test equipment.[56] Some day, these may be added to all equipment.

An indicating type of autoclave label, printed legend, or tape should be put on all packages wrapped in muslin, nonwoven material, two-way crepe paper, or paper subjected to hospital sterilization. It will indicate only that the package has been subjected to sterilization.

Internal indicators may reveal that a minimum temperature has been held for a specific time, that steam or gas contact and penetration has taken place, and that air elimination was complete. Such integrators exist and are preferably used in each package.[57] Some even show elimination of the toxic gas. Other devices only give a part of this information. All should be placed in the center of the package or that part most difficult for the sterilant to reach.

Internal biological monitors reveal that a heavy bioburden has been killed by the sterilizing method in that portion of the load most difficult to reach. Test packs of specific content, size, and location are used for this challenge to the system. They differ in placement in packing for gravity of the bundle and prevacuum steam autoclave, as well as for ethylene oxide sterilizers.

The biologic tests should be run at least weekly for steam sterilizers, and with each load for ethylene oxide.[58]

For prevacuum steam sterilizers, a Bowie-Dick test should be run daily with the first run of the day. For this, a special pack is prepared and a special test sheet or crossed tape is placed in the center of the pack. This is not a sterilization test, but will show that air has been entrapped in the vacuum sterilizer.[58]

Culture of the spore test strips must be meticulous, and presumptive identification of the spores should rule out accidental laboratory contamination. Cultures must be carried out at prescribed temperatures.[58]

Each hospital should have a recall plan that identifies the measures to be taken if any of the test procedures suggest the possibility of sterilization failure.

Standards for all of the sterilization methods and test methods are in preparation by the AAMI.[58]

Disinfection or Abridged Sterility

Sterility is a concept that may not be absolute and precise, but is so nearly so that it is a universally appreciated standard. Disinfection is as imprecise as sterility is precise. For this reason, this author prefers the term "abridged sterility."[59] This means the destruction of vegetative organisms, and includes the tubercle bacillus and *Pseudomanas aeruginosa* on surfaces. For similar destruction upon animate surfaces such as the skin and mucous membranes, the term "antisepsis" is applicable.

Abridged sterility, therefore, has certain major deficiencies. Spores are not destroyed. In most situations, spores are not pathogenic to humans, and are so only under special situations. Anthrax is not a common infection, and in our immunized world, neither is tetanus. However, our relationship with the disease-causing microbes is changing so that what appears harmless today may become a scourge tomorrow.

Of greater importance to this author, however, is the fact that we have at hand a variety of means of monitoring sterility. While the tests are not infallible, they are of sufficient reliability that they give us warning (with a considerable margin for safety) of nonsterility. At present, no such methods are available for any state less than complete sterility. Until we have a monitor that will denote the demise of all vegetative organisms, reliance on the techniques of disinfection must be empiric. This is not adequate when the risk is infection.

The following are some methods of disinfection.

Pasteurization is the application of heat for a specified period of time to accomplish a disinfection process. Its application to milk and dairy products is generally accepted. Originally, it was used only for food products. In recent years, with a need to disinfect inanimate objects with less heat than steam and more quickly than ethylene oxide would permit, it has been recommended by some for disinfection of a variety of objects, particularly in respiratory therapy.

The old boiling water tanks have just been discarded from hospital use and now the pasteurizing boiling water tank is being reintroduced. The principle differences probably lie in the improved control of temperature, more accurate timing, and the very important factor of drying. Still, the lack of any test method renders it suspect. However, with the cost-containment drives limiting the use of disposables, it seems possible that this may become a "growth" concept.

Chemical disinfectants, in general, act by the coagulation of microbial protein. They depend on the concentration of the germicide and microbial elements (bioburden) and the cleanliness of the surfaces being treated, including the physical and chemical factors surrounding the surface.

For most chemicals, the higher the concentration, the greater the lethal effect. This is not universally true, however, as 70% isopropyl or ethyl alcohol is more potent than 95%. The importance of cleanliness and disinfection has been repeatedly stressed. Clean surfaces usually have a lower concentration of microorganisms. The type of organism is also of major importance. The capsule of the tubercle bacillus protects it against many chemicals. The hepatitis virus is particularly resistant to many disinfectants.

The rate of kill is quite variable, and none kill on contact. The time factor is very important. Therefore, drying should often be somewhat delayed after soaking, in, e.g., floor disinfection.

The alcohols isopropyl and ethyl are both splendid disinfectants and antiseptics in the 70 to 95% concentrations. They kill and evaporate rapidly and leave no residue. They also combine well with many other antiseptics.

Chlorines are good disinfectants and antiseptics and are active even against viri and spores in proper concentrations and in sufficient time. They can be corrosive.

Iodine is an excellent disinfectant and is probably the strongest antiseptic that is available. New combinations have enhanced stability.

Phenolics are proven disinfectants. Recent combinations have improved stability and provided widespread acceptance in housekeeping.

Quatenary ammonium compounds have enjoyed great popularity as disinfectants and antiseptics. As they do not destroy the tubercle bacillus, they have been ascribed limitations in use.

Activated gluteraldehyde is a newer antiseptic. It is said to be sporicidal in 3 to 10 hr. It destroys vegetative organisms at a 2% aqueous solution in 20 min. It is somewhat unstable and must be relatively fresh. It must be used in a narrow range of pH (7.5 to 8.5).

Chlorhexidrine has just received Food and Drug Administration approval as an antiseptic on human skin. It is the only substance presently (1978) approved with a tincture of iodine for surgical skin preparation.

CONCLUSIONS

Sterilization with appropriate testing should be employed whenever possible. If disinfectants are to be used, they should probably be rated against alcohol because this is the cheapest and most efficient of the chemical bactericides. However, it is not actively sold, while all of the rest are touted with advertising and salesmanship.

Product efficiency is very hard to evaluate as is cost effectiveness. Someday, we may have a valid scale as simple as the phenol coefficient that will be relevant in the hospital setting. The Association of Official Agricultural Chemists (AOAC) dilution confirmation test is required by the U.S. Department of Agriculture for specific claims of germicidal effectiveness against specific vegetative organisms. For hospital use, it is carried out against three organisms, the *Staphylococcus amoeus, Salmonella choleraesuis,* and *Pseudomonas aeruginosa.* A similar test is the A.O.A.C. tuberculocidal test.

Those who are responsible for choosing hospital disinfectants would be well advised to review some of the methods that have been recommended by Pryor,[60] the laboratory section of the American Public Health Association, Spaulding,[62] Litsky,[63] etc.

REFERENCES

1. Accreditation Manual for Hospitals, Joint Commission on Accreditation of Hospitals, Chicago, 1978, 21.
2. National Nosocomial Infections Study: Quarterly Report, Center for Disease Control, Atlanta, March 1975.
3. **Altemeier, W. A., Sandusky, W. R., and Pruitt, B. A., Jr.**, Manual on Control of Infections in Surgical Patients, J. B. Lippincott Co. Philadelphia, 14.
4. **Dixon, R. E.**, Nosocomial infection: a continuing problem, *Postgrad. Med.*, 62, 95, 1977.
5. **Litsky, B. Y.**, *Hospital Sanitation*, Modern Hospital Press, Chicago, 1973, 64.
6. **Elek, S. D. and Conen, D. E.**, Experimental production of infection in man, *Br. J. Exp. Pathol.*, 38, 573, 1957.

7a. **American Hospital Association**, Housekeeping Manual for Health Care Facilities, American Hospital Association, Chicago, 1966.

7b. **Blount, R. N.**, *Housekeeping Procedures for the Small Hospital*, Charles C Thomas, Springfield, Ill., 1977.

7c. **Chase, M. L.**, *Housekeeping Management for Health Care Facilities*, Catholic Hospital Association, St. Louis, 1976.

7d. **Koren, H.**, *Environmental Health and Safety*, Pergamon Press, Elmsford, New York, 1974, 229.

8. **Pryor, A. K. and Wold, C. D.**, Follow these suggestions to make a hospital cleanable, *Mod. Hosp.*, 112, 134, 1969.
9. Official and Tentative Methods of Analysis, Association of Official Agricultural Chemists, 1960, Washington, D. C., 1960, 67.
10. **Mallison, G. F.**, Environmental Control in Hospitals: Methods of Microbiology, American Society for Microbiology, Washington, D. C., 1970, 618.
11. **Litsky, B. Y. and Litsky, W.**, Investigation on contamination of surfaces, *Am. J. Public Health*, 58, 534, 1968.
12. **Litsky, B. Y.**, *Hospital Sanitation*, Modern Hospital Press, Chicago, 1973, 75.
13. **Litsky, B. Y.**, *Food Service Sanitation*, Modern Hospital Press, Chicago, 1973, 75.
14. **Austin, P. R. and Timmerman, S. W.**, *Design and Operation of Clean Rooms*, Business News Co., Detroit, 1965, 77.
15. **Nelson, J. P.**, O.R. clean rooms, *J. Assoc. Oper. Room Nurs.*, 15, 71, 1972.
16. **Wells, W. F.**, Airborn infection, *JAMA*, 104, 1698, 1936.
17. **Beck, W. C.**, The open door in the operating room, *Am. J. Surg.*, 125, 592, 1973.
18. **Kethley, T. W. and Cown, W. B.**, What is quality of air in your operating rooms, *Guthrie Clin. Bull.*, 46, 25, 1976.
19. American College of Surgeons, Committee on the operating room environment: special air systems, *Bull. Am. Coll. Surg.*, 57, 18, 1972.

20a. **Runkle, R. S. and Phillips, G. B.**, *Biomedical Applications of Laminar Airflow*, Chemical Rubber Co., Cleveland, 1973.

20b. **Luciano, J. R.**, *Air Contamination Control in Hospitals*, Plenum Press, New York, 1977, 215.

21. **Lidwell, O. M.**, Evaluation of methods for the control of surgical sepsis, Workshop on Control of Operating Room Airborne Bacteria, National Research Council, Washington, D. C., 1975.
22. NASA, Contamination Control Handbook, NASA SP5076, Office of Technology Utilization, NASA, Washington, D. C., 1969.
23. Minimum Requirements of Construction and Equipment for Hospital and Medical Facilities, U. S. Department of Health, Education and Welfare (Health Resources Administration) 74-4000, Washington, D.C., 1977.
24. **Beck, W. C.**, Definition of microbiologic clean air, *Bull. Am. Coll. Surg.*, 61, 18, 1976.
25. **Fahlberg, W.**, Wound isolation technique, *Proc. Assoc. Adv. Med. Instrum.*, 1975.
26. **Burke, J. F.**, A new approach to isolation, *Hosp. Pract.*, February 1967.
27. **Michaelson, G. S., et al.**, Development of an Open Isolation System for the Care of Low Resistance Hospital Patients, U. S. Public Health Service, No. 43-65-999, National Cancer Institute, Washington, D.C., 1968.
28. U.S. Public Health Service, Isolation Techniques for Use in Hospitals, PHS Publ. No. 2054, Public Health Service, Washington, D.C., 1970.
29. Manual for Evaluating Drinking Water Supplies, Bureau of Water Hygiene, U.S. Public Health Service, Cincinnati, 1969.
30. General Standards for Construction for Hospital and Medical Facilities, Public Health Service Publ. No. 930-A-7, U.S. Department of Health, Education and Welfare, Washington, D.C., 1969.
31. **Beam, E. L.**, Progress report on water quality criteria, *J. Am. Waterworks Assoc.*, 54, 1313, 1962.

32. **Searcy, P. E. and Furman, T. deS.**, Water consumption by institutions, *J. Am. Waterworks Assoc.*, 53, 1111, 1969.
33. **Michaelson, G. J. and DeRoos, R. L.**, Use of the barometric loop for protection of portable water systems, *Am. Plumb. Eng.*, 3, 99, 1969.
34. **Koren, H.**, *Environmental Health and Safety*, Pergamon Press, New York, 1974, 59.
35. **Bourdillon, R. B.**, Studies in Air Hygiene, Medical Research Council Special Rep. Ser. No. 262.
36. **Wetzler, T. F. and Quan, T. J.**, Critical analysis of the microflora on toweling, *Am. J. Public Health*, 61, 377, 1971.
37. **Lancaster, D. L.**, A Reference Manual of Food Sanitation Service, Publ. No. 48105, National Sanitation Foundation, Ann Arbor, Mich., 1973.
38. American Hospital Association, Food Service Manual for Health Care Institutions, American Hospital Association, Chicago, 1972.
39. Food Service Sanitation Manual, Public Health Service Publ. No. (FDA) 78-2081, U.S. Government Printing Office, Washington, D.C., 1976.
40. **Falick, J.**, Waste handling in hospitals, *Archit. Eng. News*, 7, 46, 1965.
41. **Iglar, A. F.**, Hospital solid waste management, in *Environmental Health and Safety in Health Care Facilities*, Macmillan New York, 1973, 267.
42. Encyclopedia Americana, Clean air amendment of 1970, in The Americana Annual, Americana Corp., New York, 1971, 714.
43. Rubbish Incinerators, NFPA Bull. National Fire Protection Association, Boston, 1972.
44. **Falick, J.**, Waste handling in hospitals, *Archit. Eng. News*, 7, 46, 1965.
45. **Barbeito, M. S. and Gremillion, G. G.**, Microbiologic safety evaluation of an industrial refuse incinerator, *Appl. Microbiol.*, 16, 291, 1968.
46. **Walter, C. A.**, The surgeon's responsibility for asepsis, *Med. Instrum.*, 12, 149, 1978.
47. Standards for Basic Aseptic Technique: AORN Standards of Practice, Association of Operating Room Nurses, Denver, 1978, 3.
48. **Beck, W. C.**, Handwashing substitute for degerming, *Am. J. Surg.*, 135, 728, 1978.
49. Standards for O.R. Wearing Apparel: AORN Standards of Practice, Association of Operating Room Nurses, Denver, 1978, 3.
50. **Beck, W. C.**, Sterilization by a new technique Ultrasonics plus Chemicidal action, *Guthrie Clin. Bull.*, 48, 31, 1978.
51. Accreditation Manual for Hospitals, Joint Commission on Accreditation of Hospitals, 1978, 61.
52. **Standard, P. G., Mackel, D. C., and Mallison, G. F.**, Microbial penetration of muslin and paper wrapped sterile wraps stored on open shelves and closed cabinets, *Appl. Microbiol.*, 22, 432, 1971.
53. **Probst, H. D.**, The effect of bactericidal agents on the sterility of surgical linen, *Am. J. Surg.*, 86, 301, 1953.
54. Ethylene oxide, ethylene chlorhydrin, and ethylene glycol: proposed maximum residue limits and maximum levels of exposure, *Fed. Regist.*, 43, 27474, 1978.
55. Association for the Advancement of Medical Instrumentation Committee, *Fed. Regist.*, 43, 27474, 1978.
56. **Litsky, B. Y.**, Thermocouple-pyrometer data for evaluating in hospital packaging material, *J. Assoc. Oper. Room Nurs.*, 23, 1175, 1976.
57. **Beck, W. C.**, A new integrator for monitoring time and temperature of steam sterilizers, *Med. Instrum.*, 10, 293, 1976.
58. Association for the Advancement of Medical Instrumentation, Good hospital practice: steam sterilization and sterility assurance in preparation, *J. Assoc. Oper. Room Nurs.*, 26, 242, 1977.
59. **Beck, W. C.**, Abridged sterility: a level of disinfection, *J. Assoc. Oper. Room Nurs.*, 26, 242, 1977.
60. **Pryor, A. K.**, Evaluating hospital disinfectants, *J. Environ. Health*, 31, 118, 1968.
61. APHH Laboratory Section Committee on Microbial Contamination of Surfaces, A cooperative microbiological evaluation of floor cleaning procedures in hospital patient rooms, *Health Lab. Sci.*, 7, 258, 1970.
62. **Spaulding, E. H.**, Chemical disinfection and sterilization in the hospital, *J. Hosp. Res.*, 9, 5, 1972.
63. **Litsky, B. Y.**, *Hospital Sanitation*, Modern Hospital Press, Chicago, 1973, 117.

FIRE SAFETY

C. Roger Camplin

INTRODUCTION

When a fire occurs in one of our health care buildings we cannot sound the alarm and evacuate like many other occupancies. Our occupants are nonambulatory in varying degrees and some who are connected with monitoring and life safety are as immoveable as the building itself. The fire must be fought while the building is occupied. This requires fire fighters who are on continuous duty to handle rescue and initial attack while awaiting arrival of fire department personnel and equipment. The responsibility of this preliminary fire fighting falls upon the health care staff. Your actions in a fire emergency can be the difference between a minor incident and a tragic event.

PREPAREDNESS

Awareness and Committees

A health care facility is the type of occupancy that requires constant attention to fire and fire hazards. Elevating staff, patient, and visitor awareness to a level that will provide correct response to fire conditions is a challenge, but it is a required and worthy challenge. The safety committee or fire subcommittee requires a high level of fire awareness. This group, however structured, will come to grips with fire problems, programs, corrective actions, inspections, and all the associated fire activities. As with any decision-making body, a more intelligent decision can be made if the group is educated regarding the task at hand. Utilize fire inspectors, fire insurance representatives, or any other person or media to provide the committee with knowledge about fire and fire prevention. A multi-disciplinary committee as required by the Joint Commission on Accreditation of Hospitals (JCAH) will need to be informed if they are to make intelligent decisions.[1] Circulating articles and clippings regarding health care facility-related fires or activities is an excellent method to improve awareness.

Drills and Rehearsals

Drills and rehearsals can be used not only to test the fire plan, but as a form of continuing education for participants. In addition, the drill can be utilized as a positive reinforcement to not only provide additional training, but instill a cooperative attitude in participants (by letting them know that a mistake will be explained in a positive manner) so that a mistake is less likely to occur in another drill or in an actual fire situation (Table 1 and Figures 1 and 2). Drills required by authorities are actually the least requirement for compliance.[1] Some authorities will allow false or accidental alarms to be used as documentation of a drill if the fire plan has been implemented and critiqued.[2]

A drill should be realistic for the fire hazards associated with that specific area, i.e., flammable liquids or clothing fires in laboratories, soiled utility room or bed fires in patient care areas, and drills for wastecan fires in almost any area. The fire drill evaluation should cover all performance aspects included in the fire plan (Table 2).

Emergency Patient Relocation

A part of every fire plan should be a plan for emergency patient relocation. There are many adequate training aids that provide an assortment of carries for various types of patients.[3] An emergency patient relocation program needs to be custom designed

Table 1
FIRE FACTS FOR HOSPITAL FIRE SAFETY PLAN

When a fire occurs
- Rescue — save anyone threatened by the fire
- Alarm — turn in an alarm; pull the fire alarm and call emergency operator; maintain contact with the operator
- Close — close doors (fire doors, stairway doors, room doors)
- Extinguish — obtain proper fire extinguisher and use it

Classification of fire
- Class A — common combustibles (cloth, wood, paper)
- Class B — flammable liquids (grease, alcohol, gasoline)
- Class C — electrical (flowing current)

Fire codes
- Dr. Red — the code for "Fire"
- Dr. Green — the code for "All Clear"
- Dr. Blue — the code for "Fire Drill"

In a fire drill (Dr. Blue)
- Simulate saving anyone threatened by fire
- Report fire drill to emergency operator
- Shut fire doors and room doors
- Obtain proper fire extinguisher and describe how to use it

Note: Keep calm and do not panic. Do not unduly alarm patients. Follow emergency patient relocation plan. Know where the fire exits are. Do not use elevators in fire emergencies; elevators often fail during fires.

to fit the type of facility or area of service being dealt with. A few basic carries usually suffice for most situations. Keep the program as uncomplicated as possible; staffs remember three or four carries more readily than they do a dozen or more.

A more intense training will be required for emergency patient relocation and retraining, and drills may be required frequently to maintain proficiency. As important as the specific carries, is where and with what forethought patients are relocated. A thorough understanding of horizontal exits and smoke barriers will assist staff in making correct decisions. An emergency patient-relocation program can easily be extended into an evacuation plan when properly structured.

Fire Behavior and Classification

The fires in health care facilities that cause death, damage, and disruption are mostly medium to small fires that generate tremendous quantities of smoke. Smoke, or products of combustion, is what usually kills patients and requires patient relocation. Fire behavior varies according to the basic factors of heat, fuel, oxygen, and the uninhibited chain reaction of the combustion process.[4] How a fire progresses and when it is detected, contained, and suppressed will be the measure of a successful fire plan. A fire (other than an explosion) progresses through the fire progression curve, i.e., through time, fire increases in hazard as it progresses from incipient, smoldering, open flame and high heat conditions (Figure 3). The effects of fire on humans accumulate as the fire progresses. These detrimental factors begin with fire gases and proceed through smoke, heat, flame, and insufficient oxygen.[4] The components of fire gases and smoke are what health care facilities must be concerned with for life safety (Table 3).

Some of the problems associated with fire gases (products of combustion) and smoke

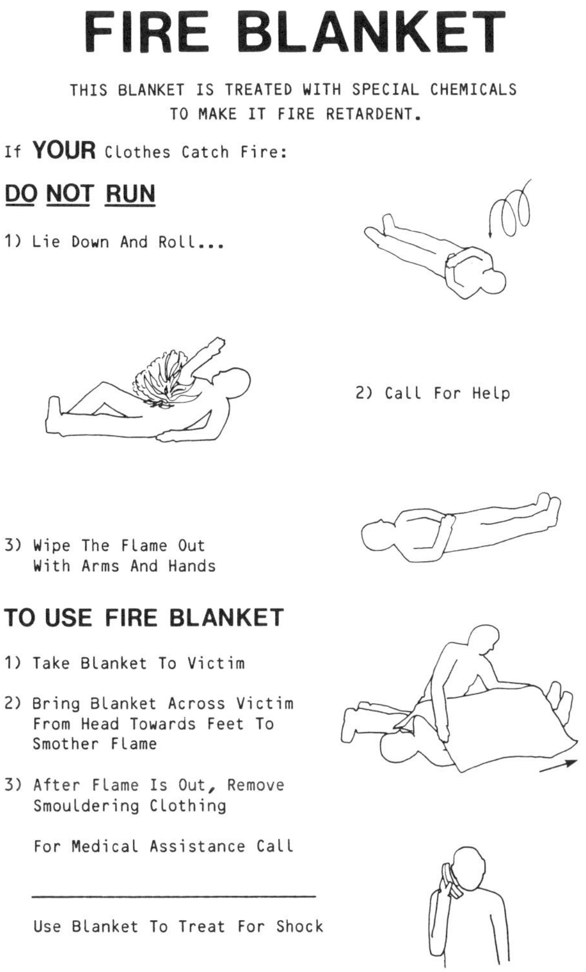

FIGURE 1. Fire blanket use poster.

are reduced visibility and the physiologically debilitating effects these products have. Materials having different properties burn with different characteristics. Basically, we are concerned with four classifications of fire: (1) Class A — ordinary combustible materials (wood, cloth, paper, plastics), (2) Class B — flammable or combustible liquids and flammable gases and greases (alcohol, ether, cooking grease, natural gas, propane), (3) Class C — fires involving energized electrical equipment, and (4) Class D — certain combustible metals (magnesium, titanium, sodium).[4] A fire may involve single or multiple classes of fires.

Fire plans must take into consideration the fire load of an area. This includes the amount of combustible contents and the classification characteristics of the possible fire. Fire detection and protection is also based upon these same fire-load factors.

Training

New Employee Orientation

The necessity and benefits of orienting a new employee, beyond those required by JCAH, should be well recognized by now.[1] The new employee is very receptive to information, is eager to learn, and will be more likely to want to do things correctly

NO SMOKING

IN CASE OF FIRE OR CHEMICAL EMERGENCY

Rescue anyone in affect area

Alarm pull fire alarm box and phone ________

Close all doors to contain smoke and fumes

Extinguish fire, if this can be done safely, if not direct fire brigade to fire

IN CASE OF FIRE OR EMERGENCY

Nearest Exit ______________________________

____

Evacuation Route, If Necessary ______________________________

____

Nearest Fire Alarm Box ______________________________

If you think you smell smoke, or need emergency assistance
Call Security at ______________

Fire Blankets may be used to smother flame, or to cover
yourself to escape through flame

Call ________ for more information, or non-emergency assistance

FIGURE 2. Chemical emergency poster

to make a good first impression in the new job than at any other time. If the correct information on fire and safety is presented in a manner that provides a creative learning environment, the new employee will be well informed and be able to respond correctly to fire violations and fire incidents by following the fire plan.

The fire plan should be described in detail with examples. Sharing with people the reasons for following requirements or plans aids in their understanding, and later in recalling the correct action. A follow-up of the fire plan that goes into the specifics of that employee's responsibilities should be conducted by the supervisor once the employee begins work.

Special Programs

The employee must be reorientated annually and continually kept informed of any changes in the fire plan due to construction alterations, building facility upgrading, or fire system changes or upgrading.[1] Again, an employee who knows that the fire doors close automatically upon activation of the fire alarm will relate to that system and be less apt to block the doors with moveable equipment, and will alert vulnerable patients to their being bumped by closing doors when the alarm is heard.

Special fire training should include a fire brigade — a select group of specially trained, knowledgeable employees that can respond to fire and safety emergencies and provide immediate assistance until the fire department arrives.[1] Also, training for employees in sensitive life safety areas (operating rooms, emergency rooms, intensive

Table 2
FIRE DRILL OBSERVER'S REPORT

DATE: TIME OF DRILL: A.M. - P.M.

OBSERVERS LOCATION:

		YES	NO
1.	DID EMPLOYEE KNOW PROCEDURES?		
2.	WAS PAGE CENTER NOTIFIED OF LOCATION?		
3.	DID FIRE BRIGADE RESPOND?		
4.	WERE ALL DOORS AND OTHER SOURCES OF DRAFTS CLOSED?		
5.	WERE ELEVATORS IN USE?		
6.	DID PAGE CENTER PAGE THE PROPER LOCATION?		
7.	WHAT WAS OVERALL RESPONSE OF PERSONNEL?		
8.	WAS THE FIRE PLAN FOLLOWED?		

COMMENTS PERTAINING TO HOW FIRE DRILLS COULD BE IMPROVED

SIGNATURE: TIME SECURED A.M.
P.M.

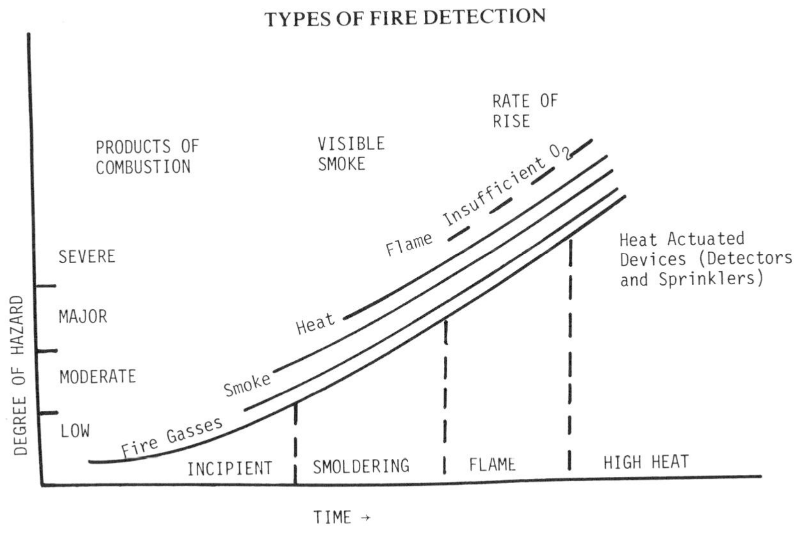

FIGURE 3. Fire progression curves.

Table 3
COMMON GASES FROM FIRES

Gases		Results
Carbon dioxide	(CO_2)	Overstimulated breathing
Carbon monoxide	(CO)	Asphyxiation
Hydrogen sulfide	(H_2S)	Respiratory and nervous system damage
Sulfur dioxide	(SO_2)	Irritation
Ammonia	(NH_3)	Irritation
Hydrogen cyanide	(HCN)	Cyanosis
Nitrogen dioxide	(NO_2)	Anesthetic
Acrolein	(CH_2CHCHO)	Irritation

care) and special hazard areas (storage, laboratories, flammable gas and liquid storage, etc.) should be conducted to provide the needed additional precautions and procedures.

The requirement for a fire blanket in a laboratory provides little protection if the fire victim attempts to run for the blanket and fans the flames into more intense burning, rather than falling to the floor, rolling, calling for help, and having someone bring the blanket to assist in smothering the flames. In the preceding example, the training is more important than the item for use.

Procedures

Several fire facts for a hospital safety plan are provided in Table 1. Each fire plan should be custom tailored for that physical facility, its occupancy, hazards, and resources. The fire plan can be general and subdivided into specific responsibilities or areas. It can also be comprehensive and specific, depending upon the above factors.

Additional procedural materials must be provided for the fire protection and detection systems that cover tests and inspections, preventive maintenance, and the taking of systems or equipment out of service. Local authorities and insurance companies frequently have requirements for fire systems that must be satisfied. As with all policy and procedures, an annual review and update, if necessary, is required.

Sources for Information and Assistance

National and regional sources for information and assistance regarding fire safety are listed in Table 4. Local and state authorities and resources cannot be listed because of space limitations, but should be sought out and utilized. In many instances, state and regional hospital associations have excellent resources that vary from libraries of books and films to seminars on fire safety. These associations are usually knowledgeable about local fire safety consultants that provide services for the health care industry.

PREVENTION

Codes and Standards

The varied codes and standards that health care facilities must comply with cause many administrators, architects, engineers, and safety persons considerable grief. In fact, there exists many "Catch 22" situations — the damned-if-you-do and damned-if-you-don't-type problem. However, there are very few problems that cannot be solved even though initially they appear unsurmountable.

Most authorities having jurisdiction (AHJ) do state that any other AHJ having a more rigid standard or code will be recognized and supported.[1,5] Most regulatory bod-

Table 4
NATIONAL AND REGIONAL SOURCES FOR
FIRE SAFETY INFORMATION

American National Standards Institute (ANSI)
1430 Broadway
New York, N.Y. 10018

Factory Mutual Engineering Association (FM)
1151 Boston-Providence Turnpike
Norwood, Mass. 02062

Department of Health, Education, and Welfare (HEW)
(Check for Regional Offices)

Joint Commission on Accreditation of Hospitals (JCAH)
875 N. Michigan Avenue
Chicago, Ill. 60611

National Bureau of Standards (NBS)
Washington, D.C. 20234

National Safety Council (NSC)
444 N. Michigan Avenue
Chicago, Ill. 60611

Occupational Safety and Health Administration (OSHA)
(Check for Regional Office)

Underwriters Laboratories, Inc. (ULI)
333 Pfingstenen Rd.
Northbrook, Ill. 60062

ies have removed or modified items that cause continued direct conflict, but on occasion, even a single code- or standard-making group will have discrepancies. Again, almost all are solvable.

Groups that impact most heavily on health care in codes and standards include, but are not necessarily limited to:

1. Occupational Safety and Health Administration (OSHA)
2. Department of Health, Education and Welfare (HEW), now Health and Human Services (HHS)
3. Joint Commission on Accreditation of Hospitals (JCAH)
4. Health Care Financing Administration (HCFA)
5. State hospital licensing agencies
6. Local fire, safety, and health agencies, etc.

Insurance company representatives and the various professional associations that survey and accredit or approve for safety and/or health must also be included. These are not listed because of space limitations and the possibility of offending a group by an unintentional oversight. Do check the various professional groups in a facility for all standard or code requirements.[6] Most of these AHJs will cite local or regional building codes, but when safety or fire is referenced, the majority will be from either the National Fire Protection Association (NFPA) or the American National Standards Institute (ANSI). Other significant agencies or associations are listed in Table 4.[2]

One can have considerable impact on these standards by becoming active in the various groups according to one's area of expertise. The standards-making process is much like the voting process: if one does not vote in an election, one cannot complain about the outcome. The same applies to the standards process: one can participate according to one's abilities or just sit back, let things happen, and learn to live with them. We will all have to live with standards and should participate in their formulation whenever possible.

Flammable Liquids

The handling and storage of flammable liquids in a health care facility has an important impact upon the safety and health of the occupants. The fire potential is serious because of the explosive or fast moving types of fires that are the rule with flammable liquids. Health hazards from vapors (fire hazards, too) are also of serious concern.

Local, state, and federal codes and standards enforced by AHJs will limit quantities of various classes of flammables usually based upon data found in National Fire Protection Association (NFPA) standards.[7] Specifics for health care facilities will usually involve laboratories that AHJs inspect based upon the NFPA 56C Standard, Laboratories in Health Care Facilities. This standard deals more directly with flammable-liquid hazards (and other hazards) in health care facility laboratories.

Beyond what AHJs require, a laboratory or other area where flammable liquids are used and/or stored (housekeeping, operating rooms, maintenance, anesthesia, research, etc.) should abide by a flammable-liquids code or safe-practice policy approved by the safety committee. The following items might be included.

Fire plan — Special plans to deal with specific hazards including rescue, alarm containment, and extinguishment.

Storage — Negative ventilation in storage cabinets for flammable liquids. Keep most hazardous items on lower shelves.

Handling — Unbreakable containers or protective containers for transport of flammable liquids. Use small amounts and follow strict procedures for transferring flammable liquids.

Refrigerators — Laboratory-safe or explosion-proof (where required, which is seldom, the explosion-proof refrigerator should be in an explosion-proof room) refrigerators for flammable-liquid storage. All refrigerators must be marked "approved" or "not approved" for flammable-liquid storage.

Waste disposal — Strict requirements for disposal of flammable-liquid wastes that meets EPA and local codes.

Inspections

Some AHJs require self-inspections of all areas on an annual basis.[1] Other AHJs will allow up to 50% of those inspections to be conducted in conjunction with other agencies and the use of that agency's report as documentation. Hopefully, all health care facilities will have recognized and implemented a self-inspection mechanism that includes adequate fire safety evaluations.[2] Checklists are usually utilized for this purpose and can be obtained from insurance carriers or other sources.[8] However, like most safety-related materials, it is usually more beneficial to construct a checklist or evaluation form designed specifically for use in a specific facility. Items pertaining to fire safety should include, but not necessarily be limited to:

1. Fire plan posted
2. Smoking policy posted and followed
3. Fire extinguishers — correct type, maintained, well placed
4. Exits — marked, clear passage, doors unlocked
5. Flammable liquids — quantities correct, stored properly, used properly, disposed of properly

6. Heating devices — approved type, proper use
7. Fire detection — correct type, maintained, well placed
8. Fire doors — correct type, operable, unblocked
9. Fire separations — without openings or violations
10. Refrigerators — clearly marked for type of storage
11. Flammable-liquid storage cabinets — quantities correct, contents correct, construction correct, vented correctly
12. Smoke separations — without openings in walls, doors operable

Hazardous Areas

Hazardous areas in hospitals must be handled in a special way and be scrutinized more severely. Historically, these are areas where fires occur and have the greatest potential to occur. The most universal source for hazard of contents, as it is referred to, is in the NFPA Life Safety Code 101, 4-2 Hazard of Contents.[5]

In a health care facility, one must be concerned with storage areas such as flammable and combustible, laundry and linen areas, laboratories, dietary and nourishment areas, and mechanical equipment areas including electrical closets. Both the construction and fire detection/protection should be equal to the hazard potential. Inspection of these areas should be more frequent and fire brigade training should be more concise. Usually, fire and insurance inspectors assist greatly in inspections of these areas based upon past incidents and losses.

Policies and Procedures

It is fair to say that one cannot be expected to perform if no directive has been given. It is also fair to say that even if a directive is given, it must be recorded and available for referral and clarification. Certain aspects of fire safety can be relegated to memory, but there are many items regarding policy, procedure, practice, etc. that will eventually get misplaced in our minds. For this reason (among others, including consistency), we must have policy and procedure in a written format. AHJs will be better able to evaluate the overall fire plan with a well-prepared policy manual as a guide. It is also handy for new employees or for providing continuity in a staff change.

PROTECTION

Alarms

Fire alarms are required in all hospital buildings and are activated by varying types of devices. New facilities or upgraded systems are required to have all heat and smoke detectors connected to the fire alarm system, as well as have the system activate smoke and fire doors that are held open by automatic release devices. Fire alarm systems usually contain the following components.

Pull stations — Manually activated fire alarm devices.

Fire warning devices — Either chimes, horns, or bells that ring, often in codes that indicate the area where the alarm originates.

Fire detectors — Heat (rate of rise, fixed temperature, or combination) or smoke (products of combustion or visible) detectors are most common in hospitals. Waterflow devices in sprinkler piping can act as detection devices also.

Control panel — The heart of the system where power to the system and system status is monitored. (Fire alarm systems are fail safe; power is always on throughout the system so if a wire or device fails, a trouble-indicator light and bell indicates the problem that requires attention.) Some newer systems are mini-computer based, are self-monitored for status, and can print out information or display it on CRT instruments.

City tie — The connection to a fire department alarm system that is legally responsible for the area or (if not locally allowed) an off-site area, is constantly attended and can relay the alarm to the local fire department.

Brigades

Fire brigades are recommended by many codes and authorities.[9] The fire brigade can be a valuable additional skill that personnel can utilize for the immediate response to fire in a health care facility. It can also provide them with knowledge that can save them and those around them at home or anywhere else. There are several sources for fire brigade training that identify the specific areas of health care fire safety.[10] Components of a fire brigade training program should include

Prerequisites — Administrative and departmental approval, physical exam.

Program — Fire brigade training program with reference manual, visual aids, hands-on-training with extinguishers and fire hoses.

Emergency patient relocation — Training manual with patient types and carries, hands-on-training.

First aid — American Red Cross first aid, CPR.

Self-contained breathing apparatus — Training manual with actual practice in smoke environment (optional).

Usually, the local fire department will willingly assist in these programs. One aspect that cannot be overemphasized is that the hospital fire brigade provides response, rescue, containment, and extinguishment until the fire department arrives and then assists the fire department as requested. A fire brigade is valuable, but does not replace the fire department.

Detectors

Fire detectors serve an extremely important function in a health care fire system.[4] Codes and authorities require them in ever increasing numbers unless a facility is fully sprinklered (a combination detection and extinguishing device).[11] Fire detectors can be valuable early-warning tools when matched to the right task. An overview of the various types and their applications would include

Heat-activated devices (HAD) — Fixed-temperature devices set to an alarm at 135°F and up, rate-of-rise (ROR) devices that respond to a rise in temperature of a stated rate (in degrees/minute) and combination devices which are fixed temperature and rate of rise.

Photo electric devices — These devices respond to products of combustion (smoke) that interfere with or diffuse a light beam focused on a source that responds to intensity changes.

Ionization devices — These detectors use alpha particles across two sources, one of which is exposed to atmosphere that allows products of combustion (smoke) to interfere, initiating the device.

Flame detectors — There are many types that are activated by various properties inherent in flames.

Sprinklers — Basically a heat detector (heat melts a special temperature-sensitive solder) that allows water to flow.

Spacing of detectors is crucial, as is matching the proper detector to the hazard. In health care facilities, detectors can be used to provide early warning, detection in unoccupied areas, activation of extinguishing devices, or release of doors. Maintenance and testing of fire alarm systems, including detection systems, is required by some authorities and necessary if one expects the systems to work when needed.[1]

Extinguishers

Fire extinguishers are required in all health care facilities and must be matched to

Table 5
PORTABLE FIRE EXTINQUISHERS[20]

Classification of fires
- A — ordinary combustibles (wood, paper, cloth)
- B — flammable liquids (grease, alcohol, gasoline)
- C — flowing electrical current
- D — combustible metals (sodium, magnesium)

Portable extinguishers

Type of extinguishant	Range	Discharge time	Use classification
Water pressure	20 ft	45 sec	A
Carbon dioxide	4 ft	8 sec	B, C
Dry chemical	8 ft	8 sec	A, B, C

Extinguishants

Type	Use classification	Extinguishing process/element removed
Water	A	Cooling/heat
CO_2	B, C	Smothering/oxygen
Dry chemical	A, B, C	Reaction interruption/chain reaction

Extinguisher conditions
- In working order
- Visible
- Not blocked
- Handy location

Proper usage
- Proper selection for class of fire
- Remove pin while holding neck of extinguisher
- Aim nozzle at base of fire
- Squeeze handle

Extinguishant application techniques

Water — the use of water fog or spray from extinguishers or hose lines absorbs the heat faster and also covers more fire area while protecting the fire fighter from the heat

CO_2 — the blanketing effect of the inert gas displaces the air and smothers the fire (a continuing sweeping motion with the extinguisher is most effective); total flooding of an area with CO_2 can cause short-term vision and breathing problems

Dry chemical — any dry chemical not reaching the hot source of the fire will tend to billow out and create a vision and breathing problem; the chemical must be applied directly to the burning area (the chemical is not toxic, but is irritating to eyes, nose, throat and lungs as any dust would be)

the area and hazard.[1] As with all safety apparatus, unless the people who will be using the equipment have been properly trained to use it, they probably will not do an adequate job and may complicate matters. The placement, type, and maintenance of fire extinguishers must be in compliance with the codes and standards applicable.[12] A map with extinguisher locations and types can aid greatly in the regular inspecting that is required. Often, security guards can visually inspect the units on their rounds. See Table 5.

Basic types of extinguishing agents and their uses on classes of fires can be obtained from many sources. A brief review would include

Water — Most common and economical, usually pressurized with air, and can be used with a hand-pump extinguisher. Also available with additives that reduce surface tension of water and soak into matresses and upholstered furniture for more thorough extinguishment. (Lowers temperature of burning materials.)

Carbon dioxide — A gas at atmospheric conditions, but compressed to a liquid state in the extinguisher. Leaves no residue, but is a potential problem in that it reduces the oxygen level in the area where used. (Replaces oxygen around burning materials.)

Dry chemical — Many types are available. Usually not toxic, but does obscure vision and impair breathing. However, is better for humans than smoke from a fire. Puts out more fire per pound than other types of extinguishers. (Absorbs heat and coats surface of burning materials.)

Halons — Effective only in confined areas where concentrations can be kept up to required percentage for extinguishment period. Usually expensive and toxic when exposed to heat of fire.

When training health care people in fire extinguishment, always emphasize the basics of how a device or method works. For example, a blanket or pillow can be used to smother a waste can fire; it removes the source of oxygen.

Fire Blankets

Laboratories in health care facilities are required to have fire blankets.[1] The purpose of this blanket is to smother the flames of a victim's clothing that is burning. Always emphasize that if one's clothes start burning, do not run, drop to the floor, and roll. Many serious burns incur when a victim attempts to run to the fire blanket. The correct procedure is to drop and roll, call for help which will bring the blanket, and apply it starting at the head of the victim and dragging it toward the feet, moving the flame away from the face. A poster should be provided at the site of every fire blanket (see Figure 1).

Fire Departments

The fire department that serves the health care facility can be as varied as the facilities themselves. Some areas are served by volunteer departments that rely upon assistance from neighboring towns or districts. Other departments, usually in large urban areas, have paid departments with multi-division response to an alarm. Whatever the organization of the local fire department is, there are certain items that will maximize their value to patients, visitors, and employees in fire emergencies. These items include

Fire inspections — Cooperate with the fire inspector and utilize him as a resource to solve problems.

Preplanning — Arrange for fire officers and companies to visit the site in order to become familiar with access, exposures, hydrants, fire department connections, high-hazard areas, etc.

Notification — Make the fire department aware of any impairment to the facility or fire systems that would effect procedures or preplans (major construction, extended shutdowns of systems, etc.).

Fire-Resistive Construction and Materials

The construction of a health care facility's structural members and interior materials will make a significant difference in code and standard compliance.[1] The Statement of Construction and Fire Protection that must be completed by an individual knowledgeable in institutional construction and fire safety, particularly in health care facilities, is likely to be the most comprehensive document available for evaluating the fire integrity of a building (Table 6).

Table 6
STATEMENT OF CONSTRUCTION AND FIRE PROTECTION

JOINT COMMISSION ON ACCREDITATION OF HOSPITALS
HOSPITAL IDENTIFICATION

Name of Hospital	Building Identification
City and State - Zip Code	(Area Code) Telephone Number

INSTRUCTIONS

1. Contents of this document shall be verified by one of the following individuals: A fire protection engineer, a certified safety professional, a qualified representative of a fire insurance rating organization, a registered professional engineer, a registered architect of the state fire marshal. Equivalent individuals are requested to describe on the next page *, for JCAH review, the training, education, and/or experience which qualifies them to verify the contents of this document.

2. The types of building construction considered in this document are based on the NFPA 220, Types of Building Construction, 1975.

3. Complete a separate Statement of Construction and Fire Protection for each building in which patients are housed overnight. A statement must also be completed for each major addition to these buildings that has different structural fire protection characteristics.

4. A rough sketch must be completed for each Statement of Construction.

5. All questions must be answered. When different levels of protection are provided, please describe the construction providing the least amount of fire protection. Indicate "Y" for "yes," "N" for "no," "NA" where not applicable, unless otherwise specified. Failure to respond to all questions completely will prevent processing.

6. List on page 2, **, all "equivalencies" granted by the authority having jurisdiction, and append copies of supporting documents.

STATEMENT VERIFIED BY

Name (type or print)	Title	Profession
Organization	Registration Number (where applicable)	State license number (where applicable)
Street Address, City, State, Zip Code		(Area Code) Telephone
Signature		Date

The smoke from fires is the greatest concern to life safety and this is why the materials used in construction and furnishing must be carefully evaluated before approval

Table 7
INTERIOR FINISH MATERIALS[5]

6-2.1.5[a] Interior finish materials shall be grouped in the following classes, in accordance with their flame spread and smoke development:

Class A interior finish
Flame spread 0-25, smoke developed 0-450. Includes any material classified at more than 25 but not more than 75 on the flame-spread test scale and 450 or less on the smoke test scale described in 6-2.1.6. Any element thereof when so tested shall not continue to propagate fire.

Class B interior finish
Flame spread 26-75, smoke developed 0-450. Includes any material classified at more than 25 but not more than 75 on the flame-spread test scale and 450 or less on the smoke-test scale described in 6-2.1.6.

Class C interior finish
Flame spread 76-200, Smoke developed 0-450. Includes any material classified at more than 75 but not more than 200 on the flame-spread test scale and 450 or less on the smoke-test scale described in 6-2.1.6

Note: Existing interior finishes complying with the above flame-spread ratings only may be continued in use.

[a] Interior finish materials as specified in 6-2.1.5 shall be classified in accordance with NFPA 255, Method of Test of Surface Burning Characteristics of Building Materials (see Appendix B).

for purchase or installation. New requirements by the JCAH for carpeting in hospitals is a further step in the flammability of furnishings that will likely become more rigid in the future[1] (Table 7). One has only to review health care facility fire experiences to see that a burnout or flashover from a single room can cause deaths both across the corridor and in rooms down the corridor, or require relocation of all patients from an area. Requirements for smoke and fire compartments that all components, doors, walls, penetration ductwork, and openings around any penetrations of the separations resist the passage of smoke or fire as required, will assist in dealing with health care facility fires. Fire and smoke separations between floors, buildings, and areas of buildings, where required, are crucial life safety aspects and should be followed explicitly.[5]

Existing health care facilities can overcome JCAH building and grounds deficiencies by utilizing the equivalency procedure. This process is derived from NFPA 101 Life Safety Code, 1976, 1-4.2, Equivalency Concepts. A further step in the equivalency direction is the National Bureau of Standards, Fire Safety Evaluation System for Health Care Facilities. The basic goals of this system include abilities to evaluate the level of fire safety in existing health care facilities relative to the level prescribed in the Life Safety Code, and to determine the equivalent of alternative systems for safety from fire for new designs, construction, or modification to existing health care facilities (Table 8). The JCAH and federal agencies indicate tentative approval of this evaluation/equivalency method which should assist health care costs in providing fire safety (see Appendix).

PROTECTION SYSTEMS

Fire protection systems are required in most situations, particularly where high hazards exist, but are also utilized to provide additional protection in equivalency proc-

Table 8
EQUIVALENCY PROCESS[1]

Application should include

Hospital	Specific section of standard Intent of standard Additional or alternative method of protection
Local authority	Acceptance of the equivalency by the authority having jurisdiction

Note: Hospital should determine if the alternate method of construction will provide equivalent protection.
Apply to JCAH engineering department for equivalency.

esses.[1] The NFPA 101 Life Safety Code allows travel distance increases, less fire resistance for laboratory enclosure, and less restrictions for glass in corridor walls, for example, when parts or all of the building is protected by an automatic fire extinguishing system (AFES). A brief review of AFESs and their applications follow.

Carbon dioxide — CO_2 systems in health care facilities are usually found in food preparation areas and consist primarily of exhaust hood and duct protection.[1,4] Redundant (backup) systems are often required by insurance providers. These systems must be designed, installed, and maintained according to NFPA 12 carbon dioxide-extinguishing systems. Advantages of a CO_2 system is that there is no residue to cleanup after a discharge of the system, a valuable asset in a food preparation area. Large quantities of CO_2 discharged in a confined area can become a health hazard to personnel because of oxygen depletion.

Dry chemical — The dry chemical system can be used in food preparation also, but leaves considerable residue and requires thorough cleanup.[4] It does provide quick fire extinguishment and little possibility of a reignition, especially from grease that is often the fuel in food preparation-area fires. Like CO_2, the dry chemical is a mild health hazard, and both obscure vision when discharging.

Halon — Halonenated extinguishing systems are usually found in data processing areas (CO_2 is sometimes used), special equipment areas (labs and radiology), flammable-liquid storage (CO_2 is also sometimes used), and even in rare book or record areas.[4] A colorless, odorless, tasteless gas that is expensive but harmless to contents best describes halonenated systems. However, the gas can be a health hazard when reacting with fire. A sealed area is required to maintain concentrations for effective extinguishment. NFPA 12B halonenated extinguishing-agent systems should be used for design, installation, and maintenance.

Sprinklers — Water sprinkler systems are the oldest and probably most recognized fire protection system.[4] The utilization of sprinklers and systems in health care facilities has been recognized basically through the Life Safety Code.[1] Sprinklers can contain and usually extinguish a fire, but do not provide the required early warning needed in patient-occupied areas. Sprinklers can be utilized in sensitive areas (operating rooms, intensive care units, etc.) when used in conjunction with a preaction system.[4] Preaction systems are dry systems that are activated by a detector in the protected area that opens a valve allowing water to fill the system and be available if a sprinkler head is activated by the heat of a fire. Using this system provides early detection for patient relocation and handling the fire before the sprinkler is needed. If the fire does escalate an activated sprinkler system is waiting.

Standpipes and pumps — Standpipes and fire pumps are valuable components in the overall fire fighting and protection system.[4] The standpipe system can provide the volume of water required by the fire fighter to quickly knock down a fire while the fire pump is supplying the pressure and volume of water required.[1] A fire pump is usually required only where other sources (water towers, city pressure, etc.) do not provide the required pressure at the highest point of use. Service to valves, hose, and pump should follow the prescribed NFPA standard.[13,14] Where fire pumps are provided, they must be on electric service having standby power.[1]

SERVICE AND PREVENTIVE MAINTENANCE

All fire safety equipment and systems must be serviced and maintained.[1] This service and maintenance should include the information usually found in a preventive maintenance program. Frequently, specialists must be retained or contracted to provide the proper service to sophisticated equipment or systems that the facilities own staff cannot adequately service. When this situation occurs, the vendor should be required, as part of the contract, to provide the documentation required to satisfy authorities.[1] Fire safety equipment and systems that could be included in this program are

- Fire alarm and detection systems.
- Fire extinguishing systems.
- Fire extinguishers.
- Fire pumps.
- Fire blankets.
- Exit lights.
- Exit doors, smoke doors, fire doors.
- Flammable-liquid storage facilities.

APPENDIX

Tables for Use in Fire/Smoke Zone Evaluation

FIRE SAFETY EVALUATION SYSTEM

Step 1: Determine Occupancy Risk Parameter Factors - Use Table 1.

A. For each Risk Parameter in Table 1, select and circle the appropriate risk factor value. Choose only one for each of the five Risk Parameters.

Table 1. OCCUPANCY RISK PARAMETER FACTORS

RISK PARAMETERS	RISK FACTOR VALUES					
1. PATIENT MOBILITY (M)	MOBILITY STATUS	MOBILE	LIMITED MOBILITY	NOT MOBILE	NOT MOVABLE	
	RISK FACTOR	1.0	1.6	3.2	4.5	
2. PATIENT DENSITY (D)	PATIENT	1-5	6-10	11-30	>30	
	RISK FACTOR	1.0	1.2	1.5	2.0	
3. ZONE LOCATION (L)	FLOOR	1ST	2ND OR 3RD	4TH TO 6TH	7TH AND ABOVE	BASEMENTS
	RISK FACTOR	1.1	1.2	1.4	1.6	1.6
4. RATIO OF PATIENTS TO ATTENDANTS (T)	PATIENTS / ATTENDANT	1-2 / 1	3-5 / 1	6-10 / 1	>11 / 1	ONE OR MORE* / NONE
	RISK FACTOR	1.0	1.1	1.2	1.5	4.0
5. PATIENT AVERAGE AGE (A)	AGE	UNDER 65 YEARS AND OVER 1 YEAR		65 YEARS & OVER 1 YEAR & YOUNGER		
	RISK FACTOR	1.0		1.2		

* RISK FACTOR OF 4.0 IS CHARGED TO ANY ZONE THAT HOUSES PATIENTS WITHOUT ANY STAFF IN IMMEDIATE ATTENDANCE

Step 2: Compute Occupancy Risk Factor (F) - Use Table 2.

A. Transfer the circled risk factor values from Table 1 to the corresponding blocks in Table 2.

B. Compute F by multiplying the risk factor values as indicated in Table 2.

Table 2. OCCUPANCY RISK FACTOR CALCULATION

	M		D		L		T		A		F
OCCUPANCY RISK	☐	×	☐	×	☐	×	☐	×	☐	=	☐

Step 3: Compute Adjusted Building Status (R) - Use Table 3A or 3B.

A. If building is classified as NEW use Table 3A. If building is classified as existing use Table 3B.

B. Transfer the value of F from Table 2 to Table 3A or Table 3B as appropriate. Calculate "R."

C. Transfer "R" to the block labeled "R" in Table 7 on page 4 of the work sheet.

Table 3A. (NEW BUILDINGS)

	F		R
1.0 ×	☐	=	☐

Table 3B. (EXISTING BUILDINGS)

	F		R
0.5 ×	☐	=	☐

Step 4: Determine Safety Parameter Values - Use Table 4.

A. Select and circle the safety value for each safety parameter in Table 4 that best describes the conditions in the zone. Choose only one value for each of the 13 parameters. If two or more appear to apply choose the one with the lowest print value.

Table 4. SAFETY PARAMETERS VALUES

PARAMETERS	PARAMETERS VALUES						
1. CONSTRUCTION	COMBUSTIBLE				NON-COMBUSTIBLE		
	WOOD FRAME		ORDINARY				
FLOOR OF ZONE	UNPROTECTED	PROTECTED	UNPROTECTED	PROTECTED	UNPROTECTED	PROTECTED	FIRE RESIST
FIRST	−2	0	−2	0	0	2	2
SECOND	−7	−2	−4	−2	−2	2	4
THIRD	−9	−7	−9	−7	−7	2	4
4TH & ABOVE	−13	−7	−13	−7	−9	−7	4

PARAMETERS	PARAMETERS VALUES				
2. INTERIOR FINISH (Corr. & Exit)	CLASS C	CLASS B	CLASS A		
	−5	0	3		
3. INTERIOR FINISH (Rooms)	CLASS C	CLASS B	CLASS A		
	−3	1	3		
4. CORRIDOR PARTITIONS/WALLS	NONE OR INCOMPLETE	<1/3 HR	≥1/3 <1.0 HR	≥1.0 HR	
	−10 (0)*	0	1 (0)*	2 (0)*	
5. DOORS TO CORRIDOR	NO DOOR	<20 MIN FR	≥20 MIN FR	≥20 MIN FR & AUTO CLOS	
	−10	0	1 (0)***	2 (0)***	
6. ZONE DIMENSIONS	DEAD END MORE THAN 100	DEAD END 30 − 100	NO DEAD ENDS >30 & ZONE LENGTH IS		
			>150	100 − 150	<100
	−6 (0)**	−4 (0)**	−2	0	1
7. VERTICAL OPENINGS	OPEN 4 OR MORE FLOORS	OPEN 2 OR 3 FLOORS	ENCLOSED WITH INDICATED FIRE RESIST		
			<1 HR	≥1 HR <2 HR	≥2 HR
	−14	−10	0	2 (0)*	3 (0)*
8. HAZARDOUS AREAS	DOUBLE DEFICIENCY		SINGLE DEFICIENCY		NO DEFICIENCIES
	IN ZONE	OUTSIDE ZONE	IN ZONE	IN ADJACENT ZONE	
	−11	−5	−6	−2	0
9. SMOKE CONTROL	NO CONTROL	SMOKE PARTITION	MECH. ASSISTED SYSTEMS		
			BY ZONE	BY CORRIDOR	
	−5 (0)***	0	3	4	
10. EMERGENCY MOVEMENT ROUTES	<2 ROUTES	MULTIPLE ROUTES			
		DEFICIENT CAPACITY	W/O HORIZONTAL EXIT(S)	HORIZONTAL EXIT(S)	DIRECT EXIT(S)
	−8	−2	0	3	5
11. MANUAL FIRE ALARM	NO MANUAL FIRE ALARM		MANUAL FIRE ALARM		
			W/O F.D. CONN.	W/F.D. CONN.	
	−4		1	2	
12. SMOKE DETECTION & ALARM	NONE	CORRIDOR ONLY	ROOMS ONLY	CORRIDOR & HABIT. SPACE	TOTAL SPACE
	0	2	3	4	5
13. AUTOMATIC SPRINKLERS	NONE	CORRIDOR	CORRIDOR & HABIT. SPACE	TOTAL SPACE	
	0	2 (0)**	8	10	

NOTE: * Use (0) when item 5 is −10.
** Use (0) when item 10 is −8.
*** Use (0) in zone with less than 31 patients in existing buildings.

* Use (0) when item 1 is based on first floor zone or on an unprotected type of construction.
** Use (0) when item 1 is based on an unprotected type of construction.
*** Use (0) when item 4 is −10.

Step 5. Compute Individual Safety Evaluations - Use Table 5.

A. Transfer each of the 13 circled Safety Parameter Value from Table 4 to every unshaded blocks in the line with the corresponding Safety Parameter in Table 5. For Safety Parameter 13 (Sprinklers) the value entered in the (People Movement Safety) is recorded in Table 5 as 1/2 the corresponding value circled in Table 4.

B. Add the four columns, keeping in mind that any negative numbers deduct.

C. Transfer the resulting total values for S_1, S_2, S_3, S_G to the blocks labeled S_1, S_2, S_3, S_G in Table 7 on page 4 of this sheet.

Table 5. INDIVIDUAL SAFETY EVALUATIONS

SAFETY PARAMETERS	CONTAINMENT SAFETY (S_1)	EXTINGUISHMENT SAFETY (S_2)	PEOPLE MOVEMENT SAFETY (S_3)	GENERAL SAFETY (S_G)
1. CONSTRUCTION				
2. INTERIOR FINISH (Corr. & Exit)				
3. INTERIOR FINISH (Rooms)				
4. CORRIDOR PARTITIONS/WALLS				
5. DOORS TO CORRIDOR				
6. ZONE DIMENSIONS				
7. VERTICAL OPENINGS				
8. HAZARDOUS AREAS				
9. SMOKE CONTROL				
10. EMERGENCY MOVEMENT ROUTES				
11. MANUAL FIRE ALARM				
12. SMOKE DETECTION & ALARM				
13. AUTOMATIC SPRINKLERS			÷ 2 =	
TOTAL VALUE	S_1 =	S_2 =	S_3 =	S_G =

Step 6. Determine Mandatory Safety Requirement Values - Use Table 6.

A. Using the classification of the building (i.e., New or Existing) and the floor where the zone is located, circle the appropriate value in each of the three columns in Table 6.

B. Transfer the three circled values from Table 6 to the blocks marked S_a, S_b, and S_c in Table 7.

Table 6. MANDATORY SAFETY REQUIREMENTS

	CONTAINMENT S_a		EXTINGUISHMENT S_b		PEOPLE MOVEMENT S_c	
ZONE LOCATION	New	Exist.	New	Exist.	New	Exist.
FIRST FLOOR	9.0	4.0	6.0	3.0	6.0	1.0
ABOVE FIRST FLOOR	14.0	8.0	8.0	5.0	9.0	3.0

Step 7. Evaluation Fire Safety Equivalency - Use Table 7.

A. Perform the indicated subtractions in Table 7. Enter the differences in the appropriate answer blocks.

B. For each row check "Yes" if the value in the answer block is zero or greater. Check "No" if the value in the answer block is a negative number.

Table 7. ZONE SAFETY EQUIVALENCY EVALUATION

					YES	NO
CONTAINMENT SAFETY (S_1)	less	MANDATORY CONTAINMENT (S_a)	≥0	S_1 [ ] − S_a [ ] = C [ ]		
EXTINGUISHMENT SAFETY (S_2)	less	MANDATORY EXTINGUISHMENT (S_b)	≥0	S_2 [ ] − S_b [ ] = E [ ]		
PEOPLE MOVEMENT SAFETY (S_3)	less	MANDATORY PEOPLE MOVEMENT (S_c)	≥0	S_3 [ ] − S_c [ ] = P [ ]		
GENERAL SAFETY (S_G)	less	OCCUPANCY RISK (R)	≥0	S_G [ ] − R [ ] = G [ ]		

CONCLUSIONS:

1. [ ] All of the checks in Table 7 are in the "Yes" column. The level of fire safety is at least equivalent to that prescribed by the Life Safety Code*
2. [ ] One or more of the checks in Table 7 are in the "No" column. The level of fire safety is not shown by this system to be equivalent to that prescribed by the Life Safety Code.*

*The equivalency covered by this worksheet includes the majority of considerations covered by the Life Safety Code. There are a few considerations that are not evaluated by this method. These must be separately considered. These additional considerations are covered in the "Facility Fire Safety Requirements Worksheet." One copy of this separate worksheet is to be completed for each facility.

REFERENCES

1. Accreditation Manual for Hospitals, Joint Commission on Accreditation of Hospitals, Chicago, 1979.
2. Safety Clinic Handbook, Joint Commission on Accreditation of Hospitals, Chicago, 1978.
3. **McGrath, R.,** Emergency Removal of Patients and First Aid Fire Fighting in Hospitals, American Hospital Association, Chicago, 1974.
4. Fire Protection Handbook, National Fire Protection Association, Boston, 1974.
5. Life Safety Code, Standard 101, National Fire Protection Association, Boston, 1976.
6. **Camplin, C. R.,** Personal philosophy on minimum standards, Midwest Area Health Care Safety Association Meeting, 1976.
7. Fire Protection Guide on Hazardous Materials, National Fire Protection Association, Boston, 1975.
8. Safety Guide for Health Care Institutions, American Hospital Association, Chicago, 1972.
9. Private Fire Brigades, Standard 27, National Fire Protection Association, Boston, 1979.
10. **Bartels, R. H., Camplin, C. R., and Polletta, G.,** *Hospital Fire Brigades/A Training Manual,* Camplin, Bartels and Associates, Chicago, 1979.
11. Automatic Fire Detectors, Standard 72E, National Fire Protection Association, Boston, continuously updated.
12. Portable Fire Extinguishers, Standard 10, National Fire Protection Association, Boston, continuously updated.
13. Standpipe Hose Systems, Standard 14, National Fire Protection Association, Boston, continuously updated.
14. Fire Pumps, Standard 20, National Fire Protection Association, Boston, continuously updated.

SAFETY IN THE HOSPITAL ELECTROMEDICAL INSTRUMENTATION SYSTEM

Paul E. Stanley

INTRODUCTION

In its Accreditation Manual for Hospitals, the Joint Commission on Accreditation of Hospitals (JCAH) recognizes the principle that "the hospital shall be functionally safe and sanitary for patients, hospital staff, and visitors."[1] Functional safety extends to the operation of all systems within the facility, many of which involve the use of electrical energy, and many that are closely coupled to patients for monitoring diagnostic or therapeutic purposes. The electromedical instrumentation system is the largest in number of components of all of the hospital systems, and, therefore, deserves special attention from the safety viewpoint.

Electrical and instrumentation safety in the hospital is most vital to safe hospital operation, yet probably overemphasized compared to many other important areas. There are two or more reasons for this anomaly. Although the use of electricity is a common experience to almost every one in the U.S., there remains a mystery about the electrical circuit and how electricity really works. The nature of even a minor electrical shock such as the "static" shock caused by the charge built up on the body by walking across a rug on a dry day or the sparks which occur from a "short" in an appliance power cord add to the mystery, and generate a degree of fear of electricity.

In addition to these factors, the lack of documented information concerning problems of electrical safety in the hospital has made the mystery even deeper. Statements were made that 1200 electrocutions occurred in hospitals each year. Later, this figure was increased, in print, to 5000 and then to 10,000 and even 20,000 electrocutions annually.[2,3] None of these figures were based on hospital records, but on anecdotal accounts in which preciseness had no part. Fear of malpractice suits, ignorance, carelessness in reporting and recording, etc. all contributed to the lack of a solid data base on which to evaluate the problem, or determine whether a problem really existed.

The result was that in the decade from 1965 to 1975 there appeared a plethora of articles dealing with the possible electric shock problem in hospitals. Some of these were the result of careful research, some pointed out that a possibility of shock did exist, and others reviewed the total picture as accurately as possible. Still others were patently inflammatory. Often, the view was expressed that only this or that wiring method of electrical system would solve a problem assumed to exist. As the debate went on, few facts become convincingly clear.

The rapid rise of the use of electrical apparatus in the diagnosis and treatment of disease has introduced the electrical system into the intimate vicinity of the patient. This, in turn, has made the subject of electrical safety of paramount importance in the safe and proper operation of a hospital; electrical shocks can occur in the hospital bed, the operating room, or anywhere in the hospital.

Even today, there is a lack of data concerning the probability of an electric shock occurrence and the magnitude of electric current which can cause injury. While reporting 55 electrical accidents (none of which were total) over a 42-month period in a large hospital, Bruner stated that "contrary to erroneous, if not willfully fabricated, reports in family magazines and the press, there has been no documented death due to electricity in a U.S. hospital in more than a decade."[4,5]

This means that using electricity safely in the hospital yields innumerable benefits to health care. Nonetheless, problems may develop due to many reasons, and attention

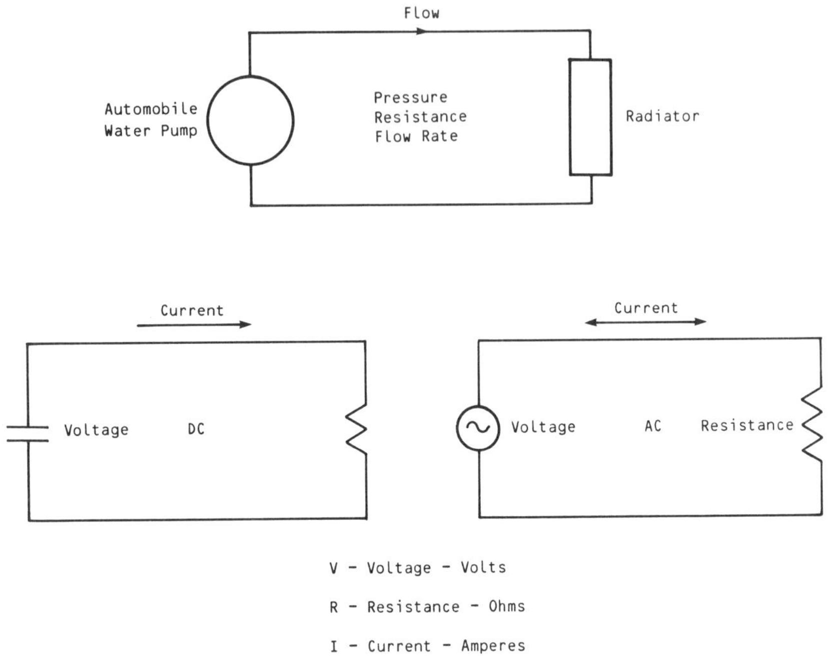

FIGURE 1. Schematic of electric circuit.

must be given to the ways in which the effects of such problems may be minimized, if not eliminated. However, such actions must not override the many other vitally important areas of safety which are required for optimal hospital care.

BASIC ELECTRICITY

Only a few basic principles of electricity will be discussed in this section of the handbook; the interested reader is urged to refer to more extended treatments.[6,7]

Benjamin Franklin and other early investigators noted that it was the flow of electricity through a muscle that caused "convulsion". This means that the important factor in electric shock is the magnitude of the current. In a crude analogy, current can be compared to the flow of water (or any fluid) in a pipe (see Figure 1). For electricity, the current is a flow of electrons in a wire or other conductor. The unit of current flow is the ampere. More often, smaller units are used in electric shock data — the milliampere (0.001 A) or the microampere (0.000001 A). Determining the magnitude of the current requires that a few other parameters describing the situation be known.

There are two requisites for the flow of an electric current: (1) a voltage source and (2) a closed circuit which includes the voltage source. The character of the voltage source is determined in part by the potential difference between its two poles. The potential differences is measured in volts, and for a dry cell flashlight battery this is 1.5 V. In the U.S., the normal voltage on the lines supplying a light or receptable in the home or hospital is 120 to 130 V. The voltage of an X-ray unit will be in the thousands or even hundreds of thousands of volts.

Also of importance in the voltage source character is its frequency. A direct current (DC) source is one that pushes continually in one direction. It may be said to be at zero frequency. Public utility current is usually at a frequency greater than zero (most commonly, 60 cps or 60 Hz).

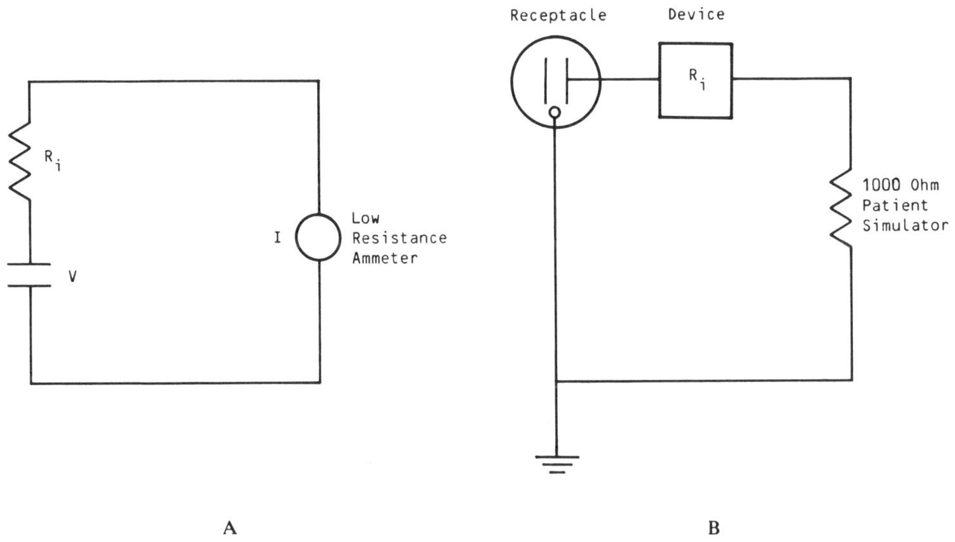

FIGURE 2. Internal resistance or impedance.

The character of the circuit must be described in terms of three elements: resistance, inductance, and capacitance. These combine into an overall characteristic called impedance. For simplicity, we shall use resistance (R) only. Resistance is measured in ohms. The current in Amperes represented by I is given by the relation

$$I = \frac{V}{R}$$

which is known as Ohm's law. The circuit may be closed by any number of elements including the human body. One resistance component exists within the voltage source itself (see Figure 2A). For example, a 1.5 V Number 6 dry cell will generate a current of more than 30 A through an ammeter, which is essentially a short circuit. This means that the resistance of the cell is

$$R_i = \frac{1.5}{30} = 0.05\ \Omega$$

On the other hand, an AA-size 1.5 V dry cell will generate less than 3 A. This means its resistance is

$$R_i = \frac{1.5}{3} = 0.5\ \Omega$$

Noted in Figure 2B is a voltage source due to "leakage" of an AC-operated lamp. It has a voltage of 120 V, yet it will generate less than 1 μA of current through a 1000-Ω "patient". By Ohm's law this means that the internal leakage impedance is 120 Ω (120 million Ω). This is so high that it may cause a voltmeter to read incorrectly perhaps only 80 V or less.

Body Resistance

It was previously noted that a human body may have a resistance of 1000 Ω, how-

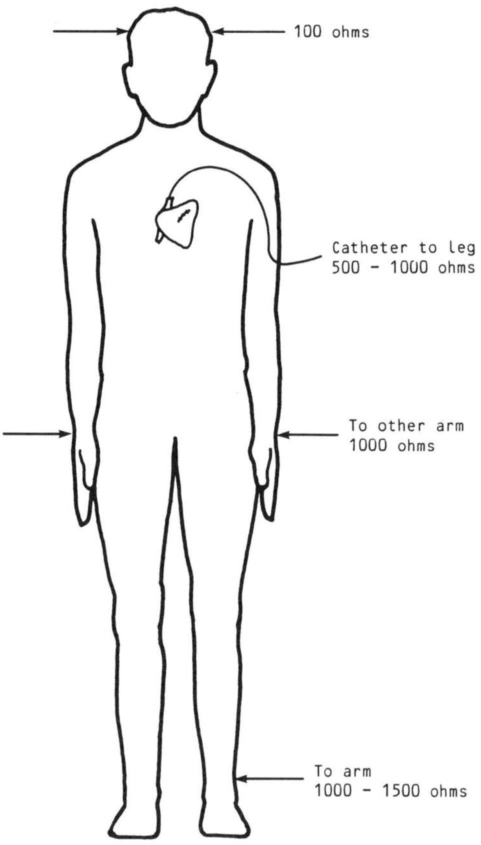

FIGURE 3. Body resistance.

ever, a precise value is difficult to specify. With the use of needle electrodes and low-voltage DC, measurements indicate that body resistance may range from 100 to 1000 Ω depending on the distance between electrodes. A conservative, average value of 1000 Ω should be used in most calculations, especially when one of the electrodes may be a cardiac catheter.

Skin resistance is a function of the thickness of the callous skin on the surface, the amount of other dead tissue, the oiliness of the surface, and the amount of moisture in the skin. For dry, calloused hands, the skin resistance may be as high as 500,000 Ω. After scrubbing with soap and a thorough soaking in water, resistance may drop to 500 to 1000 Ω or less. Similar low resistances may occur when the skin is cleansed with alcohol and covered with an electrode paste or lotion before attaching an electrocardiographic electrode (see Figure 3).

The effect of frequency on the current flow and its physiological reaction is simulated by paralleling the 1000 Ω by another resistor and a capacitor (see Figure 4).

THE EFFECTS OF ELECTRIC CURRENT ON THE HUMAN BEING

Two categories of electric shock are recognized: (1) macrocurrent shock or macroshock in which the current flow is through the body from some point on the surface; called macro because the current required to cause an effect is usually in the milliampere range or higher (see Figure 5) and (2) microcurrent shock or microshock in which the flow is through the heart muscle from a conductor in the heart through the body

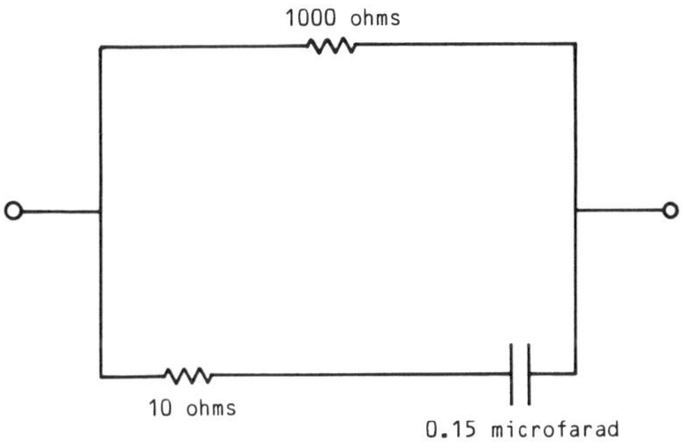

FIGURE 4. Patient impedance simulator.

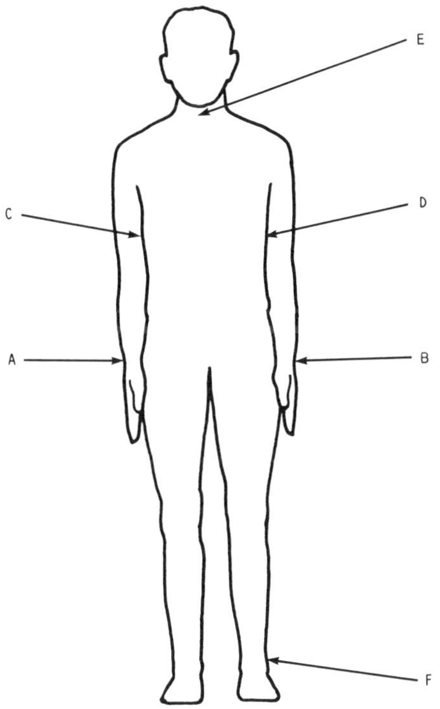

FIGURE 5. Macrocurrent shock.

to some point on the surface; called micro because the current is in the microampere range, i.e., 1000 times smaller than the macroshock range.

Macrocurrent Shock

The effect of a steady state electric current flowing through a human being is dependent upon the magnitude of the current, the frequency of the current, the weight of the subject, the duration of the flow, the characteristic of the contact (including its size and the impedance qualities of the contact surface), certain characteristics of the physical condition of the subject, the experience the subject has had with electrical shock, and whether or not the current flow was expected. Therefore, definitions of precise current levels for any shock reaction are not possible.

At the threshold of perception, the flow of electric current is recognized by a slight

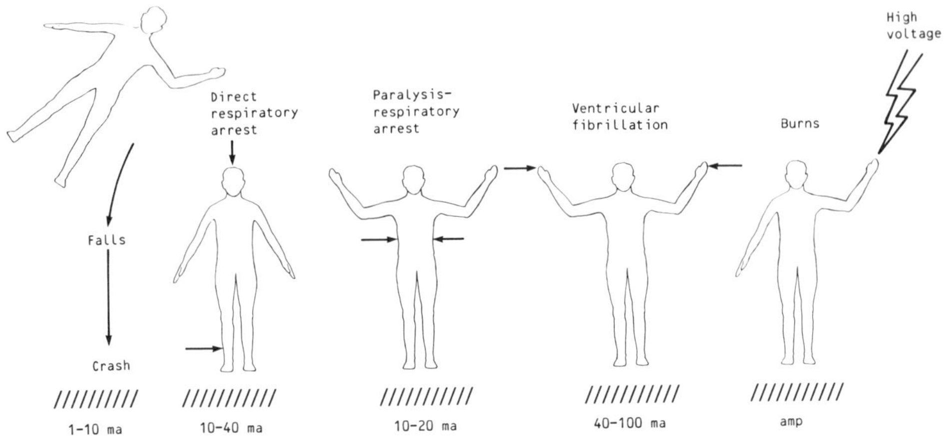

FIGURE 6. Possible effects of macrocurrent shock.

tingling or stinging sensation at the point of contact. Fewer than 1% of children and smaller adults (especially women) will detect a current of the order of 0.1 mA. Usually, this requires that the point of contact be almost needle-like and the point of insertion of the current into the body be on a particularly sensitive spot as, e.g., the underside of the arm or at certain locations on the back of the hand. For more than 50% of subjects, the threshold level will be about 1 mA. More than 99% of subjects will detect a current flow at approximately 1.5 to 1.7 mA. Normally, for a current level only slightly in excess of the threshold, the reaction will be no more than a mild surprise and probably no harmful results will occur. However, some persons may react with sufficient motion (of the arm, e.g.) that they may be said to have been startled. This will be especially true if the subject was not expecting the shock[8] (see Figure 6).

At somewhat higher levels, the reaction will be so sudden and of such magnitude that it can indeed be called the "startle reaction". This will occur when the current is of the order of 2 to 4 mA. The involuntary, sudden withdrawal of the hand from the point of contact with the current circuit (and a larger reaction throughout the whole body) may result in sufficiently violent movement to cause a fall from a ladder or a hand to be thrust into moving machinery. When the current level reaches something of the order of 4.5 or 5.0 mA, smaller adults will experience a more violent contraction of the muscles, or tetany, that is usually characterized by saying that the current has exceeded the "let-go" level. This means the subject should be grasping the conductor through which the current is flowing into his body; he will not be able to release the conductor. This reaction has been studied extensively by Dalziel and Lee who have reported that the let-go level is very much a function of the size of the individual and his experience with electric shock.[9] The person who is familiar with shock may find that although the tetany is rather severe and the pain considerable, he is able to let go at a somewhat higher level of current. For less than 1% of men, the let-go current is of the order of 20 mA, with an average value of about 16 mA. If current at the let-go level flows for a few seconds, the resultant strain on the muscle may appear as a soreness that may last for hours or even days. Currents flowing for several minutes at the let-go level may result in burns at the point of contact of the conductor with the body.

Should a current at or above the let-go level flow through the chest muscles, respiratory arrest may occur which can lead to death by suffocation if the duration of the flow exceeds 3 to 5 min. Currents of this magnitude which flow through the head into the torso for 3 to 5 sec or more may result in paralysis of the respiratory control center in the medulla oblongata of the brain. The resulting respiratory arrest will be terminated only after minutes, or even hours, during which the subject is unable to breathe for himself. If given respiratory resuscitation for the period of paralysis, he may recover without undue effects.[9]

While the let-go level for men, women, and smaller adults has been evaluated with relative accuracy, very little data exist for children. Dalziel and Lee have reported that as the current increases, children will not respond, but simply begin to cry.[9] He suggests, however, that the let-go level for children is perhaps in the neighborhood of 4.5 mA. Since it is conceivable that the tetany may cause paralysis of the chest muscles and result in respiratory arrest, the serious hazard level for children must be considered as beginning at approximately 4.5 mA.

More serious effects, including ventricular fibrillation and burns, occur at larger values of current. To understand the phenomenon of ventricular fibrillation requires a brief look at the electrophysiology of the heart.

Unlike most other muscles the heart muscle can generate the contracting process within each cell. When it does so, a random quivering of the muscle known as fibrillation occurs. However, a master control system also exists in the heart. A group of cells known as the sinoatrial node sends out a strong electrical pulse about 72 times per minute; this causes the muscles of the atria to contract in a wave-like manner. As a result, the blood is forced from the atria into the ventricles. When this wave reaches the atrioventricular node, the accompanying electrical currents trigger that node. This causes it to send out a signal to all parts of the ventricle muscles, which then contract and drive the blood out into the arteries.[10]

When a small flow of electrical current from the outside flows through the heart muscle, this paced action is interfered with and the ventricular muscle takes on a random action. The phenomenon is called ventricular fibrillation. An extraneous current of 10 to 20 μA may induce ventricular fibrillation, however, the hazard level is nearer 50 mA.

Therefore, in the use of electrical devices that come into contact with the patient, safety is achieved only if no current larger than 10 μA is allowed to flow through the heart muscle.

In the macroshock case, studies have shown that if the current flow is from left arm to right leg, e.g., a current of 100 mA/1 sec causes sufficient current to flow through the heart to almost certainly cause fibrillation. More precisely, the macroshock fibrillating level is given by the equation

$$I = \frac{K}{T^{1/2}} \text{ mA}$$

where T is the time of current flow in seconds, and K is a constant equal to approximately 100 ma/sec$^{1/2}$.

In some cases, it appears that cardiac arrest occurs when large currents flow through the chest. This situation would probably require the current to flow for some minutes so that death occurs as a result of the cessation of circulation. If the large current flow is for just a second or so, there is some probability that the heart rhythm might restart spontaneously after the current flow stops, somewhat in the manner observed after defibrillation.

If the current flow is very large due to a high voltage source, severe burns may occur in a fraction of a second or less.

Microcurrent Shock

Until recently, the gross shock situations were the only electrical hazards against

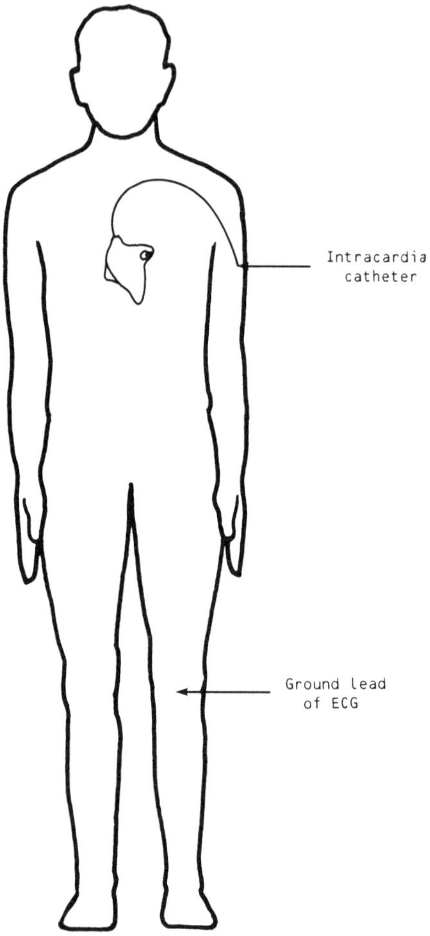

FIGURE 7. Microcurrent shock.

which care had to be taken. However, with the advent of the frequent use of conducting catheters placed directly into the heart cavities, the microcurrent shock case requires consideration (see Figure 7).

Although such cases are much more difficult to document, there has been some evidence that in past years the subtle effects of very small currents may have caused deaths. Unfortunately, as in the case of larger currents that cause ventricular fibrillation but not burns, no identifiable changes (by autopsy) are produced by these microshocks. Only circumstantial evidence (such as the presence of a cardiac catheter in the patient at death) points the accusing finger in most cases. Even then, it cannot be stated unequivocally that the cause of fibrillation was not mechanical motion of the catheter, rather than an electric current.

In 1962, Weinberg et al. published a report of studies on electrical shock hazards in cardiac catheterization.[11] They concluded that currents as low as 35 μA can produce ventricular fibrillation when the current is through the heart wall. Other studies indicate that a current as low as 12 μA/60 Hz produces fibrillation in the canine ventricle. One case is reported in which 180 μA produced fibrillation in a human being. However, the effect is very dependent on the size of the contact with the heart muscle, its location, and the medical condition of the heart.[12]

Electrical Burns

When the voltage of the current source is high, the large current which results causes joule heating of the body tissue through which it passes. Since this heat may cause blisters that increase the resistance to the point of breaking the circuit, stopping the current flow, the phenomenon is quite complicated. On the other hand, the burn may cause carbonizing of the tissue, thereby reducing the resistance. In any event, the burn will usually be quite severe and deep.

Of more concern in the hospital are burns caused by lower voltages — 120 to 130 V or occasionally 208 to 240 V, 60 Hz AC. In general, a momentary contact with the conductor carrying the voltage will result in no burn, since the current will be small. However, there have been instances of burns resulting when the subject is unable to let go and the current flows for some seconds. When the voltage is in the 3 to 10-V range, the time to cause erythema is usually 20 min or more.

In some few medical devices, a direct current is used to test the completeness of a circuit or control the apparatus. Where such devices have been used for an hour or so, a few instances of burns under the electrodes have been reported. There is evidence that these burns are more of a chemical nature than joule-heating burns.[13]

Probably the most frequent cause of electrical burns is the use of the electrosurgical unit. Nevertheless, the benefits of electrosurgery far outweigh the occasional problem. Electrosurgery involves the use of a high-frequency (500,000 to 2,000,000 Hz) voltage source. The voltage used may be as high as 5000 V in some models of electrosurgery generators; 1000 V is quite common. This combination of high frequency and high voltage provides the device the versatility to both cut tissue readily and coagulate it, thereby reducing the problem of bleeding. However, the same characteristics also provide the conditions for a greater degree of current path diversity, making the possibility that paths paralleling the desired one may exist. It is in these unwanted current circuits that burns may occur. Proper care can reduce such hazards to a minimum.[14,15]

The electrosurgical unit functions as any other electrical apparatus. There is a voltage generator and a closed circuit which includes the arc and the patient. The return of the current from the patient to the generator is achieved by the use of a special large area (8 to 100 in.^{2}) dispersive electrode to which a return cable is connected. If the dispersive or return electrode used is large enough and the return cable intact, the burn problem should be minimal.[16]

How Much Voltage?

How much voltage is required to cause death or serious injury? The answer comes from the application of Ohm's law to the previously mentioned data on resistance.

If the circuit through which the current passes is a cardiac catheter in the heart to a well-applied ground electrode on the right leg, the resistance can be of the order of 1000 Ω. A current in excess of 50 μA may be hazardous in this case. Therefore, 50 mV from a low impedance source would be a lethal voltage. On the other hand, for the calloused 500,000 Ω hands, 100 V would cause a very small current to flow and probably no harm would result. Of course, when the voltage is several hundred volts, other effects such as burns occur.

Because the hand-to-hand resistance may be as low as 1000 Ω and 1.0 mA or so may cause sudden involuntary muscular reactions that could lead to a fall or other undesirable result, a potential difference of 1.0 V or so should always be considered hazardous. An additional safety factor is introduced in the performance specifications for electrical wiring as given in the National Electrical Code.[17] For general care areas of hospitals, the potential difference between any two conductive surfaces should not exceed 0.5 V; in critical care areas, the specified limit is 0.1 V.

STATIC ELECTRICITY IN THE HOSPITAL

Static and Spark Effects on Human Beings

Although the psychological and physiological reactions to steady state alternating and direct currents have been the subject of considerable research attention, the effects of transients have received only limited study. Repeated anecdotal reports indicate that static discharges may be hazardous in microshock. Some studies have shown that the human reaction to sparks resulting from induction near extra-high voltage transmission lines may be important in setting design standards for such lines. A time vs. current relationship to be used in the design of ground fault circuit interruptors has been put forth, however, most of the work leaves much to be desired.

Deno and Zaffenella point out that their studies on the threshold of perception and unpleasantness of spark discharges has given an energy value of 0.5 to 1.5 mJ as objectionable; on the other hand, Dalziel reported the "unpleasant" shock energy as 250 mJ, a difference factor of 150 to 500 times. Deno and Zaffenella conclude that more data are needed on this subject.[18,19]

The standards proposed by the National Fire Protection Association (NFPA) and the Association for the Advancement of Medical Instrumentation (AAMI) do not address the subject of transients.

At least in part, the evaluation of the effects of transient currents is made difficult due to limitations on the response time of the nervous system of living subjects; Geddes and Baker point this out in their discussion of the strength-duration relationship for tissue excited by electrical impulses.[20] There is the suggestion that a discharge having a time constant of less than 0.1 msec might not cause any effect on living tissue.

Gibson has shown that sensation is produced in the skin as a function of the current and the number of pulses.[21] His data show that the pain threshold for 5-msec rectangular pulses repeated at 100 pulses per second, decreases rapidly with the number of pulses, from above 3 mA for a single pulse, to about 1.5 mA for 7 to 10 pulses. No work reports on spark-type (exponential decay) multiple pulses. In addition, the reported studies are very subjective and include too few subjects to assure reasonable statistical validity.

Deno has conducted studies of the "static" discharge generated by walking across a carpet under certain conditions. His data suggest that the static discharge may be oscillatory, which in the light of Gibson's work may explain why such discharges cause a response in tissue.[21]

Generation of Static Charges

The theory of the generation of static charges has been only descriptively explained for the most part. When two dissimilar insulating materials are brought into contact, the surface-free electrons tend to "wander" across the interface. If the surfaces are moved parallel to each other with considerable pressure between them, the transfer of electrons is accentuated. When the insulators are separated, one will carry a positive and the other a negative charge.[22]

Since charges of opposite signs attract, work must be done both in the process of generation of the charges and separation of the insulators. The work done appears as the energy stored on the insulators given by

$$W = \frac{1}{2} CV^2$$

where W is the work in joules, C is the capacity of insulator, and V is the voltage or potential of the charged body.

While special Van de Graff or other machines can be built to generate very high voltages by static processes, the conditions of concern in the hospital will seldom generate voltages in excess of 20 kV. More often, the limit will be of the order of 8 to 10 kV.

The capacitance of the human body to a grounded contact is variously reported as between 200 and 700 pF depending upon the nature of the surface on which the person stands, etc. This means the energy normally stored may go as high as 0.15 (150 mJ). A more likely figure is 0.01J (10mJ) as a maximum.

The discharge which occurs when a human being touches a grounded surface with a finger after scuffing across a carpet will be an exponential with a time constant of the order of 10 msec if the finger is wet. If the finger is dry, the discharge may be repetitive, often showing up to 20 separate spark discharges.

Static Discharge Hazards

In the hospital, static discharges may conceivably cause three types of hazards.

Startle

If the voltage or potential difference between the human subject and the surface touched is of the order of 1000 V or more, the peak current flow in the discharge will be high enough, and the time of discharge long enough, to be perceptible. The discharge will be felt as a sharp prick at the point of contact; if the total energy stored is high enough, i.e., if the voltage is sufficiently high, a small tetany of the arm muscle may be felt. The reaction is one of startle and may include a sudden withdrawal of the hand. The startle effect is almost completely eliminated if the contact with "ground" is made with a conductor held in the hand.

Ignition of a Flammable Mixture

NFPA 77, Static Electricity, states that an acceptable, average energy level for igniting a saturated hydrocarbon vapor in air is 0.25 mJ: "thus, a spark from a charged conductor the size of a large man might be hazardous if the voltage was a little more than 1500 V and the spark occurred between small electrodes."[23]

The existence of a saturated mixture in the operating room (except in the immediate vicinity of the patient's mouth) is highly improbable. Further, the use of nonflammable anesthetics has all but eliminated the explosion problem as far as static electricity is concerned.

Ventricular Fibrillation

Whether the human heart can be fibrillated by a static spark remains an unanswered question. Rumors or anecdotal accounts of such incidents have been few, yet quite persistent.

In April 1977, McCarty and Glasser reported that in one case they did cause ventricular fibrillation in a dog with a 6 kV discharge to the external end of a pacemaker lead from a human fingertip. This represented about 3.6 mJ; the heart had suffered infarction.[24]

On the other hand, others have found it impossible to fibrillate the canine heart with very short pulses, either from a capacitive discharge or from a rectangular pulse generator. The question, therefore, remains unresolved.

Elimination of Static

The obvious solution to the generation of static electrical charges on an insulator is to conduct and ground it. The use of conductive flooring with all furniture in the operating room connected to it by high resistance conductors, the wearing of conductive clothes and "booties" by personnel, and the use of conductive tubing connected to the patient generally serve to eliminate all static problems.

To say the least, such methods are bothersome. Since it was observed that static electricity problems were less when the humidity was high, humidification has been proposed, in fact, mandated for operating rooms.[25] However, if synthetic fabrics are used for clothing, it has been noted that higher humidity does not necessarily eliminate the problem. This is evident from data published by Sereda and Feldman showing that the conductivity of the fabric at a given relative humidity is very dependent upon the nature of the fabric.[26] It was noted that at 65% relative humidity, cotton does not take on a charge, while propylon may build-up 3800 V under the same condition.

Because static electrical charge has been a problem in clothes driers, manufacturers have developed materials which can be sprayed onto clothing to increase conductivity enough to prevent a build-up of charge. Under some circumstances, such materials may be used to prevent static problems in the hospital.

HOW HAZARDS DEVELOP IN HOSPITALS

While there is reasonable safety from electric shock in the hospital based on the records in the literature, hazardous stuations can develop. If the safety record is to be improved, their origins must be studied.

The electromedical system includes not only the instruments and devices alluded to earlier, but the electrical power supply as well. Electrical energy is usually delivered in the U.S. by a two- or three-conductor system in which one of the conductors is at the nominal potential of 120 V. (Other values may be used but this has no real bearing on the problem or its solution.) The other conductors will be at or near the potential of the earth or ground. The current normally flows from the source through the live conductor, through the load, and back through the neutral conductor to the grounded side of the source. The source may be a generator, but in the usual system it will be a transformer which reduces the voltage from the several thousand volts used in the main distribution system to the 120 V of the local. If the third or grounding conductor exists, a current will flow either from the live conductor through any circuit connected to the live conductor and any other ground contact. Since it is connected to the chassis or frame, the grounding conductor serves as a safety return for current should the live conductor accidently contact the chassis of the device.

The question to be asked now is how is it possible for a patient or operator to have access to the voltage on the live conductor? Several answers exist.

First, poor installation practices or design may leave the live conductor exposed in the wiring system or a device connected to it. In addition, the insulation may be worn away by the rubbing of the wire by a moving part, or the live wire may touch the ungrounded frame of a lamp, electric bed, or instrument. Unless the frame is connected to ground through the grounding conductor, a subject touching the frame and any ground will complete the circuit providing a conducting path through which a dangerous or lethal current may flow.

Second, whenever two electrical conductors are in close proximity, a capacitive coupling exists between them (see figure 8). Simply, this means that it is possible for a small quantity of electrical charge to pass through the insulation from one conductor to the other. If the voltage between the conductors is alternating, an alternating current will flow. Thus, if one of the conductors is the live wire of the electrical supply to a piece of equipment and it comes close to the frame of the device, a current will flow through the capacitive coupling to the frame and ground through any available path. This path could be the human body. This current is called the leakage current. For safety, the leakage current should be returned to ground through the grounding conductor. Resistive and inductive coupling may also contribute to the leakage current.

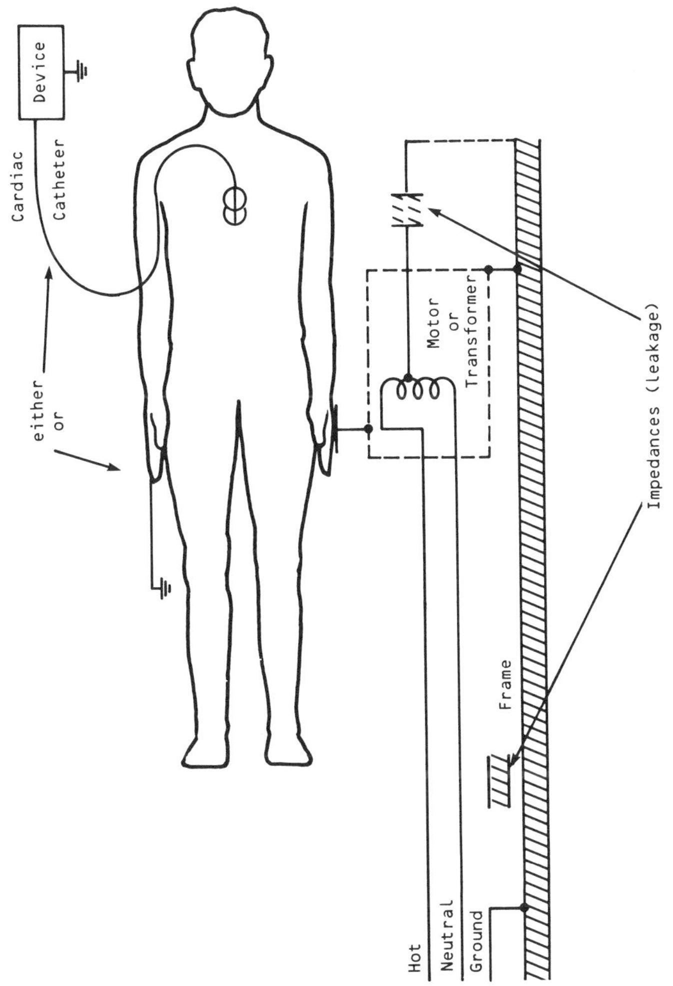

FIGURE 8. Leakage current.

Other means of coming in contact with the live conductor are numerous, however, not frequent. For example, spilling water or other conducting fluid on an instrument may provide the path. Children have been seriously shocked or even burned by putting a paper clip into the electrical receptacle while touching some grounded conductor.

The equipment used may also be the source of hazards. A very common fault in electrical equipment is the failure of the grounding conductor in the power cord. The design of many types of plugs is such that the grounding wire breaks in the plug after a few months use. When this happens, that piece of equipment is ungrounded and a hazard could exist.

The loss of grounding conductor continuity may occur in the receptacle, as well as in the cord. Because of the design of the contacts with which the ground prong makes contact, the pressure of that contact may be quite low, even zero. This means that the equipment is ungrounded. Careful attention to this design by the manufacturers of high quality receptacles has reduced the frequency of the problem. However, regular testing of the tension of this contact cannot be overemphasized. Another quite frequent source of hazardous electric shock is the failure of the personnel using the equipment to understand that misuse can result in danger. Most equipment offered on the market today is safe providing it is well-maintained and properly used. However, the simplest of devices can be hazardous if faulty operation is not recognized or the unit is misused. The general lack of understanding of the function and proper maintenance of certain sensitive equipment can transform lifeform lifesaving equipment into life-taking gadgetry.[27]

Some Case Histories

Specific examples of electrical hazards have been reported in the literature and at safety meetings.

1. A survey of 300 molded-on plugs cut off of hospital equipment such as electric beds, portable suction pumps, hypothermia machines, etc. revealed the following conditions on detailed examination: (1) 55% of the plugs had no ground prong; the ground prongs were removed because they were broken in "normal" hospital use or were bent and could not be inserted in the receptacle, and (2) 45% of the plugs had all three prongs apparently intact; visual inspection showed apparently safe plugs. When the plugs with apparently intact prongs were tested with a continuity meter, it was found that only 15% of the plugs were actually safe (i.e., there was continuity between the green conductor and the ground prong). Most of these problems have been eliminated through new designs of connecting plugs.
2. A patient was undergoing surgery when he suddenly appeared to have a rather severe, yet brief convulsion after which his blood pressure dropped rapidly as indicated by a manometer connected to an arterial catheter. The anesthesiologist attempted to listen to the patient's heart, but was shocked as his metallic stethoscope touched the patient. When it was noted as inoperative, the cardiac monitor oscilloscope was turned off; the anesthesiologist was not shocked this time. The patient's heart was in fibrillation. Investigation showed that the monitor was not grounded and that probably a transient failure in the monitor had caused approximately 40 mA to flow through the right leg of the patient and through him to ground through a head clamp.
3. A kitchen helper in a large hospital was severely shocked and suffered burns on both hands when he connected an electric hot-food cart to the wall receptacle. Since the ground wire of the three-wire power cord of the food cart was not connected to anything inside the cart, it was left ungrounded. The insulation of the neutral wire of the power cord was frayed and a 2-in. long piece of bare wire touched the metal frame, the appliance ground. Since the neutral wire is supposed to be at ground potential, this should introduce no hazard. However, an examination of the electrical receptacles of the hospital showed that many of them had the live and neutral wires reversed. Thus, when this food cart was plugged into one of these outlets, the full line voltage was placed on all its metallic parts.

   The other end of the electrical power cord had a three-prong connector with metallic reinforcement which was connected to the ground terminal of the plug. By holding this plug and inserting it into the electrical wall receptacle, the person became connected directly to ground. Simultaneous contact with a metallic part of the food cart completed the circuit through his body.

   The accident could have been avoided by inspecting both the electrical part of the food cart and the house wiring system for reversed polarity and open ground at regular intervals (preventive maintenance), and by using heavy-duty power plugs and receptacles supplied by a reputable manufacturer. Inexpensive power receptacles and plugs can be the most expensive in terms of safety. In addition, their lifetimes are usually much shorter than the better devices.
4. A 53-year-old patient was thrown into ventricular fibrillation when the controller

of his electrically operated bed was immersed in urine. The patient had elevated the backrest of his electrically operated bed to the vertical position, leaving the controller resting on his lap. He passed urine and, while attempting to return the urinal to the bedside table, spilled most of its content over his bed, thereby immersing the bed controller in the urine. The controller, in turn, carried current from a conventional 120-V grounded power line to the motor operating the bed mechanism. The patient was connected to ground by one of the ECG-monitor electrodes taped to his anterior chest wall, its connecting cable terminating at the chassis of the monitor grounded through the third wire of the power cord. Thus, current from the controller passed through the urine, the patient's buttocks, the chest electrode to the chassis of the monitor, and, from there, to ground via ground wire.

Only the careful attention of a resident who observed the appearance of a 60-Hz signal appearing on the screen of the remote monitor at the nurses station and acted immediately — disconnecting the bed from the power line and initiating proper resuscitation — prevented the accident from becoming a fatality.

This kind of accident would not occur if low-voltage bed controls and isolated patient monitor leads were used.

5. In the neurosurgical department of a 700-bed hospital, a resident was shocked while preparing to use an echo-encephalograph. His right hand was holding a metallic switch of the encephalograph and his left was on the pull of a metal drawer of the stainless steel table on which the instrument was standing.

An examination of the equipment showed that a filter capacitor in the power supply circuit of the oscilloscope had shorted, placing 300 V on the cabinet of the instrument. Grounding of the instrument through three-wire cord and the grounding prong of the three-prong connector was by-passed through the use of a three-to-two prong adaptor on the power connector, despite the fact that the electrical receptacle was of the three-prong grounded type and the adaptor was completely unnecessary to connect the instrument to the electrical power line. The rubber feet of the instrument isolated it from the steel table which was grounded by connection to the water system.

The full potential of 300 V was placed across the right arm of the victim, and his left arm to the grounded table.

Assuming the resident's body impedance to be approximately 1000 Ω a current of 300 mA or 0.3 A (20 times the value of the so-called let-go current) passed through the victim who, therefore, was unable to remove his hands from the circuit. As previously mentioned, when currents in the range of 100 mA or more pass through the chest of a human being for one or more seconds, ventricular fibrillation is most probable.

The accident could have been avoided if the instrument had been properly grounded, i.e., the three-to-two prong adaptor had not been used and/or the instrument had been conductively connected to the steel table top on which it was placed. In this case, resistance to ground through the provided ground lines would probably have been only 1 or 2 Ω, a current of many amperes would have flowed to ground, immediately opening the 1.5-A fuse of the instrument and, probably, the 20-A circuit breaker of the house power line.

6. While no accidents had been reported in the physical therapy area in a certain hospital, an examination of the wiring revealed that several of the "booths" were supplied by an "Electro-Strip" rather than an approved conduit and receptacle installation. Tests of the outlets in these booths showed that they not only did not provide good electrical connections for powering the devices to be used in the booth but that none of them provided any ground connection, although the

receptacles were of the three prong type. An examination of the receptacles throughout the hospital revealed that in half of them, the hot and neutral conductors were reversed.

An analysis of these and many other case histories of actual or potential electric shock hazards reveals that they arise from many causes: (1) careless and/or uninformed use and practices, (2) poorly designed apparatus or wiring systems, (3) careless or insufficient inspection, testing, and maintenance of devices and wiring systems, (4) failure of a component of the apparatus, particularly the grounding conductor in the power cord, (5) spillage of fluids on equipment, (6) an occasional "intentional" touching of the live conductor, especially by children, and (7) many combinations of these and other factors.

PREVENTING OR ELIMINATING HAZARDS

The electromedical instrumentation system in the hospital is very complex. It involves both the electrical wiring of the power distribution system of the hospital and hundreds of different kinds of instruments, as well as the interaction of these with physicians, nurses, patients, and other persons all of whom are fallible. However, it must function in a manner that will provide the most safety for all. This requires that electrical safety be approached in a systematic manner. There are many methods which can be used to solve the problem of safety, but only one will be discussed here. It can be epitomized by the acronym PITMED: purchasing, inspection and testing, maintenance, education, and documentation. (See Appendix A for an implementation protocol.)

Purchasing

Safety can be expected only if the equipment in a system is designed and manufactured according to good practice. Since a well-designed device may become a hazard if its components fail, appropriate attention must be given to the selection of all materials and subsystems; the entire design must be subjected to careful review before manufacturing begins. To give assurance to the quality of medical devices, the Department of Health, Education, and Welfare, under the Medical Devices Amendments of 1976 to the Food, Drug, and Cosmetic Act, was authorized to begin establishing standards and controls for medical devices. Such regulation will go far in reducing the number of defective devices delivered to health care facilities.[28,29]

Nevertheless, careful selection of instrumentation and other components of the electromedical instrumentation system is the first step in establishing electrical safety. The selection process should include a thorough evaluation of all facets of the safety problem, including the specifications of the devices considered and possible hazards which might be introduced into the overall system through the interaction of the new devices with the existing apparatus. Ease of maintenance, availability of repair parts, and the adequacy of various operating and maintenance manuals should be ascertained.[30]

Among other considerations to be given to electromedical equipment is the construction of the device. It should be so designed that when properly used there will be no danger to the operator or patient. There should be no sharp corners which scratch or cut the insulation of the power cord, thus exposing the live wires. Supports, especially scissor-type extension supports, should be designed to prevent the cutting of the power cord. Materials used should not be toxic to the patient or others under ordinary conditions. No portion of the cabinet of the device should become hot enough to cause burns or discomfort if touched by a sensitive patient.

The care given by the manufacturer to these details can be an indicator (though limited) of the care given to a primary factor in the safety design of such equipment

— the reduction of the electric shock hazard. Although a proper ground and an ungrounded or isolated electrical supply provide two levels of electrical safety, a third and very important level lies within the device itself.

Adequate insulation should be provided so that all accessible metal parts are isolated from live electrical parts. Covers over live parts should be removable only with the aid of tools, and, if feasible, automatic disconnects should turn off the power when the cover is removed. Provision should be made to easily ground the accessible metal parts. Where very high voltage occurs within the device, double insulation may be used to assure increased safety.

Similar care must be given to the design and installation of the electrical supply and grounding system to be obtained for a new portion of a hospital or updating existing systems.

It will be assumed that an adequate electrical power supply will be provided to the hospital building in accordance with good engineering practices and pertinent parts of the appropriate electrical codes. If at all possible, power should be obtained from multiple sources to minimize the probability of total failure. However, since electricity is more and more used not only for comfort and convenience, but for lifesaving monitoring and even life support systems, additional local emergency power supplies are necessary.[31] In some cases, uninterrupted power may be essential; there are functions in the hospital or equipment which cannot tolerate even a 30-sec break in power supply.

Therefore, the hospital should be organized in such a fashion that the various areas are supplied with power in accordance with need. Obviously, the laundry does not need continuous operation, but the intensive care unit must always be supplied (although it can tolerate a brief interruption while its wiring system is switched from the main source to an emergency system). On the other hand, a patient who is receiving cardiac assistance may need to be supplied continuously. It is not the purpose of this section to detail how these several sources of supply are to be obtained or controlled. They are mentioned only to point out that the need complicates the design for safety and makes it imperative that care be used in laying out and purchasing the system and all of its components.

Of utmost importance is the quality of the grounding system. In many local codes, the conduit or raceway used to enclose the circuit conductors may be used as the grounding conductor. The ground currents which flow will raise the receptacle ground only a few millivolts over the potential of the main ground bus of the system. For ordinary use, this is of no consequence; however, in the hospital, with the increased use of electrical equipment and instrumentation (some of it attached to the patient), millivolt stray potentials are undesirable and dangerous. Therefore, it is required that all circuits in a hospital be provided with a separate grounding conductor run with the circuit conductors.[17]

Whenever possible, prepurchase evaluation tests of apparatus should be conducted under the supervision of the engineering department of the hospital, and its approval should be given before the purchase order is written (see Figure 9).

Inspection and Testing

Protecting a subject from the probability of electric shock is quite simple in principle. The reduction of hazardous currents to safe levels can be achieved by:

1. Decreasing the potential difference between points of contact with a possible voltage source
2. Increasing the impedance (resistance) in the possible current path (circuit), including the insulating of conducting surfaces (see Figure 10)

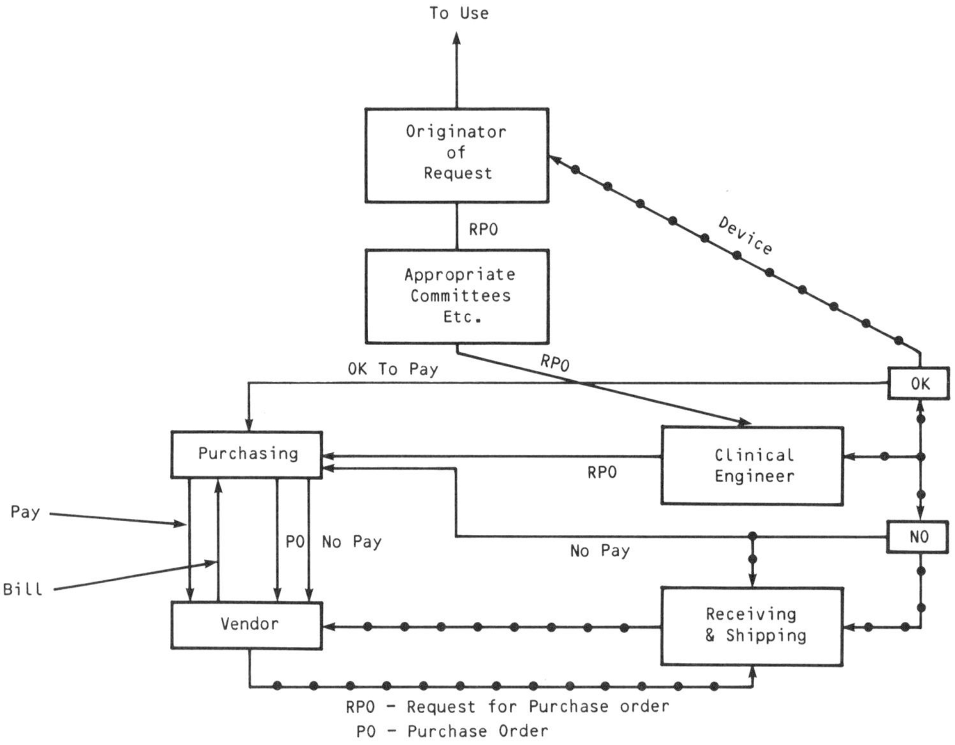

FIGURE 9. Suggested purchasing procedure.

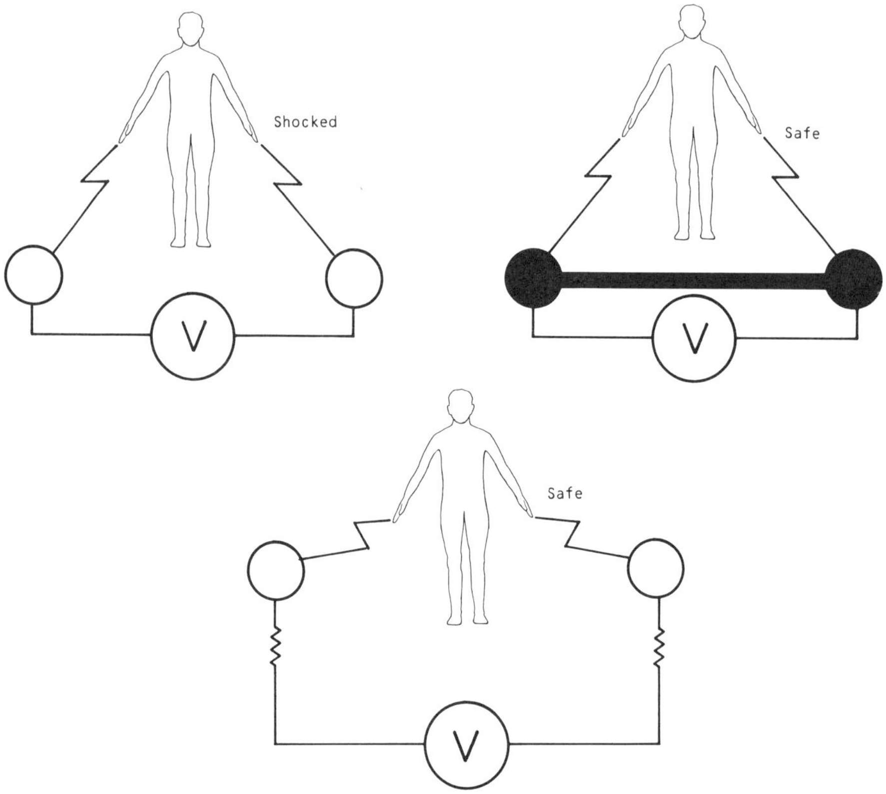

FIGURE 10. Protecting the patient from electric shock.

Implementing either of these procedures completely is virtually impossible, especially when wear and other time degradations of the system and the presence of the human element is considered. For this reason, standards of minimum performance have been established for various conditions and situations. It then remains to ascertain that the electromedical instrumentation system and all of its elements are meeting the performance standards. This may be achieved by conducting a program of inspection and tests (IT). Although combined here, they may be performed as separate functions. However, in most cases the visual inspection of the device or receptacle may be performed as part of the safety tests. In a sense, both are parts of what is often referred to as a preventive maintenance (PM) program. (See Appendix A for a protocol for the IT program.)

Whether of a new building or new device, the inspection and testing programs should begin as an incoming or acceptance inspection. A few years ago, records showed that up to 40% of new medical apparatus failed to meet specifications in some way.[32] In some cases, the fault was no more than a missing knob, but in at least one well-documented case (in the hospital files), a cardiac assist device had one of the patient leads connected to the 120-V live power conductor. Today, the quality control in medical device manufacturing has improved, but for a fully safe system, it behooves the hospital to conduct adequate inspection and test procedures on each piece of apparatus or each new section of the wiring system before allowing the unit to be used in the treatment of patients. Consider two examples where failure to do so could have resulted in tragedy. First, a new wing of a hospital was given the usual inspection and was accepted. However, when the hospital engineer started his own inspection before allowing patients to be moved in, he found that nearly one third of the receptacles were wired with wrong polarity, i.e., the live and neutral wires were reversed in their connections to the receptacles. This error does not affect the operation of equipment using the receptacles, but, for certain types of less expensive devices, it might result in having the metallic parts at 120 V so that a person touching such a device and ground could be lethally shocked.

In another hospital, the radiology department was moved to a wing with a new three-phase power supply. For nearly 3 yr after the X-ray department moved in, it was found that external grounds were required on the electrocardiographs when doing angiography (to avoid undue noise on the recordings whenever the X-ray equipment was operated). The electrical contractor failed to connect the grounding wire to the ground terminal of the distribution panel.

The inspection and testing of the electrical distribution system must include the operation of the emergency and alternate power components of the system according to NFPA 76A.[31] This portion of the test is especially important if any part of the building is to be used as intensive care or operating room facilities.

Once the electric power system has been accepted and activated, regularly scheduled testing and inspection is required to be sure that it maintains its original integrity.[1] Such inspections should begin with the terminals in the distribution panels to ascertain that all screws and nuts are tight. This might seem to be stretching the point, but one of the first reports (1960) on electric shock occurring during angiography gives the cause as the "ungrounding" of the system due to a loose connection in the main distribution panel. After tracing the grounding conductors to the receptacles, every receptacle should be checked. The frequency of such inspection and tests should be dependent upon the use of the receptacle and the immediacy of the situation. Most receptacles need to be checked only once a year, while others should be tested before every use. An example is a conscientious engineer who instituted and implemented a rule requiring a receptacle to be tested before it was used for an electrocardiogram. On the first day after the program began, a receptacle showed no ground. Further investigation showed that the ground wire was broken due to the fact that the wire had been nicked in stripping the insulation and building vibration had resulted in a fatigue failure of the wire.

In another case, a routine testing of all electric beds for leakage currents while grounded showed many of them to have such currents although the ground wires were intact. The fault lay in the poor ground contact in the receptacle. The moral here: test the pull required to remove the individual pins from the receptacle.

In older buildings, the first big item in the testing and inspection of receptacles is the location and replacement of all two wire outlets. This should be done everywhere, even in the administrator's office, if for no other reason than to eliminate all excuses for having an adaptor in the hospital. While this activity is going on, the elimination of all two wire extension cords should also be completed.

Specific tests of the integrity of the grounding conductors should include the measuring of the impedance of the ground-neutral loop and the resistance between grounding terminals and grounded conductive surfaces. Voltages between "grounds" and current flow through 1000 Ω between them should be measured.[17] After any modification or change in the electrical system, or other items which could affect the system, tests of the affected portions of the system should be made. If a receptacle is replaced, it should be tested for proper polarity after the change even though the work was done by the hospital's own trusted electrician. While it leaves much to be desired, at least the polarity of a receptacle wiring, the existence of a ground (though not its integrity), and to some extent the contact quality can be checked with some type of simple circuit tester. Finally, check both halves of the duplex receptacle. Where one half may be good, the other may have poor contact tension or may not be connected at all (especially is this true of the ground terminal).

The instrumentation and apparatus used anywhere in patient care areas should be tested in a manner paralleling that described for the electrical distribution system.[1] The incoming or acceptance inspection and tests are the beginning of a continuous program of periodic and special tests that continue until the device is retired. The program may have several classifications for the inspections and tests.

1. Beginning with the acceptance inspection and testing referred to above, this phase should include calibration and other performance tests, as well as those which are designed to determine that the device is electrically safe.
2. All patient care equipment should be tested at least semiannually, and the more critical devices should be tested quarterly.
3. Some apparatus such as that associated with cardiac surgery should be inspected and tested before each use. The extent of the testing will depend upon the criticalness of the device and time between uses, but should be as near 100% assurance of proper operation and safety as possible.
4. Any device which has been used hard, dropped, or in any way mishandled should be tested before being used, or returned to the shelf.
5. After repair, all devices should be thoroughly tested, including calibration where applicable.

All nonpatient care equipment, i.e., equipment which is not expected to come into contact with the patient or not to be involved in any way that could affect the patient's health, need to be tested annually.

While most inspections and tests will be performed by a clinical engineer or biomedical equipment technician, nurses and other hospital personnel should be aware of the need for constant attention to the electrical safety aspects of the apparatus they use. They can look for cracks in power cord insulation, broken receptacles and plugs, etc. and report such deficiencies to the proper authority.

Maintenance and Repair

Case histories accumulated by insurance carriers and others show that 50% of all failures of equipment in hospitals can be traced to inadequate maintenance. Perhaps more startling is the fact that 30% of these failures can be shown to be due to poor lubrication practices — too little, too much, or "sloppy" lubrication. Of course, much of the equipment in the hospital requires maintenance other than lubrication, but the same principle applies. The safety and reliability of the electromedical instrumentation system depends upon immediate and proper maintenance or repair when the inspection and testing program indicates the need. Hopefully, such maintenance will forestall the need for repair because the equipment has failed.

Because the equipment in a hospital ranges from the facility heating and ventilating system to water heaters to the sophistication of monitoring, maintenance of automatic clinical laboratory devices and life support apparatus is a varied and difficult activity. The education and experience required by the personnel performing the maintenance function ranges from semiskilled tradesmen to clinical or biomedical technicians and engineers with extensive preparation beyond high school. Therefore, it becomes particularly difficult for the small (e.g., less than 100 beds) hospital to have an adequate in-house staff.

The maintenance function can be carried on in a number of ways. If the hospital is large enough, no doubt the best answer is an in-house staff with the capability to handle all of the work. Other methods include using: (1) the manufacturer's service representative or service center, (2) private contractors who provide a staff of qualified personnel to perform maintenance of medical apparatus and in some cases provide maintenance service for other systems of the hospital, and (3) a shared service organization in which two or more hospitals join in the operation of a service organization suitable to meet their combined needs.[33]

A major component in the administration of a functional safety program, especially as it applies to the electromedical instrumentation system, is education. It is difficult to say where the educational process should begin. Certainly, the administrator himself must be aware that a hazard exists and that there is need for corrective measures. Many hospital engineers complain that their biggest problem is convincing their administrator that certain areas of the hospital need rewiring or whatever the problem may be. It would appear, then, that education of the administrator is the first point in the program.[34]

This effort of reaching the administrators probably belongs in the hands of hospital organizations such as the American Hospital Association (AHA). The AHA holds seminars on electrical safety especially for administrators, and aids local or state associations in conducting the same. Set up for the business heads of your hospital, this kind of meeting helps to give the administrator an appreciation of the hazard and a basis from which he can proceed to other programs.

The physician needs to be informed also. He and the engineers have produced much equipment which has contributed immeasurably to the diagnosis and treatment of disease. However, the physician may not be aware that his device can become a lethal weapon if misused or not properly built and maintained. Many are unaware of the need for grounding electrical devices or otherwise making them safe for both the operator and the patient.

Special short courses for the education of the medical staff of the hospital is the obvious answer to this problem. They must be carefully planned and to the point if the busy physician is to be a participant. To a very great extent, the responsibility for the safe use of medical instrumentation and equipment falls on the attending nurse or nursing technician of some specific designation. Usually, a specialist in the operation of the electrocardiograph may be dispatched from central services to connect a machine to a patient and take an ECG recording. The staff in the coronary care unit will have training along similar lines. Often, however, the personnel are primarily nurses by interest and training, while the technicalities of the devices are left to others. The few who take the initiative to learn more of the technical details usually will also have continued to study the material of nursing as well, and will soon be promoted to supervisory positions. Here, the nurse's attention will, of necessity, be turned to personnel problems, budgets, and other matters. If she continues her interest in intrumentation technology, it will often be only for the purpose of more intelligently writing requisitions for the new equipment.

The rank and file of her staff are, therefore, bereft of the supervisor's knowledge of technical things such as the hazards of improper use of two-wire extension cords and the failure to report any apparent malfunction of a piece of equipment. It is here, then, that the needs of in-service training become most apparent. In addition, the development of new electromedical devices is so rapid that a continuing program of instruction is needed. Often, to this must be added the rapid turnover of staff in the critical areas of the hospital.

Obviously, instruction in electromedical equipment may not need to be required for all nursing personnel; only those who may be called upon to operate it may need to take the course. On the other hand, because of the necessity to transfer personnel from one area to another at times, as many as are interested should be encouraged to participate.

Two types of courses seem to be required: one to give basic information and the first-time-over instruction, and another to refresh and update. In each, a demonstration laboratory is a valuable asset. There are many texts and audio-visual aids available for use in these instructional sessions.[7,35,36]

An important part of the safety education program is what to do if an accident does occur. No matter how carefully the electrical system has been designed, no matter how carefully the equipment has been selected and cared for, and no matter how carefully the entire electromedical instrumentation system is used, accidents will happen. It is important, therefore, to be on watch for a possible accident and to take steps to prevent a reoccurrence.

In the event that a patient or other person in the area believes he has been shocked by any piece of equipment, if the fact of a shock exists, or if there is any reason to believe that a case of ventricular fibrillation or cardiac arrest has occurred as a result of electric shock, the case should be reported immediately to the appropriate authority. If death has resulted, the area should be sealed off and the equipment in the area impounded.

An investigation in the form of a full inspection and test should be carried out on the system in use and all personnel involved should be questioned to determine completely and immediately all the facts. The results should be included in the incident report. The exact procedure should be worked out for the hospital by the engineer and other appropriate administrative staff and should be followed implicitly. The importance of this protocol cannot be stressed too highly in the educational program on electromedical instrumentation safety.

Documentation

The JCAH manual repeatedly states that "written policies and procedures shall be established" for many aspects of safety in the hospital.[1] The subject of safety in the electromedical instrumentation system is included with the several details of the scope of the safety program delineated. Such a "policies and procedure" manual is the beginning of the documentation required to assure that the hospital intends to comply with the appropriate codes and standards; records of the inspections, tests, and maintenance procedures provide evidence that it has complied.

The record system can be as simple as a file cabinet for the small hospital with relatively few pieces of equipment, to a computerized system for the larger hospital (or even for the smaller hospital if it has computer facilities).[37-39] In any case, the record will, in general, contain the same kind of information:

1. A set of manuals for each piece of equipment will be included. In some cases, two or more copies of some of the manuals, such as the operating instructions, will be needed, e.g., one for the user and one for the engineering and technician staff, for example.
2. An identifying code number for each piece of apparatus that is simpler and more easily read than the serial number placed on the device by the manufacturer will also be included. It could simply be an acquisition number starting with 00001, e.g., or it could be coded to show the usual location for the device or its type, etc. A special decal or tag identifying the hospital and carrying the number should be attached to each piece of equipment in a conspicuous place; an index file of these numbers should be maintained in a central location.
3. An equipment control record or similarly named form will be prepared when each device is ordered, and appropriate information will be entered when it is received. This record should include information on inspection, testing, calibration, and maintenance in an abbreviated though clearly identifiable manner. Such a record will gather information on what device failures, if any, are most frequent. Also, the record may help plan a preventive maintenance program, as well as serve as a guide for further purchases of similar devices
4. A standing work order will be prepared for each device which details the kinds of inspections, tests, and maintenance that are to be performed on it. By some coding device, the frequency of such regular services will also be recorded. If a card file is used, the color of the card may be used as the coding method. The form should have space in which the actual work performed can be recorded (this is transferred later in briefer form to the control record).
5. A record of all incidents of any undesirable nature which involve any part of the electromedical instrumentation system will be included in the documentation. These reports should be available to the engineering and technician staff for study as to the existence of any condition which might be related to the safety program (PITMED). (See Appendix A.)

CODES AND STANDARDS

Health care is among the most regulated industries in the U.S. More than 28 organizations and governmental agencies through over 130 committees have written some 1200 standards dealing with health care devices and practices, in addition to the pharmaceutical regulations promulgated through the Food and Drug Administration.[40] Many of these standards have been established by a consensus process in which interested associations, manufacturers, and individuals all contribute.

Electrical safety in hospitals is one of the regulated areas. Reference has been made to several codes and standards published by the National Fire Protection Association (NFPA). For many years, NFPA has served as the agency which codifies the state of the art and science of engineering in terms of appropriate practices. The result is the National Fire Codes, one section of which is the National Electrical Code (NEC). Associated with the NEC are several standards and recommended practices which have been assembled in a single package called "Basic Library of Health Care Safety".[41]

The National Electrical Code is not a law and NFPA is not a legislative body. However, its work has been so well-recognized that most of its codes are adopted by state and local governments; in this process, they become mandatory regulations or laws. Safety in the electromedical instrumentation system is covered by the NEC (NFPA 70), and standards NFPA 56A, NFPA 76A, and NFPA 76C. These codes and standards, as interpreted and supplemented by federal, state, and local agencies such as Medicare, boards of health, fire marshalls, etc. set the safety criteria for electrical power supply systems. They also provide some guidance in setting specifications for much of the electromedical instrumentation.

Other associations which have written electrical safety standards include the Association for the Advancement of Medical Instrumentation (AAMI) and the American Heart Association.[42] The AAMI standard "Safe Current Limits for Electromedical Apparatus" is approved by the American National Standards Institute (ANSI).[43]

One of the responsibilities of the safety committee of each hospital is to be familiar with the codes and standards governing all phases of the hospital operation. This responsibility extends to safety in the electromedical instrumentation system.

SUMMARY

Electrical safety in the hospital, particularly in the electromedical instrumentation system, is vital to the overall safety of the facility. Achieving electrical safety is the responsibility of the entire staff, but it is primarily the work of the clinical engineering and technician staff. Clinical engineering services may either be obtained through an in-house staff or contracted to outside agencies or shared service arrangement.

Reducing or eliminating electrical hazards may be accomplished by careful attention to five basic functions: (1) purchasing, (2) inspection and testing, (3) maintenance or repair, (4) education, and (5) documentation.

APPENDIX A: AN ITM PROTOCOL INSPECTION TESTING MAINTENANCE

INTRODUCTION

This protocol has been prepared as a minimal guide to the formation of an electrical safety and clinical engineering service in a hospital, and as the basis for a policies and procedures manual suited to the needs and methods of the hospital. It should be expanded to cover the entire electromedical instrumentation system. The forms presented are suggestions only; they may be used directly, modified to fit the patterns used by the hospital in other forms, or commercially prepared forms offered by the manufacturers of test instruments or other agencies may be used (see also the section "Safety in Special Care Units" in this handbook).

THE ELECTRICAL SYSTEM SAFETY SURVEY

The objective of the survey is to establish and implement procedures for maintaining the level of electrical safety and performance prescribed by the JCAH, the National Electrical Code, and other applicable standards. The activities of the electrical system safety program shall be coordinated with and by the hospital safety committee.

Each receptacle in every patient care area shall be inspected and tested at least annually in accordance with the electrical system safety procedure, and the results recorded on the receptacle inspection form. Recommendations for correcting unsatisfactory conditions shall be made and appropriate action taken.

When the inspection and testing survey is completed, the forms and other pertinent information shall be filed in the office of the engineering department.

Necessary equipment includes

1. Receptacle contact tension tester
2. Receptacle ground and polarity tester
3. Resistance substitution box
4. A.C. multimeter with low resistance ohmeter or a specialized test set

INSPECTION AND TEST PROCEDURES FOR NORMAL DISTRIBUTION SYSTEMS

A receptacle inspection form shall be prepared for each room or area showing the location of all receptacles and noting the type of circuit (N = normal, I = isolated, E = emergency, etc.). Each receptacle shall be checked and the results recorded on this form (see Figure 11).

For normal wiring system, power on, the following shall be determined or measured:

1. Existence of "green" wire or equivalent (NFPA 70, Art 210-5(b), 250-25 517-11)
2. Proper polarization
3. Mechanical integrity
4. Contact tension
5. Ground loop impedance
6. Voltage, neutral to grounding pole
7. Voltage grounding pole to exposed metal
8. Voltage grounding pole to all other ground poles in patient vicinity

Date of Inspection: ____________ Hospital: ____________________

Nominal Voltage: ________________ Area: ____________ Rm. No. ________

RECEPTACLE INSPECTION FORM

Sheet No. _____ Of _____

ACTION

Not Needed ☐ Needed ☐ Taken ☐

	BASIC INSPECTION								SUPPLEMENTAL INSPECTION XX				
	MECHANICAL TENSION				WIRING					Resis- tance to			
No.	OK	Defects	OK	Low	OK	Defects	Type	Line Voltage	Voltage to Building Ground	Building Ground	Ground Loop Impedance	OK	Action Needed: XXX (see reverse side)
1.													
2.													
3.													
4.													
5.													
6.													
7.													
8.													
9.													
10.													

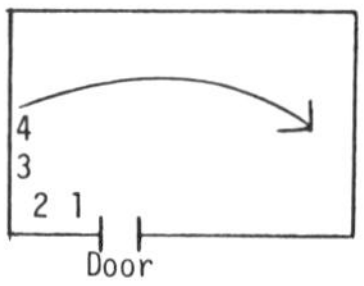

* Number each receptable only once whether single or duplex

** Use only when testing new installation or if problem exists

*** Use back of sheet for additional comments

Receptable Type: N - Normal E - Emergency I - Isolated

FIGURE 11. Receptacle inspection form.

For normal wiring system, power off, the following shall be measured:

1. Resistance, neutral to grounding pole
2. Resistance, grounding pole to exposed metal
3. Resistance between grounding poles

INSPECTION AND TEST PROCEDURES FOR ISOLATED DISTRIBUTION SYSTEMS

Isolated power system inspection and testing consists of two parts.

Part 1 — Test the line isolation monitor (LIM) by using the test button on the LIM panel. This test shall be performed at least monthly. If the test results are satisfactory, this and the date shall be recorded on a LIM test record affixed to the panel of the LIM. If unsatisfactory, Part 2 of the test shall be performed, and recommendations for immediate correcting of the condition shall be made.

Part 2 — The entire isolated power system shall be inspected and tested at least semiannually in the following manner, and recorded on the appropriate form (see Figure 12).

First, each receptacle supplied by the system shall be inspected and tested for mechanical integrity and tension.

For power on, the following tests and measurements shall be made on the LIM system:

1. Measure and record LIM current
2. Test push button for sounding alarm
3. Inspect general integrity
4. Measure and record the current from each line to ground which causes alarm.

Hospital: ______________________
Date: ______________________

ISOLATED POWER SYSTEM INSPECTION FORM

Location Manufacturer

Model Serial No.

Type: Dynamic☐ Static☐ Alarm level ________ mA

ACTION
Not Needed☐ Needed☐ Taken☐
Removed From Service
See notes reverse side)

3
2
1
Door

A. Inspect and test each receptacle supplied by the system and record on receptacle inspection form and attack to this form.

B.1. Power On

a. LIM Meter current ____________

b. Push button test ____________

c. LIM general integrity

d. Current Line to ground to course alarm

Line 1 ________ Line 2 ________

e. Resistance Line to ground to course alarm

Line 1 ________ Line 2 ________

B.2. POWER OFF

a. Resistance between line and ground.

Line 1 ________ Line 2 ________

b. Resistance between receptacle ground pole and building ground.

Receptacle No.	1	2	3	4	5	6	7	8	9
Resistance									

FIGURE 12. Isolated power system inspection form.

For power off, the following tests and measurements shall be made on the LIM system:

1. Measure and record resistance between each line and ground
2. Measure and record resistance between grounding pole and building ground and other exposed conductive surfaces
3. Measure and record resistance between grounding poles of the receptacles

EMERGENCY POWER SYSTEMS

Testing

The emergency power system of the hospital shall be exercised underload on a regular basis for not less than a 30-min period at intervals of not less than 30 days, or in accordance with manufacturers recommendation. An appropriate permanent record of the test shall be maintained, containing date and time of test, duration of run, time required to start and provide power, current and voltage readings, and any pertinent remarks concerning the functioning of the system.

All preventive maintenance, including other inspections and repairs, shall be recorded along with the exercising test records.

GENERAL PURPOSE

ELECTROMEDICAL INSTRUMENTATION

INSPECTION, TEST AND INVENTORY RECORD

Hospital ______________________ Date ____________

Item ____________ Mftr.____ Type__________

Hospital No. ___________ Serial No. ____ Date Purchase ______

Visual Inspection

1. Plug:
2. Cord and strain relief:
3. Case exterior:

Interior:

4. Groundage Resistance
5. Leakage Tests - current in ma

	Off		Operating Correct Polarity		Operating Reverse	
	From	To	From	To	From	To
		I(ma)		I(ma)		I(ma)
1.						
2.						
3.						
4.						
5.						
6.						
7.						

6. Other Inspections and Tests   Inspected by

Recommendations   Date

FIGURE 13. General purpose electromedical instrumentation inspection, test, and inventory record.

EXTENSION CORDS AND ADAPTORS

The use of extension cords shall be kept to a minimum. Only extension cords made and tested by physical plant or clinical engineering personnel shall be permitted. All such cords shall be made of 16 gauge conductors or heavier (JCAH Functional Safety and Sanitation, Standard II).

Testing

All adaptors and extension cords shall be tested on the same schedule as the receptacles of the electrical power system of the hospital, or at least annually.

MEDICAL INSTRUMENTATION SAFETY SURVEY

All new electrically operated medical devices shall be tested when received, and all existing equipment shall be tested as part of a survey of the electromedical instrumentation system. Initially, a general test and inspection procedure may be used and the results recorded on the general purpose form. The results of this survey provide a complete inventory of the hospital instrumentation and establishes a basis for a continuing program. Appropriate information shall also be entered on a maintenance record. An inspection, testing, and maintenance standing order shall also be prepared. As the

ELECTROMEDICAL INSTRUMENTATION

INSPECTION, TESTING AND MAINTENANCE RECORD

EQUIPMENT ITEM	MANUFACTURER
HOSPITAL NUMBER	MODEL AND TYPE
DATE PURCHASED	SERIAL NUMBER
VENDOR	VENDOR ADDRESS
DESCRIPTION	
NORMAL LOCATION IN HOSPITAL	

DATE	OK/FAULT	ACTION TAKEN	TIME	PARTS COST	REMARKS	OK BY

FIGURE 14. Electromedical instrumentation inspection, testing, and maintenance record.

program develops, forms for specific apparatus may be devised to suit the hospital program (see Figures 13 and 14).

Equipment

Necessary equipment include

1. Receptacle polarity tester
2. Leakage current meter and switching box or special test set
3. Multimeter
4. Additional equipment as required
5. Hand tools

Inspection and Test Procedures

1. **Attachment plug** — Inspect and note condition of plug. Check to see that it is a three-wire plug and that all three blades are intact.
2. **Line cord and strain reliefs** — Check overall condition of power cord for breaks or cracks in the insulation (particularly at the points where it connects to the plug and the chassis). Examine strain reliefs at both ends of the line cord (and at both ends of any other cord on the device), and note any conditions that require replacement.
3. **Case** — Clean the exterior. If the interior is accessible, remove any dust.
4. **Grounding resistance** — Test continuity between grounding pin and equipment chassis with ohmmeter to be sure resistance is no greater than 01.5 Ω. To insure that there are no breaks in the line, the cord should be flexed at both ends while this test is being conducted.
5. **Leakage current** — The receptacle to be used shall be tested to determine if it has been properly wired (i.e., of correct polarity and adequately grounded). The

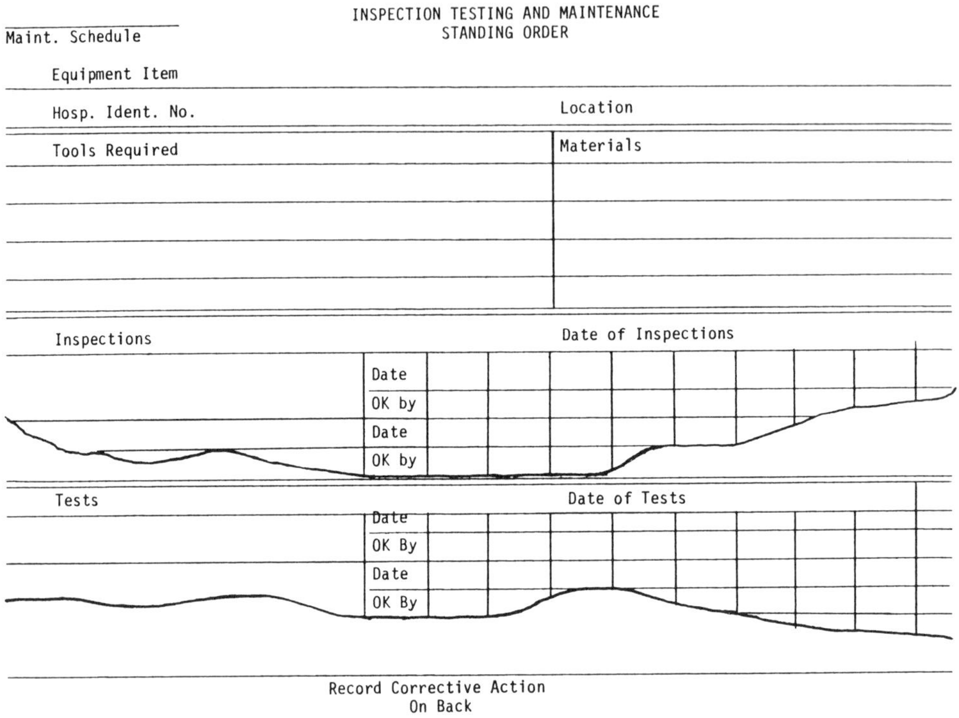

INSPECTION TESTING AND MAINTENANCE
STANDING ORDER

Maint. Schedule

Equipment Item

Hosp. Ident. No. — Location

Tools Required — Materials

Inspections — Date of Inspections

Date
OK by
Date
OK by

Tests — Date of Tests

Date
OK By
Date
OK By

Record Corrective Action
On Back

FIGURE 15. Inspection testing and maintenance standing order.

leakage current between equipment chassis and ground, including the leakage current in the grounding conductor, shall then be measured in both the off and operating positions for each of the following wiring modes: grounded, correct polarity; ungrounded, correct polarity; and ungrounded, reversed polarity.

6. **Other inspections and tests** — This space is to be used to record the condition, operation, and performance of features that may be unique to the device being tested.

MAINTENANCE RECORDS

A running record of the inspection, testing, and maintenance of each piece of apparatus shall be recorded on a form which is so labeled.

To facilitate regular tests, inspections, and maintenance of all apparatus, a standing order for each device shall be prepared and placed in an appropriate shop file (see Figure 15).

ELECTRICAL SYSTEM REMEDIAL ACTION

When inspection of the electrical system reveals a defective component (receptacle, etc.) that defect shall be noted and remedial action taken in the following manner:

1. A service request shall be prepared for each defect, and approved according to hospital procedures (see Figure 16).
2. Corrective action shall be taken by the workman assigned to the job. After the repair is finished, the affected receptacle(s) shall be tested by checking polarity and tension.

Enter number of main chassis or module

SERVICE REQUEST

	Control Number

FROM	Date	Time
Department	Location	
Person Making Request / Telephone Ext.	Verbal Request Placed ☐ Yes ☐ No	

Item

Problem (Brief statement of malfunction or failure, other devices involved, conditions and time of occurrence, whether constant or intermittent fault, if human error was contributory, etc.)

Approved	Date

Person Assigned

Work Performed

Signed	Date Completed

FIGURE 16. Service request.

3. When the work and testing is completed, the action taken shall be noted on the requisition form, signed and dated by the workman, and entered into the appropriate receptacle inspection form.

Instrumentation Remedial Action

When the medical instrumentation survey or any other inspection reveals that a device is defective in some way, it shall be appropriately tagged, and remedial action taken in the following manner:

1. A service request shall be prepared for each defect, and approved according to hospital procedures.
2. If the defect can be corrected by the hospital staff (e.g., replacement of power cord or repair of electrical bed), the action shall be taken by the workman assigned to the job. After the repair is finished, the action shall be noted on the repair requisition form, signed and dated by the workman, and the information entered into the appropriate maintenance record.

POLICY ON THE USE OF PERSONAL ELECTRICAL EQUIPMENT

Electrical equipment (radio, shavers, etc.) brought in by patients shall be permitted to be used only after such equipment has been inspected, tested, and approved by the clinical engineering service in the manner described in this handbook. Electrical equipment (radios, shavers, etc.) owned by employees of the hospital shall not be permitted in patient care areas of the hospital.

Electrical apparatus, instruments, and devices used in diagnosis and treatment, but not owned and listed by the hospital, again shall be used only after such equipment has been inspected, tested, and approved by the clinical engineering service in the manner described in this handbook.

INCIDENT REPORTING

For an electrical system and instrumentation safety and effectiveness program to work satisfactorily, every incident involving the items included in the program must be recorded. The incident reporting form furnished by the American Hospital Association, or a similar form, should be used. If a person has received or believes he has received a shock from a piece of equipment, a report shall be made.

The incident report may be used to initiate a service request with follow-up as previously described, including recording on the appropriate form and filing.

LIMIT VALUES ON MEASUREMENTS IN ELECTRICAL SAFETY SURVEY

1. Leakage current in ground wire of power cord or from exposed metal surfaces to ground: devices likely to touch patients, including beds — 100 μA; devices not likely to touch patients, e.g., floor polishers — 500 μA; and from patient leads to ground or between leads — 50 μA
2. Resistance of grounding conductor in power cord — 0.15 Ω
3. Voltage between conductive surfaces in building structure or from conductive surfaces on equipment to electrical ground — 40 mV

FREQUENCY OF TESTS

1. Clinical devices — at least semiannually or as needed
2. Nonclinical apparatus including electrical beds — at least annually or as needed (in critical care areas, the tests should be at least quarterly, or more often if problems are observed)
3. Electrical system including receptacles — at least annually or as needed
4. Any device, receptacle, or other electrical apparatus should be tested after a report of possible shock or other incident; repair or replacement; hard use (dropping, etc.); the device or a part of it appears to be worn; or before being used after receipt from manufacturer

All questionable apparatus should be tagged as not to be used.

GENERAL REFERENCES

Cromwell, L., Weibill, F. J., Pfeiffer, E. A., and Usselman, L. B., *Biomedical Instrumentation and Measurements,* Prentice-Hall, Englewood Cliffs, N.J., 1973.

Diefenderfer, A. J., *Principles of Electronic Instrumentation,* W. B. Saunders, Philadelphia, 1972.

Fleming, D. C. and Feinberg, B. N., Eds., *Handbook of Medicine and Biology, Sections A, B, and C,* Vol. 1, CRC Press, Boca Raton, Fla., 1976, 1978 and 1980.

Jacobsen, B. and Webster, J. G., *Medicine and Clinical Engineering,* Prentice-Hall, Englewood Cliffs, N.J., 1977.

Ray, C. D., Ed., *Medical Engineering,* Year Book Medical Publishing, Chicago, 1974.

Spooner, R. B., Ed., *Hospital Instrumentation Care and Servicing,* Instrumentation Society of America, Pittsburgh, 1977.

Webster, J. G. and Cook, A. M., *Clinical Engineering,* Prentice-Hall, Englewood Cliffs, N.J., 1979.

REFERENCES

1. Accreditation Manual for Hospitals, Joint Commission on Accreditation of Hospitals, Chicago, 1979.
2. **Walter, C. W.,** Electrical hazard in hospitals, *Hosp. Pract.,* 5, 53, 1970.
3. **Nader, R.,** Nader says 5000 killed in hospitals, *South Bend Tribune, (Indiana),* June 18, 1970.
4. **Bruner, J. M. R., Aronow, S., and Cavicchi, R. V.,** Electrical incidents in a large hospital: a 42-month register, *J. Assoc. Adv. Med. Instrum.,* 6, 222, 1972.
5. **Bruner, J. M. R.,** Hospitals, *J. Am. Hosp. Assoc.,* 49, 15, 1975.
6. **Karselis, T.,** *Descriptive Medical Electronics and Instrumentation,* Charles B. Slack, Thorofare, N.J., 1973.
7. **Roth, H. H., Teltscher, E. S., and Kane, I. M.,** *Electrical Safety in Health Care Facilities,* Academic Press, New York, 1975.
8. **Dalziel, C. F.,** The threshold of perception currents, *Electr. Eng.* 73, 625, 1954.
9. **Dalziel, C. F. and Lee, W. R.,** Reevaluation of lethal electric currents, *IEEE Trans. Ind. Gen. Appl.,* 4, 467, 1959.
10. **Thomas, H. E.,** *Handbook Biomedical Instrumentation and Measurement,* Reston Publishing Co., Reston, Va., 1974.
11. **Weinberg, D. L., Artley, J. L., Whalen, R. E., and McIntosch, H. D.,** Electric shock hazards in cardiac catheterization, *Circ. Res.,* 4, 467, 1959.
12. **Roy, O. Z.,** The parameters of fibrillation for 60 Hz current applied directly to the heart, annual meeting of the Association for the Advancement of Medical Instrumentation, Las Vegas, May 23, 1979.
13. **Leeming, M. N.,** Low voltage direct current burns *JAMA,* 9, 1681, 1970.
14. High Frequency Electricity in Health Care Facilities NFPA 76C, National Fire Protection Association, Boston, 1975.
15. Health Devices, Plymouth meeting, Emergency Care Research Institute, Pennsylvania, June-July 1973.
16. **Battig, C. G.,** Electrosurgery burn injuries and their prevention, *JAMA,* 204, 1025, 1968.
17. National Electrical Code (NFPA 70), National Fire Protection Association, Boston, 1978.
18. **Deno, D. W. and Zaffanella, L. E.,** Electrostatic effects of overhead transmission lines and stations, in *Transmission Line Reference Book, 345 KV and Above,* Electric Power Research Institute, Palo Alto, Calif., 1975, chap. 8.
19. **Dalziel, C. F.,** A Study of the Hazards of Impulse Currents, *AIEE Trans.,* 72, 1032, 1953.
20. **Geddes, L. E. and Baker, L. E.,** *Applied Biomedical Instrumentation,* John Wiley & Sons, New York, 1975.
21. **Gibson, R. S.,** Requirements for the Use of Electrical Stimulation of the Skin, Proc. Int. Congr. on Technology and Blindness, American Foundation for the Blind, New York, 1963.
22. Institute of Physics in London, Static electrification: a symposium, *Br. J. Appl. Phys.,* Suppl. 2, 1953.
23. Static Electricity (NFPA 77), National Fire Protection Association, Boston, 1977.
24. **McCarty, R. J. and Glasser, S. P.,** The arrhythmogenic effect of static electricity on the dog heart, *Am. Heart J.,* 93, 496, 1977.

25. Inhalation Anesthetics (NFPA 56A), National Fire Protection Association, Boston, 1973.
26. **Sereda, P. J. and Feldman, R. F.**, Electrostatic charging on fabrics at various humidities, *J. Text. Inst.*, 55, T288, 1964.
27. **Stanley, P. E.**, Monitors that save lives can also kill, *Mod. Hosp.*, 108, 119, 1967.
28. The Medical Device Amendments of 1976 (Public Law 94-295), Amendment of the Food, Drug and Cosmetics Act, May 28, 1976.
29. Good manufacturing practice regulations for manufacture, packing, storage and installation — medical devices, *Fed. Regist.* 42(40), 11, 998, 1977.
30. The Acquisition and Maintenance of Medical Equipment, U.S. Department of Commerce, December 1975.
31. Essential Electrical Systems for Health Care Facilities (NFPA 76A), National Fire Protection Association, Boston, 1977.
32. **Ben-Zvi, S.**, The lack of safety standards in medical instrumentation, *Trans. N.Y. Acad. Sci.*, 31, 737, 1969.
33. **Dodson, B., Jr. and Latimer, B. W.**, *Strategies for Clinical Engineering Through Shared Services*, Carolinas Hospital and Health Services, Inc., Charlotte, N.C., 1976.
34. **Ostrander, L. E.**, Presentation of the clinical engineering role to hospital administrators, *J. Clin. Eng.*, 4(1), 11, 1979.
35. **Arnold, B. E. and Pacela, A. F.**, Audio Visual Aids for Hospital Safety Programs, Quest Publishing Co., Diamond Bar, Calif., 1976.
36. **Link, L. J. and Feinberg, B.**, *Electrical Safety in Hospitals*, American Sterilizer Co., Erie, Pa., 1976.
37. **Cameron, H. R.**, Preventive Maintenance in Clinical Instrumentation, Presented at annual meeting of AAMI, March 1975, Boston, MA.
38. **Neuberg, J., Hunt, D., Budkin, A., and Katchis, L. J.**, An automated electrical safety and preventive maintenance program, *J. Clin. Eng.* 4, 71, 1979.
39. **Schwartz, L.**, A computer-assisted preventive maintenance system, *J. Clin. Eng.*, 4, 66, 1979.
40. **Pacela, A. F. and Arnold, B. E.**, The Guide to Biomedical Standards, Quest Publishing Co., Diamond Bar, Calif., 1976.
41. Basic Library of Health Safety, National Fire Protection Association, Boston, continuously updated.
42. Standards for a Cardiac Catheterization Laboratory, Circulation XLII, American Heart Association, 1970, 557.
43. Safe Current Limits for Electromedical Apparatus, Association for the Advancement of Medical Instrumentation, Arlington, Va., 1975.

THE EMERGENCY ROOM

Paul R. Seidlitz

INTRODUCTION

During the past 30 years, the utilization of emergency departments has grown. The reasons for this growth have been the cause of a great deal of discussion and heated debate. Some of the factors that may account for this growth are

1. Since World War II, the emphasis in medical education has been on specialization and this specialization has led to the disappearance of the general practitioner.
2. Patients now expect sophisticated treatment in a hospital rather than at home.
3. There has been a dramatic rise in the accident rate from high-speed driving and the use of alcohol and/or drugs.
4. Increased longevity has increased the number of elderly in the emergency department.

Admittedly, many of the patients seeking treatment in an emergency room do not require this level of care and/or treatment and even though there have been efforts to educate the public, there are still large numbers of patients seeking treatment in the emergency room. In general, there are two reasons why people go to the emergency room for treatment: (1) it is the appropriate site for the condition and (2) other sources of care cannot be used.

The American public is exposed to a great deal of health education material and while some of this material is not always accurate, magazine articles and television programs do stimulate the public to action. When a patient comes into an emergency department, he feels that his appearance should cause everyone to "jump into action" because that is how it is done on television; it does not matter that his symptoms are vague and he has had them for several days. He wants immediate service.

When one considers other sources of care, we must remember that a patient may come into the emergency department because alternate sources of care do not exist in his/her area or if they do exist, they are not accessible when the patient needs treatment. Also, the patient may not want to use the alternate source of treatment (see Figure 1). The publication in 1966 of Accidental Death and Disability: The Neglected Disease of Modern Science (the Division of Medical Science, National Academy of Sciences) is considered by many to be the most single-provoking stimulus to improve emergency services. This publication stressed the difference competent initial medical care, efficient transportation, and active treatment could make in survival rates. With this stimulation came expenditures to improve many emergency departments, and with this improvement came increased utilization as the public became aware of the service. All emergency rooms are used appropriately some of the time and as long as alternate sources of medical care are not accessible to the patient when he/she needs this care, the emergency department can expect to continue to treat the nonemergency patient. The hospital emergency department can expect to continue its role in treatment of critically ill or injured patients as well as the "convenience" patients.

EMERGENCY ROOM ORGANIZATION

Hospital emergency departments also are prepared to meet disaster situations that can and do occur when we least expect or want them. Emergency rooms are equipped

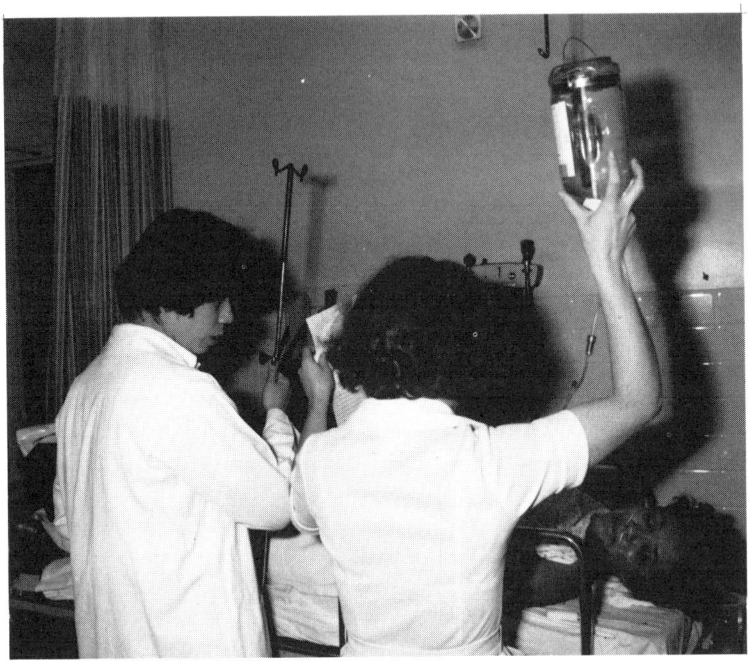

FIGURE 1. The emergency department staff may be the first experience the patient will have in the hospital. (Courtesy of Steven Carey and Allan McLean, Rush-Presbyterian-St. Luke's Medical Center.)

to handle this type of situation partly because of the increased utilization, partly because of public awareness of the service, and partly because of legislation. The Highway Safety Act of 1966 contains a standard that states must demonstrate an intent to develop an effective emergency medical services program. This standard has been reviewed and updated to include training of the ambulance personnel. In 1969 the Department of Transportation published the Requirement for Ambulance Design and Equipment, and with the General Service Administration (GSA), developed federal specification for ambulance design.

In January 1972, the President of the U.S. directed the U.S. Department of Health, Education and Welfare to develop new ways to organize emergency medical services, and later that year $8.5 million in contracts were awarded to develop model EMS systems. In 1973, the Emergency Medical System Act (PL93-154) was adopted. The act provides for assistance and encouragement for the development of comprehensive area emergency medical services. In 1974, the Public Health Service provided $26.6 million for this program. One of the requirements of the Joint Commission on Accreditation of Hospitals (JCAH) is that the hospital "must inform the community it serves of its capabilities and limitations in handling a disaster" (see Figure 2).

All of these factors have had their impact on emergency-department utilization. Taxpayers are aware of how some of their money is being spent. They want only the best for themselves or their loved ones and if they do not get the service, there are serious legal implications.

PHYSICIAN-PATIENT RELATIONSHIP

Medical malpractice suits are increasing at an unprecedented rate and most claims are based on the following factors:

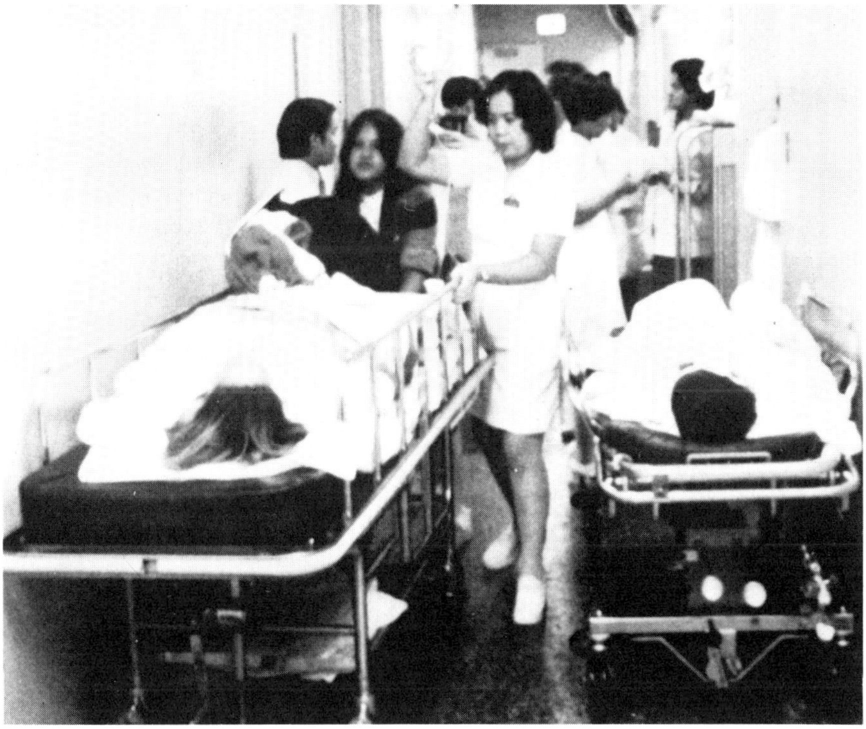

FIGURE 2. The emergency department can be exceptionally busy. (Courtesy of Steven Carey and Allan McLean, Rush-Presbyterian-St. Luke's Medical Center.)

1. Unsatisfactory relationship with the physician
2. A poor result
3. A bill the patient considers excessive

Kindness, consideration, and sensitivity to the patient sets the tone for a good relationship. This is not only true for the physician in the emergency department, but the staff that is assigned to the emergency department as well. A patient who respects and trusts his physician and the staff assigned to assist in his/her care and treatment will not mistrust or misunderstand the actions being taken. However, when the physician and emergency-department staff are abrasive and insensitive, this will breed mistrust and a lack of confidence.

Poor Results

On occasion, a poor result may be due to negligence on the part of the physician or staff. However, a patient may bring on a suit because he/she does not understand exactly what the end result may be. This often occurs if the physician and/or emergency staff does not fully inform the patient. A recent malpractice study conducted by HEW showed a high rate of diagnostic trauma error in incidents of trauma occurring in the emergency room. This is the result of many cases being handled quickly and on the basis of limited information. This could be applied to other conditions as well. The patient may be reluctant to disclose all of the facts about his/her injury or illness. This makes the treatment process very difficult, sometimes impossible. Patients may be discharged from the emergency department before their medical complaint has been completely relieved. They must understand that the emergency department is for initial treatment only. For additional care, a followup in a physician's office or clinic is necessary.

Excessive Charges

While hospital costs are high, so are the demands for quality care. The problem that occurs in this area is the patient's belief that his/her insurance will cover all charges. Patients must understand that they are liable for all hospital/medical bills not covered by insurance. Of these last two problem areas, poor result and excessive charges, the physician-staff relationship with the patient can help reduce or increase the incidents. If the physician-emergency department staff is crude, abrasive, and insensitive, the patient will not feel free to disclose all of the facts and symptoms of his illness/injury and when he receives his bill, he will think it excessive, and when he looks at the result, he will remember how he was treated and he will sue. Claims investigators report that when they interview patients, one of the first things the patients talk about is how badly they were treated when they entered the emergency room. There are many legal problems encountered daily in the emergency department. The emergency-department staff are advised to become thoroughly acquainted with local statutes and regulations and to use common sense when there is no specific regulation. Some of the more common legal problems follow.

Informed Consent

A patient must be fully informed of any proposed procedure. This information must include an alternative and the risks. In a true life-and-death situation, if the patient is unable to give his or her consent and there is no family available, the emergency-department physician may start the necessary life-saving measures. This can also apply to minors. If the threat to life is not immediate, consent from next of kin should be obtained before definitive treatment is started, assuming the patient is not able to give his/her consent. It has been generally accepted that when a patient enters the emergency department under his own power for treatment, consent is implied. This does not mean the emergency-department staff can just abandon reason and do what they wish, but that they can proceed with some basic procedure. Before going on to the more complicated situation, informed consent should be obtained (see Figure 3).

In one case, a patient came into the emergency room complaining of a severe case of hiccoughs. This situation had gone on for several days and he had been to his own family physician. Since he was not satisfied with the results of his visits and received no relief, he walked into the emergency department of a large metropolitan hospital. He was greeted by the ward clerk who asked why he was present in the emergency department, and when he explained, the ward clerk listened attentively. This patient was taken into an examination room where a nurse asked him to undress. The nurse remained, offered whatever assistance she could, and when he was comfortable on the examination table, she took his vital signs and obtained a brief history. The ward clerk entered the examination room and took down the necessary information, i.e., name, address, next of kin, insurance information, etc. After a wait of a few minutes, the emergency-department physician entered the room, asked pertinent questions about the reason the patient was there, and listened attentively. Blood tests and X-rays were ordered after some explanation was given as to the whys of these procedures and the patient consented. After the tests results were received, a provisional diagnosis was made and the results and diagnosis were reviewed with the patient. Admission as an in-patient was advised and insisted upon. When the patient received his bill for emergency-department service, his only comment was that the service he had received was worth twice the price. He felt that he had been treated exceptionally well and had been kept totally informed about what was going on and why. He did have some negative comments about his in-patient stay relating to lack of informed consent.

AUTHORIZATION FOR MEDICAL and/or DIAGNOSTIC PROCEDURES

Name________________________________ Case No. ________________

I, the undersigned, a patient in Hospital, hereby authorize and consent to the administration of such medical and surgical diagnostic and therapeutic procedures to

____
(myself or relationship)

as may be deemed necessary by the physicians or physician in charge of me.

Witness______________________ Signed ______________________
(For Procedures) (Patient or nearest relative)

Date ______________________ Relationship ______________________

AUTHORIZATION FOR SURGICAL PROCEDURES

I specifically consent to the performance of the surgical operation known as ____

____

to be performed by Doctors ________________________________

I also authorize such additional operations or procedures as are considere therapeutically necessary on the basis of findings during said operation.

I also consent to the administration of such anesthetics as are indicated in the judgment of the anesthesiologists and physicians in charge of me.

"The nature and purpose of the operation, possible alternative methods of treatment, the risk involved and the possibility of complications have been fully explained to me. No guarantee or assurance has been given by anyone as to the results that may be obtained."

Witness______________________ Signed ______________________
(For Procedures) (Patient or nearest relative)

Date ______________________ Relationship ______________________

FIGURE 3. Informed consent form.

Leaving Against Medical Advice

The patient does have the right to refuse treatment and it would not be morally or legally correct to detain this person against his/her will. In the emergency department, some nonemergency patients may become upset and leave because they have had to wait for what they believe is an extraordinarily long period of time. As long as the patient has a clear understanding of the consequences of this action, he/she should be permitted to leave. If the patient is not capable of understanding the consequences of leaving against medical advice, a court order may be necessary, assuming the patient's family has not been contacted or is unwilling to consent to the prescribed treatment. The emergency-department staff must clearly document what steps were taken, and, if possible, have the patient sign a release form.

There are instances where patients have left against medical advice and were taken to another emergency room for treatment. In one case, the patient expired and in another case, the condition was found to be serious. In both cases, it was clearly documented that the patient left against medical advice.

Police Cases

Many of the patients brought into the emergency department have been transported by the police department. The police may request copies of the medical report as well as status/condition reports. They may also request the patient's personal property. While emergency-department personnel should cooperate as much as possible, a certain amount of discretion is necessary. Local authorities must be contacted for the correct guidelines. Occasionally, during routine examinations, a concealed weapon or drugs may be discovered. A security officer and/or police officer should be summoned immediately. Emergency-department personnel must use a great deal of care when removing drugs or weapons from the patient.

Patient Property

One of the most frequent problems that occur in the emergency department is missing property belonging to the patient. Patients come to the emergency department in a number of different ways — police department, fire department, private ambulance, friends, or walk-in. In a busy emergency room, it is possible for the patient's personal property to become lost. Many hospitals have made payment for lost property because of the public-relations image of the institution even though there was a doubt the patient had the missing item. A good practice is to inventory the patient's personal objects and offer the "safekeeping" of valuables. In this way, there can be no doubt about what the personal effects were at the time of admission. There are several cases where this procedure was applied and resulted in the hospital not paying. A truck driver had collapsed and was taken, unconscious, to an emergency room. When the patient regained consciousness, he indicated he had over $1500 cash. A personal-effects inventory had been taken and no such sum of cash was listed. Investigation revealed that the driver had been playing cards, lost heavily, and attempted to cover his losses. Proper documentation of personal effects is a must. Hospitals are required to make their capabilities available; when in-patient services cannot be provided, the patient must be transferred. Of extreme importance is the patient's condition before the transfer is accomplished. The Emergency Medical Service Act provides for area-wide emergency plans that will afford the patient the best possible care. Before the patient is transported, the receiving hospital must be notified, the patient stabilized for transport, and all pertinent medical information assembled. The level of support necessary during transport must be determined. If a physician must accompany the patient, arrangements for that physician must be made. The patient must be monitored throughout the transfer and the appropriate treatments continued.

TRAINING

Personnel working in the emergency department must be properly trained for their responsibilities. In many cases, the nursing staff will be the first to see and assess the patient's condition and they must know what the correct response is for any given consideration. There must be regular in-house in-service programs, as well as attendance at outside seminars and workshops dealing with emergency medicine. No matter what the program, the physician in charge of the emergency department should find the programs acceptable and meet the needs of that particular emergency department (see Figure 4).

The training program should include the following:

1. Recognition, interpretation, and recording of the patient's signs and symptoms
2. Cardio-pulmonary resuscitation
3. Related life-support procedures
4. Parenteral administration of fluids, blood, and drugs
5. Management of sepsis

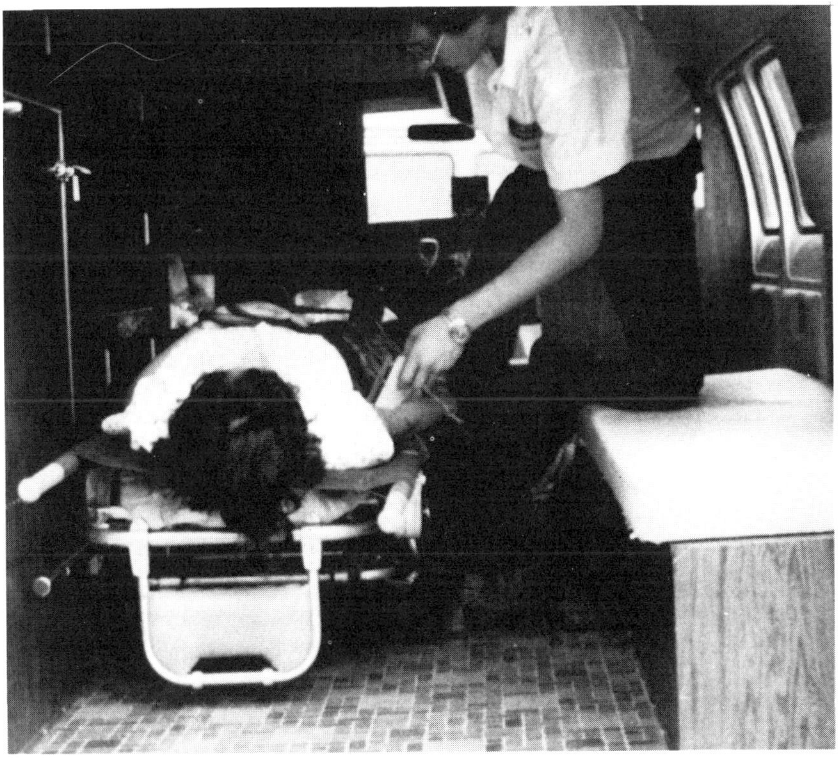

FIGURE 4. The critically injured patient can expect to be transported in an ambulance with the latest equipment and attended by a well trained technician. (Courtesy of Steven Carey and Allan McLean, Rush-Presbyterian-St. Luke's Medical Center.)

6. Care of the burn patient
7. Initial management of injuries to extremities
8. Initial management of injuries to the central nervous system
9. Effective and safe use of electrical and electronic equipment
10. Prevention of cross contamination
11. Recognition of the mental and social needs of the patients

Attendance at all in-service programs must be documented and made part of the personnel file.

POLICIES AND PROCEDURES

One of the best methods of assuring a high level of care is through the establishment of written policies and procedures. These policies and procedures must be reviewed at regular intervals with all members of the emergency department. The policy and procedure should have the following elements:

- Location and storage of supplies, drugs, equipment
- Procurement of supplies, drugs, equipment
- Infection control measures (see Figure 5)
- Procedures to be followed in the event of equipment failures
- Relevant safety practices such as care and use of electrical equipment, smoking policy, use of oxygen, care of the violent patient

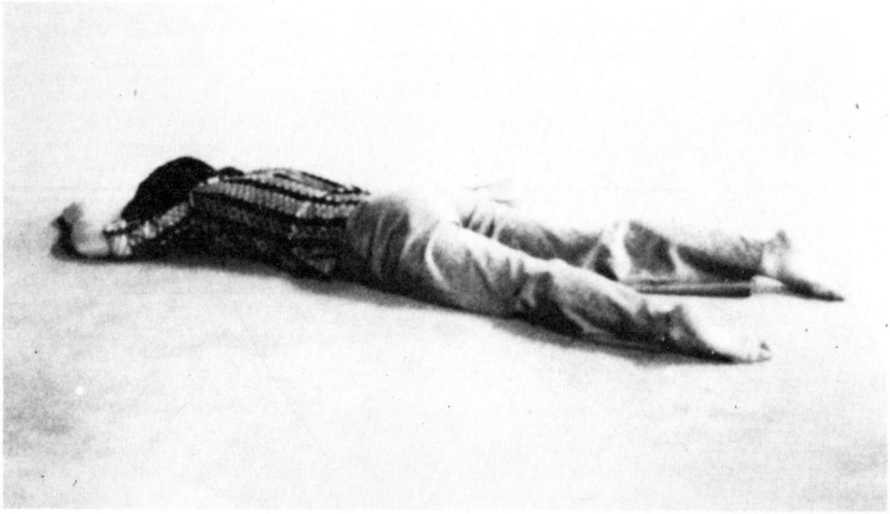

FIGURE 5. The injured patient is more susceptible to infection and every effort must be made to assure the infection will be controlled. (Courtesy of Steven Carey and Allan McLean, Rush-Presbyterian-St. Luke's Medical Center.)

- Visitor control
- Dispensing of medications
- Handling of patient's valuables
- Role of the emergency department in mass-casualty management, fire-emergency plan, severe-weather plan, civil-disorder plan, electrical-failure plan, bomb-threat plan
- Specify scope of treatments permitted in the emergency room
- Specify who may perform the special procedures (other than physicians) and under what circumstances
- Transfer of patients
- Emergency treatment of patient exposed to radiation
- Treatment of suspected rape victim
- Treatment of suspected child abuse
- Management of pediatric emergencies
- Management of "Dead on Arrival"
- Management of patient under influence of alcohol or drugs
- Precautions to be taken to protect unconscious or irrational patients

There must be provisions for safeguarding the patient's medical record and assuring its confidentiality. We want our patients to tell us about themselves and the only way to assure this is by making certain that only authorized individuals have access to this information. The medical records administrator must be involved whenever establishing policies and procedures for the medical record. Included in this policy should be the following:

1. When the patient's personal physician will receive the report
2. Safeguarding the confidentiality of the record
3. Release of information
4. Transfer of patient
5. Consent for treatment

The emergency department should be easily accessible not only from the outside, but from within the hospital. This will permit the rapid admission of patients as in-patients, as well as permit the rapid transportation of needed supplies and equipment. All equipment in the emergency room should be checked and serviced in accord with the hospital's preventive maintenance program. The equipment should be of the same quality as used equipment throughout the facility and should be suitable for the patients treated.

DISASTER PLANS

The hospital emergency department is usually the focal point of activity during a disaster (Mass Casualty Crisis). The emergency department will experience a sudden in-flow of patients and must be ready to meet this situation. The disaster plan must detail how the staff will be augmented in such a situation, as well as detail how additional supplies and equipment will be obtained. Since such a situation places an extreme demand on the staff and the hospital resources, each hospital must assess its capabilities and its limitations. Some areas require that a hospital be prepared to send a medical team to the disaster site. For many hospitals, this is not realistic because if they send a team, the facility may not be able to adequately treat the victims of the disaster (see Figure 6).

Communication with the disaster site is essential because this permits the hospital to prepare for the incoming patients. This ability to communicate will also permit the free exchange of information as the situation changes or information is obtained about a specific aspect of the disaster. During a recent disaster, the ability to communicate with the site became critical. At approximately 7:45 a.m., a chemical truck deposited its load at a factory. The driver was told where to place his load of chemicals. Unknown to the driver, he was told to place his chemicals in the wrong location. The result was a violent chemical reaction and the generation of a highly toxic gas. There were over 60 individuals in the plant at the time of the incident. There were many unconscious victims who were transported immediately to the area hospitals. The first patients that arrived were saturated with this gas and some of the emergency-department staff complained of burning eyes, difficulty in breathing, and a choking sensation. The disaster site was notified via radio and information about the chemicals was requested. Within a few minutes, the identification of the chemicals as well as the toxic gas was received. The medical teams at the site began decontamination procedures that were continued in the emergency department. The emergency staff exposed to the situation were in no real danger since much of the gas had dissipated by the time the patients were received. This information did assist the emergency-department staff with the treatment of the casualties.

In other disaster situations, the emergency department may be called upon to provide emotional support to the victims and relatives of the victims. An example of this occurred in April 1979, when an apartment building caught fire. The incident occurred at 3:30 a.m., and the residents of the building were taken to the area hospitals. None had been burned, but suffered mainly from exposure and/or mild smoke inhalation. The real challenge to the emergency-department staff was in the emotional support of individuals who had lost everything in the fire. Some of the people had medical conditions requiring maintenance medication each day. The area hospitals were prepared to meet this type of emergency. They had a plan which mobilized many of the community agencies. By noon, all of the residents of the building had been placed in temporary lodging, had clothes, and their family physicians contacted for the maintenance dose of drugs the selected patients required. This had all been thought out in advance.

The emergency department can be the center of a great deal of activity. In many

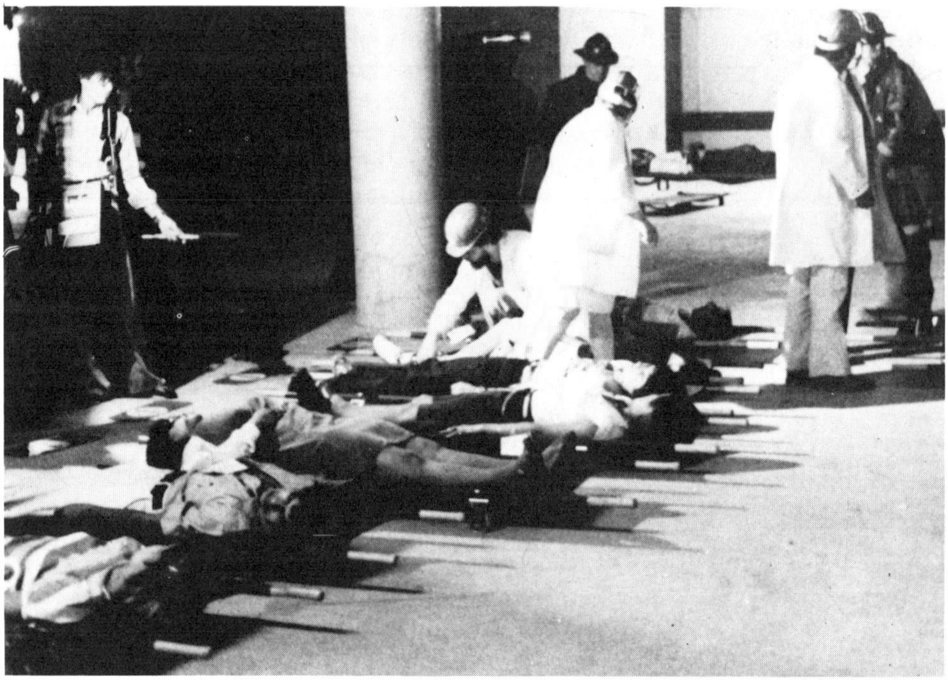

FIGURE 6. A disaster will bring together the resources of the community and the hospital to aid the patient. (Courtesy of Steven Carey and Allan McLean, Rush-Presbyterian-St. Luke's Medical Center.)

cases, it may be the patient's first introduction to the facility. A well-trained emergency-department staff can deal with all types of patients in all kinds of emotional states. Patients and relatives of patients expect only the best, and depending on how the patient is received, their reaction will be based upon their perception of the treatment received.

The spotlight is always on the emergency room and its staff. Not only hospital administrators, but the public is always watching.

CONCLUSION

The emergency-department staff is a special breed of individuals. Its members must have better-than-average technical skills, a better-than-average ability to adapt, and good public relation and communication skills. The emergency room can be quiet one moment and filled to capacity the next. The patients can be cooperative and speak slowly and clearly, or they can be uncooperative, and getting each piece of information is a challenge. The patients can be quiet and sedate or they can be highly combative. No matter what happens, no matter how often it happens, no matter what, the emergency-department staff is there doing its best for the community it serves.

OPERATING ROOM SAFETY

James H. Moore and Barbara Lea Webb

INTRODUCTION

The operating room and what happens there brings into focus the complex interaction of the surgeon, the anesthesiologist, the nurse, and a cadre of paramedical professionals all working toward the goal of helping the patient feel better. Behind this "front line" of medical professionals are several layers of administrative, technical, and legal personnel who direct through rules, standards, and laws precisely how the patients are to be cared for while in the operating room.

A portion of the guiding rules that must be addressed constantly by surgical personnel are those dealing with the various aspects of safety, both to the patient and to themselves. As with the surgery, where many skills and talents are brought to bear on the problem at hand, so it is with safety within the surgical area — safety of the room, equipment, procedure, and supplies used in the surgery — all must be under control. All must be monitored, documented, and accepted to be of value to the ultimate beneficiary — the patient.

The ultimate person responsible for the safety of the patient and the personnel is generally not well-defined. Some of the responsibility is vested with the surgeon, some with the support personnel, and some with the administrative body of the hospital. That there are operating rooms with low incidence of safety problems that can be contrasted with those operating rooms with greater safety problems suggests the entire situation can be brought under control and maintained.

The purpose of this chapter is to explore some of the various areas of safety within the surgical suite, point out some of the problems, discuss possible solutions, and suggest various ways of dealing with the responsibility for these areas of safety.

THE ENVIRONMENT

The area encompassed by the four walls, floor, and ceiling that defines the actual operating room, contributes significantly to the relative success of the surgical procedures performed there. An area cramped with personnel and equipment not only causes ineffective operation, but brings the personnel and equipment into closer proximity of the patient, thereby increasing the risk of infection, accident, and confusion by those in the room. By contrast, an area that is large enough to have adequate room for all the equipment and personnel necessary for the surgical procedure and that is adequately lighted and air conditioned, should contribute noticeably to the success factor of the surgeries performed there.

In the 1970s the surgical suite underwent one of the greatest changes of time. Open heart and organ transplant surgery both required significantly larger areas, as well as more cooling capacity to offset the increased heat load generated by more complex equipment and a greater number of personnel per room. Laminar flow "clean" rooms for reconstructive surgery requiring deep incisions and lengthy "open" times came into being. Multiple medical gas outlets for air, oxygen, and nitrogen were demanded for additional equipment and the patient. Recently, anesthetic gas-scavenging systems have become common in operating rooms to help protect personnel from continued exposure to trace amounts of anesthetic gas.[1] Each of these additional services also contribute to the necessity for an effective safety program within the surgery area. Each of these various systems serving the operating rooms require some brief explanation about their general operation before the specific problems of each relating to operating room safety can be addressed. These systems are discussed generally to promote a common understanding of some of the problems experienced by those who are involved in surgery.

Air Handling and Conditioning Systems

These systems and the equipment that make up each one generally are located in mechanical rooms above or to the side of the actual operating room. The only portion visible within the operating room is usually the inlet and exhaust grills that direct the air into the room. Several distinct problems with these remote systems can be diagnosed by careful observation of key indicators within the operating room. These will be discussed once the operation of the system has been briefly explored.

Air-conditioning systems process astounding amounts of air which is directed into individual operating rooms to cool or warm the equipment, personnel, and patient located there. This processing of air consumes considerable amounts of energy in the form of heat or cooling to the appropriate coils within the unit and powering of a fan or fans that direct the air to the individual rooms. Within the air conditioning system, several physical problems can exist that compromise the cleanliness of the air being directed into the operating room.

Units on some hospitals have had the air intake located within a few feet of such undesirable outlets of contamination and odor as laboratory hood exhaust, incinerator stack, morgue exhaust, toilet exhaust, and other surgical exhaust fans. The solutions to some of these problems require considerable effort and designing by engineering personnel, then considerable expense, to relocate as efficiently and easily as possible. Other problems can be found immediately inside the unit where the first particle filters are located. Many of the filters placed in the air stream to clean it of dirt, dust, and other matter can be found torn, broken, and heavily clogged due to misuse, or completely gone because of inattention. The result is the various heating and cooling coils located further downstream being clogged with dirt, leaves, scraps of paper, insects, and the like, severely limiting the ability of the air handling unit to provide any conditioning at all to the air that manages to pass through it. Little imagination is needed to see the effect these conditions have on the quality of care that is provided to the patient in the operating room.

Beyond the fans that move the air to its final destination are usually the HEPA or absolute filters that do the final cleaning of the air. Sometimes these are misfitted in their support frames leaving gaps beside them through which the air flows — bypassing the filter section completely — negating any effect the filters might have on the air going to the operating rooms.

Problems caused by this type of neglect or abuse usually can be spotted in the operating room by closely examining the condition of the ceiling or wall outlets for the air conditioning both within the rooms and in the hallway. Any accumulation of dirt on the ceiling surfaces immediately adjacent to the outlet diffuser means bypassed or ineffective filtering, and will require immediate and expensive correction. This condition, usually indicative of filtering compromise throughout the system, may not exist at all. Instead, continuing complaints from nurses, surgeons, and others about the "too hot" or "too cold" conditions within the operating rooms, particularly on extremely hot or cold days, may indicate clogging problems in the heating and cooling coils of the system. Attempts by hospital maintenance personnel to clean the coils may be somewhat successful in correcting the situation. A more positive approach is to have a company that specializes in high pressure cleaning of air handling unit coils contracted to clean the coils. These companies usually are quite willing to demonstrate their competence, and will take airflow readings before and after cleaning if requested to show the improvement attained by cleaning. While they are cleaning the coils, they can also high pressure clean condensate drip pans located directly beneath the chilling coils. These drip pans are a source of dirt and bacteria and should be cleaned routinely by the maintenance personnel. Once cleaned, new filters installed and all leaks closed, the remaining job is the cleaning of the ducts (if necessary) leading to the operating rooms. This should place the air-conditioning units in top operating condition. If the filters are maintained properly, the units can be kept in this condition indefinitely.

Another problem can be noted in the operating room with the air-conditioning system is the amount of lint build-up on the exhaust grills within the room. If an accumulation of lint is noted on the exhaust outlet grills within the operating room or hallway, this usually indicates the exhaust fans are working fairly satisfactorily, but the housekeeping efforts within the room require increased attention to keep these free of lint build-up. Allowing this lint build-up to continue will gradually close off the route the air being pumped into the room has to get away. This will result in stuffy rooms and perhaps complaints from staff about doors that bang shut and are difficult to open because the rooms are overpressured. The air that now cannot leave via the designed route, has no place to go except to make its way out via corridors, doorways, and other places within the surgical area. There are no filters on the exhaust system described above, however, clogged grills or nonoperating exhaust fans can cause tremendous inconvenience to those who work in the area.

HUMIDITY

To maintain a comfort level within the operating room that optimizes the varied effects of cooling and moisture of the air, requires the air to have moisture maintained at a 50% relative humidity level at all times during use. From this, several side benefits are obtained. First, moisture within the air permeates the surgical drapes, gowns, and other surgical materials, allowing these to more easily conduct static charges generated by them to the common grounding system of the operating room. This reduces the opportunity for sparks to be generated that would ignite any flammable gases being used as anesthetics. This risk is predominately in a small area around the patient's head when the anesthetic gas is being administered, nevertheless, it is a distinct risk that can be minimized. Second, it prevents the discomfort and risk associated with the involuntary jerking away of a finger, arm, or leg when a static spark occurs between a person and a highly conductive metallic object. Third, the incidence of nosocomial infections are reduced when surgeries are performed in environments where the relative humidity is maintained at a 50% level or higher.

The maintaining of the 50% relative humidity requires water to be removed from the air in summer and added in winter. Thus, the mechanical conditioning equipment performs year-round and is not as subject to start-up failures and nonuse. To assure the equipment is properly operating, a daily record log of the relative humidity in each room should be kept. Although this practice is an unpleasant chore usually assigned to a person who knows little about what he is recording, it can be beneficial. By assigning specific humidity limits (i.e., minimum 45%, maximum 60%) that, if exceeded, require immediate notification of supervisory personnel in surgery and maintenance, the program can be made to work.

The easiest method of providing relative humidity readings is to install wall-mounted direct relative humidity gauges in each operating room. These can be calibrated or checked for accuracy by maintenance personnel using a sling psyscometer at semi-annual or annual intervals. If specific limits are given on the anesthesiologist's record, they can also notify supervisory personnel when an out-of-limit condition is noted. This provides a check on the person given the primary responsibility of recording the humidity each day, and tends to discourage the "dry labbing" of humidity readings.

Further, this may be an advantage to the anesthesiologist who, in case of liability for malpractice or accident, may want to have the assurance and record that the operating room was within specific humidity limits during a particular surgical procedure.

This keeping of a humidity log is a requirement of the Joint Commission on Accreditation of Hospitals (JCAH), so its creation is not an option for the surgical administration.

EQUIPMENT

Electrical Safety

The equipment used in the surgical suites represents a cross-section of the spectrum of equipment used within the entire hospital. All of it must perform as flawlessly as possible to enable the work by the surgeons, anesthesiologists, nurses, and others to be as easily and precisely accomplished as possible.

In another section of this handbook, the subject of electrical safety within the hospital is covered in some detail. What is said here is meant to augment that, shaping it into some special cases within the operating room, as well as supplement what is stated in the electrical safety section.

Microshock

Briefly, the limits of microshock are that it is assumed to be less than 500 to 700 μA or just below the level of perception or tingling for the normal, healthy adult. The lower range of microshock is 10 μA, although levels of 20 μA are generally considered the lowest levels that could possibly cause fibrillation of the heart under worst-case conditions. Generally, however, microshock currents above 100 μA are considered dangerous, while those below 100 μA should be treated with precaution.

Microshock currents are made up of the small leakage currents inherent in all electrical power equipment. With well-maintained equipment, these small currents are drained away by grounding conductors connected to all the equipment. These grounds are subject to wear just as the equipment; if not inspected and tested periodically, they will break. This goes unnoticed because the equipment will continue to operate satisfactorily without a ground wire. This does provide a danger situation to the patient; the small leakage currents previously drained away by the ground wire, now accumulate on the metal enclosure of the equipment. These stray leakage currents will take the path of least resistance to get to the ground, whether that be through the patient, surgeon, nurse, tube or whatever. Should they pass through the patient's heart, it may cause fibrillation if applied for significantly long (1 to 10 sec), and is of large enough value (75 to 500 μA).

The hazard of microshock in the operating room is as real as it is in any other area of the hospital. The advantage here, however, is the more vigilant eye being kept on the patient by the surgical team during a procedure. Equipment to manage the negative effects of fibrillation is available once the diagnosis has been made. Microshock is a very elusive type of hazard, primarily because it cannot be felt, cannot be seen, and cannot be easily measured. Lastly, microshock cannot be determined or proven by any presently known pathological means.

Macroshock

This type of electrical shock is far more commonly reported, primarily because it can, by definition, be felt at its weakest level, and causes physical body or equipment damage at its higher levels (above 10 A). Macroshock incidents that are reported usually indicate lack of good maintenance, preventive or corrective. Power cords that are split and partially broken, damaged A/C plugs and receptacles, and damaged or misused medical equipment are all found as reasons for the incidents.

Radiofrequency Burns

The third type of electrical shock or hazard is caused by high-power radiofrequency (RF) electrical energy used with electrocautery equipment. Usefully directed, this energy provides "bloodless" cutting of tissue, and fulgration of specific organs within the body that are accessible either by surgical procedure or through a natural opening.

Radiofrequency energy has the characteristic of traveling the path of least resistance without necessarily passing through a physical conductor. If the two points of the intended pathway for the RF current are close enough together, the energy will bridge the gap utilizing the principle of capacitive coupling, and continue on its path of least resistance.

Electrocautery utilizes the principle of concentrating high levels of energy at a point where the cutting is to take place, then passing this same energy on its return path from the patient to the equipment through a large area plate usually placed on the hip, thigh, or under the buttocks.

Generally, the energy, which is controlled by the surgeon via a foot on-off pedal, causes its greatest problem when the pathway from the patient is interrupted or is highly resistant to the return flow of energy. When this occurs, the energy may return via any other available pathways, e.g., the operating table, the monitor leads, or even the physician. While some of these return paths are fairly large in area, others such as the EKG or EEG leads are quite small. These small areas require a high density of current to flow per unit area of skin, resulting in heating of the area enough to cause a burn.

The best method to reduce burns caused by electrocautery is to have equipment that is well-maintained, and personnel that are well-trained and can recognize when a hookup has not been properly made. Placement of the dispersive, indifferent, or body electrode is the most important procedure. Bony areas of the body should be avoided and good contact with as much of the electrode plate and body as possible is an absolute must. Placing the electrode plate where good blood flow and circulation reduces heat build-up caused by current flowing through the body-electrode plate interface is strongly recommended.

Generally, the small electrodes used for EKG and EEG monitoring should be located as far away as physically possible from the active cutting tip, as this prevents "short circuiting" of the active energy to the EKG equipment via the electrodes, rather than the cautery energy exiting through the large indifferent plate.

Isolation Transformers

Initially, the continued use of isolation transformers in the surgical area was thought to be a primary method of protection to the patient from all types of electrical shock, both microshock and macroshock. This later proved to be invalid and other methods of protection were developed. Among these methods were better isolation of electronic circuits, better-designed equipment, and more awareness of the hazards by anesthesiologists.

Suction Equipment

Most surgical rooms have in-house suction available at a wall outlet or outlets within the room. For more complex cases, the number of outlets available may be less than the number needed. This requires an auxiliary suction pump to be brought in to provide the amount of suction needed. With the addition of a suction pump, another possible contributor to the hazard of either micro- or macroshock in the operating room is introduced. The risks of electrical hazard increase greatly once the column of fluid from the patient to the machine is continuous. This fluid pathway is a good conductor of electrical current, and may direct hazard current either into or out of the patient depending upon the source. A well-maintained machine is basically an electrical motor with a vacuum pump attached. The design of the pump places a large reservoir (3ℓ) in the vacuum line between the patient and the vacuum pump. Under usual circumstances, this arrangement maintains isolation between the patient and motor. In actual operating room situations, this ideal situation is often compromised by the urgency of the procedure being done or the untoward condition of the patient. The result is that the reservoir fills to the top and the contents are sucked into the vacuum pump itself. After this happens, several precautions are necessary as the possibility of electrical shock to the patient now increases greatly. Some of the first indications of potential problems are a fuzzy trace on electronic monitoring equipment and a nonfunctioning suction machine.

Once this has occurred, the equipment must be disconnected, removed from the operating room, and sent immediately to the maintenance area for complete teardown, cleaning, and relubrication. The normal body fluids also act as good "degreasers", quickly destroying the lubrication of the parts within the vacuum pump. If the unit is allowed to sit for any length of time (1 day), the parts will rust and seize internally causing additional damage.

One precaution that should be established as policy within the operating room is the decontamination of the unit such as this prior to sending it for repair. If the unit will not work adequately enough to be flushed with water, a notice should be placed on the request for repair warning the repair person to take adequate and necessary precautions while repairing the unit in order to prevent being unnecessarily exposed to a contagious disease.

Electrical Safety Program

Electrical safety within the operating room can be attained in much the same way electrical safety can be attained in the patient areas of the hospital. First, a good preventive maintenance program that has the backing and support of both the physician and administrative staff of the hospital is necessary. Second, with this program should go an active education program to update and educate those who have to use the equipment daily in how to take care of it and how to determine when it needs attention. Third, a program that encourages follow-through of the various problems and complaints voiced by the users of the equipment, the operating room personnel and the staff physicians, is mandatory to its success.

The program of maintaining the equipment in good operating condition and good repair is vital to the hospital and to the surgeons. To not be able to use an operating room because a particular item of equipment is not available means the patient, the hospital, and the surgeon all suffer. All too often, the best of maintenance programs are doomed at the beginning by the attitude of some surgeons and surgery administrators, e.g., "That piece of equipment is too vital and too necessary to be taken out of service now; we will let you know when we are through with it." Needless to say, the technician usually never gets told when it is available to be checked and tested.

To surmount this problem requires tenacity, tact, and some ingenuity on the part of the technician, perhaps with the help of a reliable surgical technician within the surgery area. A more productive and usable way to solve this is to put a biomedical equipment technician in surgical scrub clothes in the surgery area at specific times (before the day shift starts and until the start-up problems have been handled) to make tests on the equipment when it is available (assuming the permission of the surgical administration is obtained first). This has side benefits that are useful to the program, too. Physicians, nurses, and surgical personnel understand technically far too little about the equipment they use each day, and are eager to learn more about the why and how of individual items of equipment provided for them to use. This eagerness can be turned into profitable use by the technician who takes time to explain why the equipment works electronically or mechanically as it does and how they (the surgical personnel) can test it simply and safely on their own to determine if there is indeed a problem or just a poor connection with a piece of equipment.

This area of education will achieve more good will and productive information among the several different specialties working within the operating room than any other method. Communication of problems, be they electrical safety, mechanical safety, etc. always flows better between those who trust and respect each other's particular skills than it does between independent, separate groups.

By holding short briefing sessions with the service representative, operating room personnel, and biomedical equipment technicians on the new equipment brought into the surgery suite, the apprehensions of using it are reduced. To then follow-up these sessions with additional sessions that explain and discuss some of the recently encountered problems serves to inform and educate the entire nursing support group. New personnel hired from the outside may be very experienced on other types of equipment. While similar, this equipment may not be exactly like to type being used in your hospital. To have these briefing sessions in the new employees' beginning days of work allows them to be much more productive and confident, and less on-the-job procedural errors are passed along and fewer serious mistakes are made.

Finally, the follow-through with the director of surgery concerning the problems within the area is important to the safety program. Getting support for the things that have to be done from a jurisdictional aspect will go far in promoting and motivating personnel to do the tasks necessary to help them do a better job. Nothing quenches the initiative to do a job well faster than a procedure or tests that those doing it do not understand.

Surgical personnel are interested predominantly in the patient's well-being and how the things they must do benefit that patient. To add needless-looking paperwork or humdrum checkout procedures without some semblance of their immediate importance to the patient, will be futile.

MEDICAL GASES

Generally, the modern operating room will have outlets at least for oxygen. In the latest surgical rooms, nitrogen, nitrous oxide, medical-grade compressed air, and vacuum may be available at wall outlets in addition to oxygen. Each of these are supplied with the idea of providing a more convenient source of the individual gases in each room rather than in bulky, space-consuming, difficult-to-manage individual tanks. Also, the hospital can provide the appropriate medical gas at less ongoing expense when centralized storage facilities are used that allow bulk purchases of the various gases. This is a distinct advantage, however, there are a number of precautions that must be taken continuously to prevent these advantages from being eaten up in waste, and at the same time adding to an occupational hazard.

Leaking Outlets

Each outlet installed in an operating room was usually located by a workman (following the guidelines of the engineer) at a point that did not physically interfere with the location of any other electrical or mechanical system wiring or piping. The result usually obtained is that the outlet is almost too far or too high or too low from where the cords and lines must reach between it and the patient area of the operating room. This continuous "almost too much" causes constant wear and abuse to the outlet. In spite of manufacturers' advertising, all equipment will wear and become loose prior to failing. The same goes for wall-mounted medical gas outlets.

After 1 to 2 years of good use, the outlets will wear internally to the point where they will leak minute amounts of gas even after all equipment has been removed from them. This small leakage, when multiplied by the number of outlets in the operating rooms as well as the hospital, can result in base usages that get larger each year. Initially, these leaks appear to be of little concern, however, if the logic of the situation is extended to all the other gases that may be leaking from room outlets, the problem can become serious. Rather than becoming a simple problem of economics, the problem becomes one of occupational safety.

Leaky Anesthetic Gas Machines

The National Institute of Occupational Safety and Health (NIOSH) has established recommended levels of 25 ppm nitrous oxide (N_2O) as target levels to be reached in reducing occupational exposure to waste anesthetic gases and vapors.[2] At one university hospital, researchers found the average levels of N_2O of 20 operating rooms were 19 ppm at 5:30 a.m.[3] This problem was found to have two sources, the central N_2O "quick connect" outlets, and the leakage from anesthesia machines.

After leak testing the various fittings on the anesthetic gas machines and repairing the wall outlets, the base average leakage level was reduced to 0.2 ppm with a total range of 1.0 to 2.0 ppm for an entire year. This report serves to illustrate a usually overlooked source of expense and potential occupational hazard within the operating room. Few maintenance men check these outlets until the leak can at least be heard or even felt. By that time, much valuable gas has been wasted.

Testing

Anesthesiologists do not regularly test or inspect their machines to the extent necessary to assure good, tight, leak-free fittings. Having manufacturing representatives make periodic service or inspection calls may not correct all the problems with a leaky gas machine either. Further, with the use the average anesthetic gas machine receives, it is practically impossible to keep a machine leak-free from one service visit to another.

This leads back to the hospital, to monitoring and controls. If the funds are available, and a technically knowledgeable person is available to conduct the tests regularly, the hospital can do the monitoring work in-house. Other alternatives would be contracting with a servicing organization responsible for preventive maintenance of anesthetic equipment. Should neither of these two alternatives be available, a positive leak-prevention program should be established by the hospital operating room and maintenance personnel to regularly replace the "quick connect" outlets. Making simple "soap tests"* of these outlets regularly will indicate the ones that require repair. The same soap test can be used on the various joints and fittings of the anesthetic gas machines to determine where loose connections, defective washers and other problems need attention to stop the leaks.

While the monitoring and programs to preventing leaks in an anesthetic system has not attained the same attention by the various code-making groups as has electrical safety, the potential is present. While electrical safety has much to do with patient safety, medical gas safety deals primarily with those within the operating room, not the patient.

Gas Scavenging

To demonstrate concern for the safety of the personnel within the operating room, several groups are urging the installation or modification of equipment to provide gas

* A 10% solution of any liquid detergent such as Joy®, Ivory®, etc. in water makes an inexpensive testing solution. Commercially prepared products that can be used to do the same test are also available.

scavenging. This technique removes excess anesthetic waste gases that leave the closed anesthetic loop via the "pop-off" valve. However, the capacity of this system is limited to an average withdrawal capacity, and cannot usually handle the large peak bleed-off volumes necessary at certain times within a procedure.

Regardless of their effectiveness and ability to scavenge waste anesthetic gases, these systems serve little use if not properly connected directly to the gas machine loop. Once removed from the machine, their ability to withdraw potential waste gases is severely limited because the scavenging hose will only accept a certain amount of gas per unit time. If that gas is highly concentrated as it is when it comes directly from the "pop-off" valve, the scavenging system is quite effective in keeping the concentration of anesthetic gas down. If the gas being drawn through the scavenging line is the same concentration as the air throughout the operating room, then its ability to reduce the concentration within the room is not as great as the conventional air handling system because of its smaller size. Unfortunately, this scavenging system will not significantly affect the concentration level caused by hidden or obscure leaks. Since hidden or obscure leaks continue their leaking when the operating room is not being used, the concentration of anesthetic gases such as N_2O will continue to be kept high since they are not being significantly diluted by the circulation of fresh air into the operating room.

Older air conditioning systems that use 100% outside air are more effective in reducing spot concentrations than the newer recirculation systems. These new systems allow the air to be recirculated within the operating room area and tend to spread and equalize the concentrations throughout the various rooms they serve. Thus, for example, leaks that may occur in only one outlet in one operating room will be spread throughout each operating room served by a particular air handling unit, thus raising the overall concentration within all the rooms.

Gas Outlet and Machine Control Program

To bring this problem under control requires a specific program of equipment repair, air monitoring, and good technique. As mentioned previously, this program should contain four basic parts:

1. Scheduled testing of all wall-mounted "quick connect" outlets by trained personnel
2. Frequent and routine (every 4 to 6 months) leakage testing of all the equipment used by the anesthetists
3. Air monitoring of each operating room and hallway with quality survey equipment
4. Upgrading and maintaining individual gas administrative technique to avoid or reduce the possibility of unnecessary gas spill in the operating room

This program monitors itself to some degree, as routine surveys of the operating rooms and hallway (part three) will indicate worsening conditions that can then be addressed. The indications of increasing residual anesthetic gas levels should prompt action to repair outlets and do detailed leak checking on gas machines. Once this routine has been established, the final step can be undertaken to improve anesthesia administrative skills (part four) using data accumulated during the surveys.

These and other problem areas can be most effectively dealt with by education of the user initially using outside sources such as vendors or others. These sessions need not be elaborate or lengthy, but should strike on the problems encountered and their solutions.

LIGHTING

The safety aspects of lighting within the operating room are centered around three areas: enough light for the surgeon to see adequately, burns because of the heat produced by the light heating articles, and the mechanics of the lighting fixtures and their support.

The fundamental problem in the operating room procedure of field lighting has been getting the light into the various cavities of the body where the surgeon can see what he wants to. Once the light is in the cavity, the ultimate is refining the content of that light to enhance the actual colors. To provide this adequate lighting within the cavity where the surgeon is working has (until recently) been supplied by incandescent lighting sources. A recommended level of lighting by the Illuminating Engineering Society Lighting Handbook of 2500 footcandles is about the limit of lighting that can be provided on one spot easily without overly large bulb assemblies.[4] To attain the higher illuminating levels requires other, more efficient methods of light production. Most general high-level illumination levels are into ranges of 4000 foot-candles, although some recently developed sources can produce up to 10,000 foot-candles of illumination.

To attempt to meet the problem of getting adequate light into a cavity generally requires auxiliary lights to be brought onto the scene. These lights, although effective for many situations, also bring with them several hazards. Because they are moved from room to room, they have much more wear and tear placed on them than those fixed within a room. This wear and tear shows up as power cords that are worn and frayed with various types of adaptors for the different types of areas they are used in. These need to be checked often because the cords are subject to being broken, walked on, and run over with heavy equipment.

Further checking may reveal that a larger than specified bulb has been installed either to increase the amount of energy or simply because that was the only size available at the time the other one went out. These oversize bulbs produce much more heat than the fixture was ever designed to dissipate.The result is that the surrounding metal enclosure becomes too hot to touch. Unfortunately, this is taken care of by putting a surgical towel over the reflector, thereby creating another hazard, that of fire or at least smoke within the room.

In most operating rooms, the traditional incandescent lighting fixtures are standard devices. These require little maintenance other than bulb replacement, however, they do require that some attention be given to their support mechanism and any reflector that they may have. The support of the light should be shaken periodically to determine if there is any play or loosening of bolts or welds that hold the assembly to the building structure. Any unusual play or looseness should be checked and reported immediately. If the support poles or pipes penetrate the ceiling, a regular check should be made to prevent the plaster of the ceiling from being ground into a fine powder by the movement of the support pole as it moves, dropping dust onto the surgical field.

The reflector of one of the popular types of surgical lights has a coating that passes the heat-producing portions of the light produced into the room, while reflecting the light part of the energy onto the operating field. These coatings can fail after use, and also begin to allow the light energy to pass into the room, rather than reflecting it onto the patient. To determine when this has or is occurring on an individual basis is difficult without the use of a light meter. Once the deterioration involves several reflectors, the determination is not as difficult. Usually, it begins when the surgeon complains about the low light level even though the bulbs in the lights may have just been replaced and the reflectors cleaned. Generally, one will find by observation that the operating room that used to have a warm orange glow above the lights and a sharp blue glow on the field, now has a predominantly blue glow over the entire room. This requires replacement of the reflectors in order to return to the normal operation of the lamp.

INFECTION CONTROL IN THE OPERATING ROOM

In the operating room, infection control is the responsibility of every member of the surgical team, the support personnel, and the administration for the area. From the surgeon to the person who cleans the floor, if one member is not conscientious and willing to perform his assignment well, a patient's life will be endangered.

The control of infection is of high priority and depends on a wide range of procedures being properly implemented at the proper time with the necessary quality of effort expended. Traffic and communication control, proper aseptic techniques, instrument, sponge, and needle counts, and environmental control are all areas that contribute to or detract from infection control. Improving only one of these areas will not necessarily improve the whole infection control program. For example, the sterilization of goods and supplies is one aspect of aseptic technique and disinfection of the operating room environment is another, while antisepsis of hands and arms of operating room personnel, along with proper use of scrub apparel is still another asepsis technique to help lower the risk of infection to the patient.

Many of these areas are treated in detail in the literature and will not be discussed here except to outline specific areas that should be considered in evaluating specific programs.

Traffic

Wheel and walking traffic within the operating room must be controlled to prevent the spread of bacteria from outside the operating rooms into the area. A four-zone traffic-control concept is the most effective way to identify the various functions for each of these areas.

The "protective area" provides a place for the transition of people from outside the surgery area to enter into the boundaries of the operating rooms. This area includes the patient reception area, the locker rooms, lounges, and surgical offices.

Inside this boundary is the "clean area" that includes patient holding areas, clean storage areas, scrub areas, and recovery rooms. This area is the final transition point prior to entering the sterile area.

Within the "sterile area" are the operating rooms and the sterile supply-storage areas. Specific control procedures and techniques must be enforced within this area to maintain it as bacteria-free as possible for the patient.

Finally, a "dirty area" must be defined that provides for disposal of all utilized materials and linens from the surgical sterile area. This area, and the previous ones, must be arranged to allow the progressive flow of supplies and personnel from one area to another. In no case should dirty materials be taken through the sterile or clean areas, nor should incoming traffic in the protective area be exposed to the flow of material from the dirty area.

Communication Control

To maintain the flow of personnel, patients, and supplies into and out of the operating room will require good communication among the various functions within the surgical area.

A system that uses two control desks functions well with a large number of operating rooms, while smaller operating suites may have to use slight modifications of this plan. The external desk is the control point that directs patient and personnel flow while screening incoming telephone calls. The internal desk controls and directs the activities within the operating room area itself. This desk or control point is responsible for expediting blood for transfusions, positive patient identification and physician notification, and the hour-by-hour needs of the various operating rooms.

For large numbers of operating rooms, this internal communications desk function may have to be split into two or more areas to divide the responsibilities and provide for an effective flow of patients into and out of the available operating rooms. Regardless of the size, however, the concept remains valid and must be modified slightly within each particular operating room situation to function smoothly.

Blood Transfusion

Blood for transfusion within the operating rooms should be maintained in a controlled environment at optimal temperatures until released for use. It should be transfused into the patient through a sterile, pyrogen-free transfusion set that has a filter capable of retaining precipitates and coagula potentially harmful to the recipient. If a given number of transfusions are to be given to the patient during an operative procedure, one of two methods can be used: (1) only request transfer of blood from the blood bank to the operating room at the time it is to be administered, or (2) by-placing a maximum of 6 units of blood, and three frozen Koolit® packages inside a styrofoam ice chest. The ice chest should be adequately insulated to maintain a thermometer temperature within the chest of 10°C for 3 hr in the ambient 70°F temperature of the operating room. With the ice chest procedure, blood is readily available to the anesthesiologist at any given time.

Careful identification of the recipient and the blood container is essential. Prior to transfusion, the transfusionist shall sign the transfusion form indicating that information identifying the container with the intended recipient has been matched, item by item, in the operating room in which the recipient is having surgery. Each unit of blood should have a special label attached to the blood container. The information on the label should include patient name and signature, patient hospital-registration number, and date of donation as well as blood type.

Blood should not routinely be warmed before its transfusion. However, warming of blood toward body temperature is appropriate during transfusion in reasonable qualifying situations, such as in rapid or massive transfusion. At such time, warming of blood should be accomplished during its passage through the transfusion set. The warming system must be equipped with a visible thermometer, and, ideally, with an audible warning system. Blood may not be warmed above 38°C and once it is warmed, it must not be added to the blood prior to, or during, a transfusion. Only sodium chloride injection U.S.P. (0.9%) should be administered with transfusion.

LEGAL ASPECTS

The importance of careful handling and accurate labeling of specimens and tissue biopsies cannot be overemphasized. The surgical outcome for many patients is dependent on the laboratory report. Procedure policies of the hospital must be familiar to the personnel entrusted with specimen care and equipment counts.

Safety measures must be defined and observed in the handling of sponges, instruments, needles, and specimens during a surgical procedure. The legal liability of the surgeon, the hospital, and the employee places much at stake and it cannot be passed over lightly. Much has been written about each of these areas from all positions, and it will only be discussed briefly here.

A key factor to consider during the development or updating of surgical procedures is the standardization of equipment and supplies for better control through review by administrative, surgical, and legal representatives, before changes are made to procedures.

Listed below are brief summaries of count procedures with the general reasons why they are necessary, and procedures to include in an overall surgical protocol.

Needle Counts

Surgical needles vary considerably in shape, size, point design, and diameter, depending on the surgical procedures being performed. They may be curved or straight, or the point may be round or have a trocar (cutting edge).

The surgeon is often distracted by the procedure and cannot remain aware of each and every needle he uses. Hence, it is the responsibility of the scrub nurse to see that each needle she hands the surgeon is returned to her before handing him another.

When lost in a patient's incision, a needle causes the same adverse body reaction as does any foreign object. The needle creates a special danger, however, because it can penetrate into other organs near the operative site. With this hazard so great, a needle count is a must in all cases.

A needle count should be taken at the time the needle is handed into the sterile field. Another should be taken at the first line of closure, followed by a recheck as the skin is closed. Finally, the needle count must be recorded in the patient's surgery record.

Sponge Counts

Accounting for all sponges used in an operative procedure is done to prevent the loss of a sponge in the patient and the same subsequent adverse body reaction as mentioned above.

A sponge count falls into several parts:

1. The first count is performed by those who assemble the sponges in packages, be it hospital personnel or commercial suppliers.
2. The second and third counts are made by the scrub and circulating nurses at the time the sponges are handed into the sterile field. The circulating nurse records the count on the operative record.
3. The fourth count is made as the first line of closure sutures is placed.
4. The fifth count is made as a recheck as the skin is closed.

When a hollow organ is opened, an additional check of the count is made as the organ is closed.

Instrument Counts

It is not uncommon for an instrument to be lost during an operative procedure. This is particularly important in the present day of surgery, where many instruments are small and many are used at one time during a procedure.

The hospital employee who assembles the instrument set counts all items according to standards, then signs his own name on a designated slip kept with the set of instruments. The scrub nurse rechecks the count during arrangement of the instruments on the sterile field and at the beginning of wound closure.

EMPLOYEE ASPECTS

The constant aim of optimum patient care must be the primary objective in the minds and actions of all persons involved in care of the operative patient. Accepted standards of conduct, honesty, and observation of policies, rules, and regulations must be practiced by all personnel at all times.

Personal Hygiene

Personal hygiene is of the utmost importance. The following evidence of it should be expected from each employee:

1. Daily bath
2. Skin free from cuts, abrasions, or lesions
3. Hair clean and controlled under a turban
4. Nails clean, well-trimmed, and free of polish

Upper respiratory infection in any person in the operating room is a source of infection for the operative patient. The nose and mouth are a source of bacteria, hence, talking should be limited, and sneezing, coughing, and laughing should not occur in the operating suite.

Wearing Apparel

The wearing apparel for all persons working in the operating room suite should be made of cotton or a material that has been treated to prevent static spark generation. The outfits may be one- or two-piece garments; whatever one's preference, they should fit well, without loose, flopping folds or shirttails, which are a source of contamination. Most importantly, surgical wearing apparel should never be worn outside the operating suite, regardless of the impressionistic value it may have to the personnel.

Footwear should be of the style of a well-fitting support for the feet. Conductive footwear is mandatory in anesthetizing locations and where anesthetic gases are used. Because of the danger of static spark generation, all persons working in the operating room must regularly test the conductivity of their own footwear by means of a conductometer located outside the operating room area, but within the clean areas of surgery.

Headgear is a means of preventing free hair from falling into the sterile area, or the hair shedding of contaminants. Within the clean and sterile area of the operating room, all persons must wear a headpiece. The headgear should be disposable, and should cover the long front hair, the side and back of the head, and facial hair. The head cover should provide effective ventilation and comfort, yet be close enough in texture to prevent penetration of hair or escape of dandruff. The outer edges of the headgear should fit snugly and securely by means of elastic or ties.

Disposable face masks should cover the face and mouth of each person entering the operative suite. The mask must fit snugly, as air must filter through it rather than escape around it. Masks should be changed frequently in order to maintain effective bacterial barriers. Masks should never hang under the chin or be pushed up onto the forehead between cases, but should be discarded.

PATIENT ASPECTS

Mental Preparation of the Surgical Patient

At no other time during the patient's stay in the hospital is he confronted with the fearful situation of being totally unable to help himself or voluntarily control his physical being. Factors that contribute to the patient's fears are his family and his concern for them, unknown factors as to what is going to transpire while in the operating room, and what to expect postoperatively.

These fears and apprehensions are very real to the surgical patient, and if not properly handled can, in some cases, cause unnecessary danger to the patient before and after surgery. Preoperative visits by a qualified R.N. from surgery can psychologically prepare the patient for the actual surgical procedure. As a general rule, surgical procedures carry with them a greater degree of psychic stress for the simple reason that the patient is able to appreciate the results of what is to be expected by the preoperative visit.

An organized plan for teaching the patient what he will need to know is of prime importance. The plan must be flexible enough to permit individualized teaching. Facts that need to be discussed with the patient are (1) a definition and explanation of his surgical procedure, (2) what the patient may expect in the recovery room or intensive care unit, and (3) what the patient's responsibilities in self-care will be upon his return to the unit after surgery. The nurse should inform the patient that he may not remember every detail that is presented to him, however, he will be able to recall his instruction as necessary in the course of his postoperative care.

Always keep in mind, the patient may have difficulty in understanding the instructions given if the nurse is too technical in her terminology. The instructions and explanations should be in simple terms, perhaps involving the patient's family as well to make certain all the questions are accurately answered and discussed.

At no time should a nurse enter into a preoperative visit with the idea of rushing through the topic to be discussed. She must be a good listener, as well as a good teacher.

Positioning the Patient

The responsibility of positioning the patient for surgery is one of the most important functions in the operating room. The responsibility is with the circulating nurse, the anesthesiologist, and the surgeon.

In positioning a patient, comfort and safety for the patient is of vital concern, as the anesthetized patient is unable to help himself.

Principles to be observed are

1. Proper respiratory functioning should be maintained. Pressure on the chest could inhibit free exchange respiration.
2. Unimpaired circulation must be insured. Pressure on any part of the extremities could interfere with venous blood flow.
3. Muscle and nerve must be protected from pressure. Improper positioning over a prolonged period of time could cause serious injury or paralysis.
4. Individual physical condition of the patient should be of major concern. The very thin, elderly, obese, and indigent patients need particular attention to prevent additional complication to recovery.

Skin Preparation

The purpose of skin preparation preoperatively is to render the skin as clean and free of bacteria as possible without causing irritation or damage to the skin. This preparation area must be wider than the proposed incision would seem to require because of the possibility of an unexpected extension of the incision. A disposable safety razor should be used, along with a soap solution. Shaving must be against the grain of the hair shaft to effect a clean, close shave. Scrapes, abrasions, and cuts during a skin preparation can be uncomfortable for the patient and may be a means of infection to the postoperative patient. Every precaution must be used to prevent nicking of the skin, as this allows infection to start preoperatively.

When a prep should be done will vary at different hospitals. Some surgeons prefer the prep to be done the evening prior to surgery, while others prefer the prep to be done the day of the surgery. Regardless of when the prep is done, the head nurse or nurse in charge is ultimately responsible for its adequacy.

Draping of the Patient

The purpose of drapes is to establish a barrier against migration of bacteria within the drape when it may become saturated with body fluids. The drape is utilized to decrease contamination of the patient's surgical wound and to render all surfaces in close proximity to the patient ''sterile''. Moisture is the means by which the bacteria can most easily move in the textile drapes. When these drapes are used, a double thickness must be present in order to prevent a moisture breakthrough.

Nonabsorbent disposable drapes are superior as bacterial barriers. These drapes are soft, lint-free, lightweight, compact, readily sterilized, nonirritating, static-free, and moisture-resistant. The lightness of these drapes prevents heat retention by the patient, and because of their moisture-resistant properties, it is rarely necessary to reinforce them with additional multiple layers.

SUMMARY

In the world of the operating room, safety is the responsibilty of every member of the team, from the surgeon who performs the operation to the person who cleans the floor. If one member of the team is not conscientious and willing to perform his assignment well, a patient's life could be endangered. Thus, safety in the operating room is of a high priority to insure that the patient's postoperative recovery be achieved in the minimum amount of time.

Regardless of the architectural design to control infection, effective hospital and operating room control must be carried out by all levels of personnel directly or indirectly related to the operating room suite. Control programs involve methods of housekeeping and maintenance of all facilities, cleanliness of air in the suite, and of the skin and apparel of patients, surgeons, and personnel, sterility of surgical equipment, strict aseptic technique, and careful observance of all the staff to well-defined and implemented written procedures, rules, and regulations.

Finally, the most important person in this team, the patient, must be cared for with a sincere, dedicated concern by all personnel. He is the one the entire operating room was established for in the first place.

GENERAL REFERENCES

Adler, G. R., Electrical safety in the operating room, *J. Am. Assoc. Nurse Anesth.*, 44(6), 619, 1976.

Birch, A. A., Collapse of an operating room table, *Corresp. Anesth.*, 49, 62, 1978.

Fahlbery, W. J., Fundamentals of hospital safety in the operating room, *Hosp. Top.*, 54(2), 19, 1976.

Gonsep, D. I., Design hazards of electrosurgical devices, *Med. Instrum.*, 10(2), 130, 1976.

Laufman, H., Trends in operating room devices, *Med. Instrum.*, 10(2), 98, 1976.

Sabo, B., Hazards of macroshock, microshock in the o.r., *J. Assoc. Oper. Room Nurs.*, 24(5), 892, 1978.

Schneider, A. J., Patient monitorage in the operating room — an anesthetist's viewpoint, *Med. Instrum.*, 10(2), 105, 1976.

Seawalt, S., Eight steps to implementation of a count system, *J. Assoc. Oper. Room Nurs.*, 28(6), 1098, 1978.

Whitcher, C., Monitoring occupational exposure to inhalation anesthetics, *Anesth. Anal.*, 56, 778, 1977.

Altemeier, W. A., *Manual on Control of Infection in Surgical Patients*, Lippincott, New York, 1976.

Ballinger, W. F., *Alexander's Care of the Patient in Surgery*, Mosby, St. Louis, 1972.

Cromwell, L., *Medical Instrumentation for Health Care*, Prentice-Hall, Englewood Cliffs, N.J., 1976.

Gensberg, F., *A Manual of Operating Room Technology*, Lippincott, New York, 1966.

LeMaintre, G., *The Patient in Surgery: A Guide for Nurses*, W. B. Saunders, Philadelphia, 1975.

Roth, H. H., Teltscher, E. S., and Kane, I. M., *Electrical Safety in Health Care Facilities,* Academic Press, New York, 1975.

Standards for Blood Banks and Transfusion Service, American Association of Blood Banks, Washington, D.C., 1978.

Webster, J. G., *Medical Instrumentation,* Houghton Mifflin, Boston, 1978.

Weinburg, D. I., *Engineering in the Practice of Medicine,* Williams & Wilkins, Baltimore, 1967.

REFERENCES

1. **Whitcher, C., Piziali, R., Sher, R., et al.,** Development and Evaluation of Methods for the Elimination of Waste Anesthetic Gases and Vapors in Hospitals, GPO Stock No. 1733—007, U.S. Government Printing Office, Washington, D.C., 1975.
2. Criteria for a Recommended Standard — Occupational Exposure to Waste Anesthetic Gases and Vapors, HEW Publ. No. (NIOSH) 77-140, U.S. Department of Health, Education and Welfare, Public Health Service Center for Disease Control, National Institute for Occupational Safety and Health, Cincinnatti, 1977, 194.
3. **Lecky, John H.,** The mechanical aspects of anesthetic pollution control, *Anesth. Analag.,* 56, 71, 1977.
4. Illuminating Engineering Society, *IES Lighting Handbook,* Illuminating Engineering Society, New York, 1972, chap. 12.

SAFETY IN SPECIAL CARE UNITS

David H. Gordon

SCOPE

This chapter deals with safety problems encountered in certain patient areas of the acute care facility. These areas will be referred to as special care units.

A special care unit is one in which the nature of care provided is either very specialized or intensive, or both. The staff-to-patient ratio in these units is relatively high, sometimes approaching one-to-one, and the patients are acutely ill. A special care unit may be multipurpose, treating a wide variety of critically ill patients, or specially designed and staffed to treat patients in specific diagnostic categories. Special care units typically include those listed below:

- Coronary care unit
- Respiratory care unit
- General medical intensive care unit
- Surgical intensive care unit
- Pediatric intensive care unit
- Neonatal intensive care unit
- Shock-trauma unit
- Burn unit
- Postoperative recovery room
- Renal dialysis

Many of the safety problems faced by special care units are similar or identical to those not only in other areas of the hospital, but in other industries as well. We must consider the safety of all occupants (permanent as well as transient), including patients, medical staff, nursing staff, other hospital support staff, and visitors. The emphasis of this chapter, and the emphasis in real life, is on patient safety simply because patients are the people least able to fend for themselves in the face of hazards. To compound matters, they are also the population with the most exposure to hazards; frequently, they are invasively connected to physiologic monitors, life support equipment, and other diagnostic and therapeutic aids produced by our high-technology society.

This chapter recommends specific policies and practices in each of several categories. The detailed rationale for some of these recommendations, particularly in the areas of electrical safety and infection control, is omitted because this support material is discussed elsewhere in the manual.

The illustrative examples used throughout the chapter, including case histories and sample policies and procedures, are taken from real situations. The frequently referenced "Metro Hospital" does not, in fact, exist; the examples attributed to this facility either do or did occur at one of six facilities with which the author is familiar.

SAFETY AND EFFECTIVENESS

While this entire manual is devoted to safety, it must be emphasized that the concepts of safety and effectiveness must be operationally integrated if the safety effort of the hospital is to be successful. This applies equally to facilities, equipment, and biological considerations. Functional integration of effectiveness and safety is best achieved through application of fail-safe design principles. Ideally, when a failure occurs in a fail-safe system, the user is automatically notified, the patient, staff, and equipment are all protected, and system effectiveness remains virtually unchanged. More practically, when a hazard arises the faulty equipment or system should either harmlessly shutdown (lose effectiveness), or when this is inadvisable, the user should be automatically warned of the hazard, and/or a backup system should automatically engage. A familiar example is the emergency power generator system. In the most common application, sensing devices detect loss of electricity from the local power company, and within 10 sec an on-site diesel-powered generator is brought on line to power those devices and systems required for adequate operation of the hospital for the duration of the power failure.

An extension of the fail-safe concept convinces us that, wherever possible, we should not depend on human involvement simply to assure safety, especially when that involvement does not also assure equipment or system effectiveness. As an example, it was the policy of one hospital some years ago to supply each portable ECG machine with a grounding cable on a retracting reel. The cable was fitted with a large spring-loaded battery clamp and instructions were printed on the machine in big red letters telling the user that the clamp was to be affixed to the nearest water pipe or radiator before using the machine on a patient. Otherwise, the instructions said, the patient might receive an electric shock. Months after this policy went into effect, a patient did receive a shock; the battery clamp had not been attached to anything. On reflection, no one was really surprised that the warning had gone unheeded. The ECG technicians had used the machine for years with and without this "safety feature", and to the best of anyone's recollection, no one had ever received a shock. Furthermore, and most importantly, effectiveness of the machine was sometimes degraded when the cable was attached as instructed; at best, performance was usually unaffected, i.e., effectiveness was not assured by safe procedures.

A much better approach to achieve the intended purpose — effective grounding of the machine — is to provide properly grounded receptacles, properly wired plugs, and scheduled service of both plugs and receptacles to assure continued integrity of the grounding system. The burden of this aspect of electrical safety should be placed where it is most likely to succeed — in a clinical engineering department. Wherever possible, the clinical staff should be relieved of safety-related tasks that do not impact their day-to-day operation.

FACILITIES SAFETY

The Physical Environment

The American Hospital Association and the National Safety Council have jointly published the valuable Safety Guide for Health Care Institutions.[1] The guide notes that falls are the predominant cause of patient injuries, and with the exception of accidents unique to the operating room, falls and improper handling of materials are responsible for the majority of accidents that disable hospital personnel.

Patients, nursing staff, resident and visiting physicians, support staff, and visitors are all susceptible to injury from falls in or around the critical care area. The special care unit, particularly in a teaching hospital, tends to sustain an enormous amount of traffic: CCU patients coming from the emergency room, or in transit to or from the cath lab; the postcardiac surgical patient enroute from the operating room with an entourage of nurses, surgeons, anesthesiologists, and frequently much equipment including a ventilator, one or more drainage pumps and one or more infusion pumps or bottles hanging from i.v. poles, and physiologic monitoring equipment. People are given ample opportunity to trip over each other, equipment, power cords, and patient connecting lines.

Proper facilities design coupled with safe operating practices, preventive maintenance and continuing education will minimize accidents due to falls and collision. Reduction of accidents due to improper handling of materials is best accomplished through the learning and practice of correct technique. In the Special Care Unit this primarily relates to the lifting and transferring of helpless patients by the staff. Proper patient handling techniques are described elsewhere in this handbook.

Design Considerations

Accident prevention begins in the design phase of facilities and is perpetuated through preventive maintenance and staff education. The safety effort must carefully consider each of the items listed below in the design of new special care units.

Traffic control — Wherever possible, special care unit corridors should only serve the traffic necessary for the unit to function efficiently; the corridors of the unit should not be a major thoroughfare for other hospital functions. The objectives here are fourfold. First, minimizing traffic through the unit decreases the potential for a falling or collision injury. Second, the special care unit staff is busy enough with the tasks of direct patient care; adding the distractions of irrelevant traffic can only degrade safe and effective staff performance. Third, reducing traffic aids in controlling the spread of infection. Finally, we must consider the psychological impact of various kinds of traffic on patients in the unit. Intuition and first-hand feedback from coronary care unit patients tells us that their constant exposure to other critically ill patients, particularly those appearing to suffer from physical trauma, is distressing.

Corridor size — Corridors should be wide enough to minimize congestion during peak traffic periods. The 1976 Life Safety Code (paragraph 10-2.2.5.2) specifies that "aisles, corridors, and ramps required for exit access or exit in a hospital or nursing home shall be at least 8 feet in clear and unobstructed width." This section of the code deals with exit contingencies during emergencies, particularly fire, but the principle applies to routine safety enhancement. Corridors leading to, and within, the special care unit must not be obstructed by trash carts, linen or other supply carts, or power cords. Permanent potential obstructions, such as water fountains, should be recessed. During safety inspections, the most frequent excuse offered for corridor obstructions is lack of adequate storage space. Thus, design of new facilities must include an adequate allowance for storage, particularly for areas providing critical care, which, by necessity, are supply- and equipment-intensive. In paragraph 10-2.2.5.4, the Code states that "any room, and any suite of rooms...of more than 1,000 square feet shall have at least 2 exit access doors remote from each other." Most special care units are larger than 1000 ft^2, and thus require two exit doors. For safety in day-to-day operation, these two doors should not encourage traffic through the unit. The door at one end of the unit could, for instance, handle routine operations traffic, while the other door could be for emergencies (fire, etc.) only.

Floors — Floor materials in and around a special care unit should be clean, dry, slip-resistant, and, in the case of carpet, permit easy transport of wheeled patients and equipment. The American Carpet Institute points to numerous studies indicating that carpet tends to hold less bacteria than tiled areas and tends to reduce the spread of bacteria.[3]

Patient rooms — Special care unit rooms should be sized to promote safe and effective patient care, and should be located such that all patients in the unit can be seen from a central nurses' station. The U.S. Department of Health, Education and Welfare requires a minimum clear area of 120 ft^2 in each intensive care unit single-bed room.[4] Intensive care rooms which are smaller than the suggested minimum overcrowd too easily, making it impossible for the staff to have safe and easy access to the patient. Single rooms much larger than 150 ft^2 offer little advantage to direct patient care. HEW also requires that all beds be arranged to permit direct visual observation by the nursing staff: "Viewing panels shall be provided in doors and walls for nursing staff observation of patients. Curtains or other means shall be provided to cover the viewing panels when the patient requires visual privacy. Glazing in viewing panels shall be safety glass, wire glass, or clear plastic to reduce the hazard from accidental breakage except that wire glass is required in glazed openings to corridors or passageways used as means of egress for fire safety purposes." In addition, the Joint Commission on

Accreditation of Hospitals (JCAH) requires that "direct or indirect visual observation by unit staff of all patients shall be possible from one or more vantage points."[5] This strong emphasis on patient visibility in special care units is mandated by the functional requirements for effectiveness of treatment and safety in patient care.

Safe Practices

Accidents will occur in the most well-designed facility without collateral safe operating practices. The following considerations are not unique to the special care unit, but deserve particular attention due to the increased risk to both patient and staff in that environment.

Corridors, passageways, patient rooms, and ancillary facilities — Within the special care unit, these must be kept as free and clear of clutter as possible. Obviously, with fewer things to trip over, there should be fewer tripping and falling accidents.

Storage and supply areas — These should be well-organized. The intended location for each item should be appropriately labeled, and an easy-to-understand inventory location guide should be conspicuously posted in each supply room. An "out-of-stock" log should be available for the staff to use as inventory is depleted.

Compressed gas cylinders — These (most commonly O_2) need particular attention in the special care unit. They should be properly capped and stored and secured by a chain or strap. The contents of each cylinder should be properly identified by both label and color code. Do not, however, rely solely on color code, as variability exists between manufacturers. Also, cylinders should never be left in a corridor or passageway, even if properly secured. A violent strike by a bed or machine in transit can cause a serious accident. In addition, gases should never be stored where they could be subjected to extreme heat. The resulting high pressures within the cylinder can cause an explosion, with the cylinder becoming a lethal projectile.

Body mechanics — Exercise care in lifting patients or transferring them from bed to stretcher, chair, or weighing scale. (See section in this handbook on proper body mechanic techniques.) With helpless patients, always have at least two persons perform such tasks. To prevent inadvertent disconnection, added care is required with patients connected to ventilators, invasive monitoring equipment, and infusion lines.

Patient falls — Use bedrails, and, if necessary, restraints to prevent patient falls or other self-harm when the patient's condition is such that these are deemed necessary.

Patient equipment — Locate the bedstand and nurse-call controls so that they can be safely used by the patient. The patient should not have to stressfully reach for these items.

Medication — Follow hospital standards in the administration of i.v. solutions and in dispensing medication. Another section in this handbook notes that the probability of medication errors is higher in special care units than anywhere else in the hospital. The controls required to prevent such errors must be comprehensive and well-understood by the entire staff.

Patient, staff, and visitor education — This is central to the issue of accident prevention. Special care unit staff meetings should always include a review of accidents as part of the educational process, and policies and procedures should be continually subject to the revisions required to prevent future misadventures.

The Electric Power Distribution System

The National Electrical Code

Safety, installation, and performance requirements of the electric power distribution system are specified by local authorities. These requirements are generally based on (or duplicate) the National Electrical Code, NFPA 70.[6] Some of its requirements or recommendations for critical care areas are shown below.

517-84. Critical Care Areas.

(a) Each patient bed location shall be provided with a minimum of six single or three duplex receptacles, and grounded to the reference grounding point by means of an insulated copper equipment grounding conductor.

(b) Each patient bed location shall be supplied by at least two branch circuits, one or more from the Emergency System. At least one shall be an individual branch circuit. All branch circuits from the normal system shall be from a single panelboard; all branch circuits from the Emergency System shall be from a single panelboard. Emergency System receptacles shall be identified, and shall also indicate the panelboard and circuit number supplying them. Exception: Branch circuits serving only special-purpose receptacles or equipment in Critical Care Areas shall be permitted to be served by other panelboards.

(c) Each patient bed location shall be provided with a patient grounding point, grounded to the reference grounding point by means of an insulated continuous copper conductor, not smaller than No. 10, running directly to the Reference Grounding Point or by means of a conductor permanently connected to the grounding conductor of a nearby power receptacle. The patient grounding point shall contain one or more jacks, approved for the purpose. See Section 517-82.

(d) The equipment grounding terminal bars of the normal and Emergency System panelboards shall be bonded together with an insulated continuous copper conductor, not smaller than No. 10.

(e) One or more room bonding points shall be provided, and shall be grounded to the reference point by means of an insulated continuous copper connector, not smaller than No. 10.

(f) Exposed conductive surfaces in the patient vicinity shall be connected to the room bonding point(s) or the reference grounding point by continuous copper conductors, or conductive building structural members having conductance at least equal to AWG No. 10 copper wire. The bonding conductors, if installed, may be arranged centrically or looped as convenient. Exception: Small wall-mounted conductive surfaces not likely to become energized such as surface-mounted towel and soap dispensers, mirrors, and so forth, need not be connected to the Room Bonding Point.

(g) Any of the grounding and bonding points in Section 517-84 (c) through (f) shall be permitted to be combined into a single point.

(h) One patient bed location shall not be served by more than one reference grounding point.

517-90. Additional Protective Techniques. Isolated Power Systems.

(a) The isolated power system shall be approved for the purpose and so designed and installed that the systems meet the provisions and are in accordance with Section 517-104. Exception: The audible and visual indicators of the line isolation monitor shall be permitted to be located at the nursing station for the area being served.*

Regarding Section 517-84(a), the author cautions that the minimum requirement of six receptacles per bed location may not be enough in units where a great many powered devices are used, such as in a postcardiac surgery intensive care unit. Ten receptacles are more realistic for these locations. It is further recommended that each bed location be served by at least three branch circuits in areas where life support devices are extensively used. Ideally, one circuit breaker per receptacle is preferred. In one instance, a short circuit in a reading lamp tripped a circuit breaker, disabling power to a ventilator. Tragedy was narrowly avoided by an alert member of the nursing staff. With individual circuit breakers, the incident would not have occurred.

Use of grounding jacks to assure proper grounding of portable equipment is of questionable value. Periodic inspections of both the equipment and receptacles should be the first line of defense against inadequate grounding since the cables connecting the grounding point to the equipment introduce serious tripping and falling hazards.

Isolated power systems (IPS), while permitted in critical care areas by the Code, are initially expensive and provide no protection for microshock hazards, although they do protect against macroshock. Maintenance costs are higher than for grounded power systems, and IPS are frequently not considered cost-effective. The reader is referred to Health Devices, Volume III (pages 239 to 263, August-September 1974) for a full discussion of the pros and cons of isolated power systems.

* Reproduced with the kind permission of National Fire Protection Association 70, National Electrical Code, National Fire Protection Association, Boston, 1977.

A Safe Electrical Environment

The Joint Commission on Accreditation of Hospitals (JCAH) states the following:

> A continued effort shall be made at all levels to provide an electrically safe environment within the hospital. All personnel must be instructed that the use of electricity introduces the hazards of burn, shock, explosion, fire, and power failure, with the possibility of injury, disability, or death, and damage to or malfunction of equipment or facilities. Written policies and procedures shall be established for, but not be limited to...Systematic, periodic evaluation of the electrical power distribution systems and all electrical and electronic non-patient care equipment. Evaluation shall be made of all elements of electrical power distribution systems, including receptacles, following new construction, renovation, or replacement, and at least annually thereafter. Receptacle inspection shall include testing for polarity, quality of ground, and mechanical security.[5]

The same document also requires that all inspections, action taken, and recommendations be documented in writing.

The program guidelines recommended by the JCAH are comprehensive; written policies and procedures, required implementation, and thorough documentation with appropriate internal distribution are all included. In practice, written policies are easy to generate, but written procedures and enforced implementation are often difficult for all hospitals to achieve in all patient areas. Where fiscal constraints and limited manpower resources prohibit full implementation, it is recommended that strong emphasis be placed on special care units, emergency rooms, operating rooms, and cardiac catheterization laboratories where patients are particularly susceptible to hazards associated with the power distribution system.

In one large teaching hospital, for example, there are well over 10,000 receptacles in all patient care areas. Special care areas (those treating critically ill patients) receive quarterly receptacle inspections. Intermediate care areas receive annual inspections, and areas where electrically operated devices are not routinely used for patient care are inspected only every 5 yr. All patient areas, however, employ U.L.-approved hospital-grade receptacles.

The following policy was developed by a hospital in 1978. It is based on JCAH guidelines requiring procedures, implementation, and documentation and assigns specific functional responsibilities. Such a policy appears in the safety committee minutes of the hospital and is approved by its medical board.

POLICY
POWER DISTRIBUTION SYSTEM AND NONCLINICAL EQUIPMENT: SAFETY AND EFFECTIVENESS

General

It is the policy of Metro Hospital to assure that the electrical power distribution system, as well as all electrical, electromechanical, and electronic nonclinical equipment, remain safe and effective.

Application

All elements of the electrical distribution system are included. All nonclinical electrically powered equipment, both fixed and mobile, are also included. Nonclinical equipment encompasses building, dietary, and entertainment equipment, as well as electric beds, lamps, and similar items.

Acceptance Testing

All new elements of the electric power distribution system, as well as all applicable equipment, shall be evaluated for safety and performance prior to being put into service. It shall be the responsibility of the engineering services department to assure that such acceptance testing is performed in accordance with applicable safety standards, codes and regulations, and manufacturers' specifications. Acceptance testing procedures and results shall be documented.

Scheduled Service

Elements of the power distribution system and all applicable equipment shall be periodically evaluated for safety and effectiveness and calibrated or repaired if required. Primary emphasis shall be placed on those items serving critical care areas. Tests shall be performed in accordance with written procedures based on applicable safety standards, codes and regulations, and manufacturers' specifications. The testing interval shall be specified. It shall be the responsibility of the engineering services department to assure that scheduled service procedures and testing intervals are established and that all procedures and work are documented.

Procedures for conducting an electrical safety inspection in special care units are contained in Appendix A. These procedures were developed in 1970 and have been revised annually. The procedures are practical, detailed, provide for good documentation of results, and require only moderate technical skills for implementation.

Emergency Power

Special care units must continue to provide life support and patient monitoring in the event of electric power failure, i.e., the electrical power distribution system must be fail-safe. For this reason, an autonomous source of emergency power is required. Such generators are expensive, space-consuming, and noisy. They must be large enough to permit the hospital to function adequately for the duration of the emergency, but need not power the luxuries and conveniences afforded by the normal power system. Therefore, in the design phase of special care units, careful attention must be paid to deciding which circuits are to be connected to the emergency power source. Consider the following incident.

In the respiratory care unit of one hospital, all life support and monitoring circuits were designed into the emergency power system, but the nurse-call system was not. Power failed for 3 hr late one evening when the census was high and the unit was short-staffed. The result in this case was some added inconvenience for the nursing staff, but a catastrophe could have occurred. The next day, the engineering department connected the nurse-call system power supply to an emergency circuit.

The National Electric Code fully describes requirements for the installation, operation, and maintenance of emergency power systems.[6] Loss of normal power must be detected and the emergency source brought on line within 10 sec of power failure. Receptacles connected to the emergency power source should be appropriately identified, and the staff should be familiar with which receptacles can be used during failure of the normal power system.

Heating, Ventilation, and Air Conditioning

Heating, ventilation, and air conditioning (HVAC) systems for special care units and all other areas of the hospital must provide an air supply at specified temperature, humidity, exchange rates, recirculation rates, and filtration levels. Minimum HEW requirements for temperature and humidity are shown in Table 1.[4] Compiled from the same source, Table 2 specifies pressure relationships and ventilation requirements, while Table 3 specifies filtration efficiencies.

All HVAC system components must be installed in accordance with local regulatory requirements. The JCAH requires policies and procedures similar to those required for the electrical power distribution system.[5] HVAC equipment is usually large and expensive, and, in the author's judgment, the hospital is wise to follow the lead of commercial industry in keeping its mechanical systems in good working order via a comprehensive preventive maintenance program for safety, clinical effectiveness, and economic reasons.

Table 1
TEMPERATURE AND HUMIDITY REQUIREMENTS FOR CERTAIN CLINICAL AREAS[4]

Area designation	Temperature		Relative humidity (%)	
	°F	°C	min	max
Operating rooms	70—76[a]	21—24[a]	50	60
Delivery rooms	70—76[a]	21—24[a]	50	60
Recovery rooms	75	24	50	60
Intensive care rooms	75—80[a]	24—27[a]	30	60
Nurseries unit	75	24	30	60
Special care nursery unit	75—80[a]	24—27[a]	30	60

[a] Variable range required.

Table 2
GENERAL PRESSURE RELATIONSHIPS AND VENTILATION OF CERTAIN HOSPITAL AREAS[4]

Area designation	Pressure relationship to adjacent areas	Minimum air changes of outdoor air per hour supplied to room	Minimum total air changes per hour supplied to room	All air exhausted directly to outdoors	Recirculated within room units
Nursery unit	P	5	12	Optional	No
Recovery room	P	2	6	Optional	No
Intensive care	P	2	6	Optional	No
Patient room	E	2	2	Optional	Optional
Patient room corridor	E	2	4	Optional	Optional
Isolation room	E	2	6	Yes	No
Isolation room-alcove or anteroom	E	2	10	Yes	No
Medication room	P	2	4	Optional	Optional
Soiled workroom or soiled holding	N	2	10	Yes	No
Clean workroom or clean holding	P	2	4	Optional	Optional
Toilet room	N	Optional	10	Yes	No
Bedpan room	N	Optional	10	Yes	No
Bathroom	N	Optional	10	Yes	No
Janitors' closet	N	Optional	10	Yes	No
Sterilizer equipment room	N	Optional	10	Yes	No
Linen and trash chute rooms	N	Optional	10	Yes	No
Clean linen storage	P	2	2	Optional	Optional

Table 3
FILTER EFFICIENCIES FOR CENTRAL VENTILATION AND AIR CONDITIONING SYSTEMS IN GENERAL HOSPITALS[4]

		Filter efficiencies (%)	
Area designation	Minimum number of filter beds	Filter bed no. 1	Filter bed no. 2
Sensitive areas[a]	2	25	90
Patient care, treatment, diagnostic, and related areas	2	25	90[b]
Food preparation areas and laundries	1	80	—
Administrative, bulk storage, and soiled holdings areas	1	25	—

[a] Includes operating rooms, delivery rooms, nurseries, recovery rooms, and intensive care units.
[b] May be reduced to 80% for systems using all-outdoor air.

Table 4
STATION OUTLETS FOR OXYGEN AND VACUUM (SUCTION) SYSTEMS[4]

Location	Oxygen	Vacuum
Patient room for adult medical, surgical, and post-partum care, and for pediatrics	A	A
Examination and treatment room for nursing unit	B	B
Patient room for intensive care	C	C
Nursery and pediatric nursery	A	A
General operating room	F	F
Cystoscopy and special procedure room	D	D
Recovery room for surgical and obstetrical patients	E	E
Delivery room	F	G
Labor room	A	A
Treatment room for emergency care	D	D
Autopsy room	—	D
Anesthesia workroom	—	D

Note: A = one outlet accessible to each bed (one outlet may serve two beds); B = one outlet (portable equipment for the administration of oxygen and suction may be considered acceptable in lieu of fixed outlets); C = two outlets for each bed or provide one outlet with Y-fitting; D = one outlet; E = one outlet for each bed; F = two outlets; G = three outlets.

Medical Gas Systems

Requirements for medical gas systems — air, oxygen, and vacuum — vary with different special care units. The minimum requirements of HEW are listed in Table 4 for oxygen and vacuum. Installation requirements for vacuum systems are specified by the Compressed Gas Association in their Pamphlet No. P-2.1; NFPA 56A and 56F specify installation requirements for nonflammable medical gas systems.

Scheduled service of compressors, suction pumps, and outlets is required to assure ongoing system safety and effectiveness. Without periodic lubrication of outlets, for instance, system leaks can severely strain pumps or compressors. These outlets generally require special lubricants to prevent seal degradation and ensure biocompatibility. Consult the manufacturer for details.

Valves should be conveniently located for access by the engineering staff, but not so accessible as to invite sabotage or mischievous behavior by young or ill-bent visitors. In addition, the 1974 Occupational Safety and Health Act (OSHA) specifically provides that oxygen "storage containers, piping, valves, regulating equipment, and other accessories shall be protected against physical damage and against tampering."[7]

Contingency plans must be prepared in the event of electric power failure, and, in the case of water-cooled machines, loss of water pressure. Sufficient portable suction pumps must be available to supply the needs of all special care facilities, as well as operating rooms. Tanks of medical oxygen and air must also be available, with members of the appropriate staff (engineering or respiratory therapy) trained in connecting the tanks into the central gas systems.

It is also recommended that each special care unit using the central system have visual and audible alarms actuated by significant changes in operating pressure. Scheduled service procedures must include verifying performance of the alarm system.

Water

Complete water loss in the special care unit is obviously disastrous to both the general safety and effectiveness of patient care. For these reasons, the JCAH specifies that a backup capability be available in the event of primary system failure. This author cautions the special care unit to consider all implications of water loss, including shutdown of steam autoclaves and possible loss of central vacuum and compressed air supplies. Backup supplies can be stored in-house, or standby contracts can be arranged with outside vendors. In addition, water temperature at the hot water outlet must be high enough to serve its function, but not so high as to cause burns. A maximum temperature of 110°F (43°C) is specified by HEW.

CLINICAL EQUIPMENT

General

During the last 15 years there has been an enormous increase in the quantity and variety of devices used in the diagnosis and therapy of critically ill patients. The last 10 years has seen an increasingly widespread concern for the safety of the patient whose environment has become crammed with all sorts of machines to monitor his every variable, sustain his respiration, cool or warm him, infuse all manner of fluids, and even resuscitate him when his heart fails. This concern for patient safety is reflected throughout the hospital community. It is probably the fundamental reason why the new field of clinical engineering has grown so rapidly. Clinical engineering departments are one of the very few new features to be found on hospital organization charts in decades.

Old literature has been revised. In 1976, the JCAH began requiring hospitals to develop a comprehensive program for the safe application of electrically powered clinical devices. The Medical Device Amendments of 1976 allowed the Food and Drug Administration (FDA) to ban or recall hazardous or potentially hazardous devices. The American Society for Hospital Engineering of the American Hospital Association has published (1978) "A Hospital Recall and Reporting System for Medical Devices." In 1971, the Emergency Care Research Institute (Philadelphia) began publishing "Health Devices," a consumers' report for the health care industry.

The proliferation of clinical equipment, its relative complexity, and recognition of the risks associated with its use all contribute to the need for a special effort to assure safe and effective application.

The Need for a Comprehensive Program

In this author's experience, most incidents involving clinical equipment are associated with one of two basic operational weaknesses. These are

1. The user does not fully understand operation of the device and/or the hazards associated with its use (or the user acts hastily and forgets to pay attention to detail).
2. The device has been abused in routine use and/or it has not been properly maintained.

Spontaneous equipment failures certainly do occur, and equipment exists that is not as inherently safe as it could be, but in the main, the two reasons cited above constitute the majority of clinical equipment problems. This is particularly true in hospitals where educational and scheduled service programs are not fully developed.

Hospital-wide policies, procedures, and services for dealing with safety and effectiveness of clinical equipment must be developed and implemented. These must be firm enough to comply with applicable external standards, yet flexible enough to be tailored to the needs of individual special care units.

The JCAH requires development of, and compliance with, a program intended to minimize hazards associated with the use of electrically powered clinical devices.[5] Portions of these recommendations appear below. It should be emphasized that the principles involved apply equally to all clinical devices, not just electrically powered ones.

> A continued effort shall be made at all levels to provide an electrically safe environment. All personnel must be instructed that the use of electricity introduces the hazards of burn, shock, explosion, fire, and power failure, with the possibility of injury, disability, or death, and damage to or malfunction of equipment or facilities.... Written policies and procedures shall be established for, but not limited to... special precautions that must be taken when the care of a patient requires the use of any type of electrically operated device.... Method and frequency of testing verification of performance- and use- specifications, for all electrical and electronic patient care equipment, based upon established safety requirements, performance criteria, and manufacturers' claims. Such testing and verification shall apply to both fixed and mobile equipment, with particular emphasis on life-support equipment, such as respirators, defibrillators, physiological monitoring systems, infant incubators, and warmers .... All new equipment shall be so evaluated prior to its use. The testing interval... shall be consistent with the manufacturer's recommendations, standards promulgated by recognized technical organizations, and frequency of use. In no case shall the testing interval exceed 6 months. The requirement for written records of all inspections performed on electrical and electronic systems and equipment, including any action taken or recommended. Development and implementation of an effective system for determining current leakage, ensuring proper grounding and other device-safety requirements, and providing appropriate corrective measures.[5]

As in the case of the electrical power distribution system, the JCAH approach to safety and function is comprehensive; written policies and procedures, implementation, and documentation are all required. Note that safety and effectiveness (performance) are tightly linked. It can easily be argued that a device which does not perform according to the specifications of a manufacturer is, by default, unsafe even though shock, burn, or other conditions secondary to unsafe equipment are absent.

Two case histories are presented below which illustrate what can and frequently does happen in the absence of a comprehensive program for equipment safety.

Case History No. 1

The clinical engineering department of County Memorial Hospital was called at 7:30 a.m. and informed that at 2:30 a.m. on the same morning a 67-year-old white male neurosurgical patient had arrested. During the resuscitation attempt, the patient was subjected to numerous defibrillation shocks from three different defibrillators. It was alleged that none of the machines worked.

Inspection of the machines by the clinical engineering department revealed a loose lamp holder on one machine and crushed insulation on the power cord of another, but both of the machines were functionally sound. The third machine, which happened to be the one first used on the patient, was in perfect condition. Functional testing of all machines included repeated discharges into a test load at various power output settings.

Interview of all parties present at the attempted resuscitation, including seven nurses and two physicians, revealed two crucial facts. First, the patient had not been continuously monitored; thus, the exact time of arrest in relation to the start of resuscitation protocol could not be ascertained. Second, everyone involved concluded that the machines had malfunctioned because the patient did not "jump" when the shock was delivered.

Retrospectively, it was concluded that enough time had elapsed between the arrest and its discovery that neuromuscular response to the shock was not possible. (This author is not aware of any published work which estimates the time between cessation of circulation and neuromuscular dissociation, but it is probably not much more than 10 min.)

Several lessons were learned from this incident. First, the clinical engineering department should have been "on call" 24 hr/day to respond to emergencies, or alleged emergencies. Second, the medical and nursing staff should have been alert to the possibility that the patient was in fact dead on discovery of the arrest. Third, all defibrillators at County Memorial were placed on a monthly performance verification schedule to assure that conditions like the loose lamp holder and frayed power cord would be corrected by a trained technical staff before more serious problems developed.

Case History No. 2

A nurse in the surgical intensive care unit at Heelum Hospital called the biomedical electronics department to report intermittent, but unresolvable 60Hz interference on the ECG presentation of a recent cardiac surgery patient.

On investigation, the biomedical equipment technician (BMET) noted that the patient was surrounded by electrically operated equipment, including monitors, a ventilator, three infusion pumps, and a chest drainage pump. The nurse and BMET selectively unplugged each device and found that the drainage pump was the culprit; the trace cleaned up as soon as the pump was unplugged. A replacement pump was installed and the original one carefully inspected. Ground wire current was measured and found to go to zero intermittently. The power plug was opened: the screw attaching the ground wire to the grounding prong was missing, and the ground wire was intermittently touching the hot terminal, thus raising the metal case of the pump to full line potential. Fortunately, this radiating antenna interfered with the patient's ECG; the presence of the interference inspired the nurse to call for help.

Three important points are noteworthy. First, the nurse's response to the electrical interference was both valid and fortunate. Second, the plug was improperly installed. Had an equipment acceptance test program been in effect, this defect would have been detected. Third, routine scheduled service would also have detected the fault.

Components of a Comprehensive Program

Policies

As suggested earlier, a comprehensive equipment safety program for each special care unit begins with the umbrella policies, procedures, and services provided by central administration. An example of a policy statement designed to comply with JCAH standards is shown below.

POLICY
CLINICAL DEVICE SAFETY AND EFFECTIVENESS

General

It is the policy of Metro Hospital to assure that all powered clinical systems and devices are as safe and effective as possible when they are properly used for their intended purpose.

Application

All systems and devices, both fixed and mobile, which are used by medical, nursing, or technical staff in the diagnosis, therapy, or other aspect of direct patient care, and which are either electrically, pneumatically, or otherwise powered, are included. Also included are all accessories to such equipment, as well as all equipment used to calibrate, repair, or otherwise assure the proper performance and safety of clinical equipment.

Acceptance Testing

All applicable systems and devices shall be evaluated for safety and performance prior to use for patient care. It shall be the responsibility of the Director of the Department acquiring the equipment to assure that equipment is not used for patient care prior to a technical evaluation. The clinical engineering department, or any other facility approved by the safety committee, shall either perform acceptance testing or certify that such acceptance testing has been performed in accordance with applicable safety standards, performance criteria and manufacturers' specifications. Acceptance testing procedures and results shall be documented.

Scheduled Service

All applicable equipment shall be periodically tested for safety and performance and recalibrated if required. Tests shall be in accordance with written procedures based on established safety requirements, performance criteria, and manufacturers' specifications. Frequency of testing shall be specified; in no case shall the testing interval exceed 6 months. It shall be the responsibility of the director of the department owning the equipment to assure that applicable equipment is tested. The clinical engineering department, or any other facility approved by the safety committee, shall be responsible for establishing written procedures and testing intervals. All procedures and work performed shall be documented.

Note that the policy, while broad, assigns specific functional responsibility for each major point addressed, including acceptance testing and scheduled service.

Procedures

Written policies demonstrate the initial commitment of hospital management to the concept of providing a program for safe and effective equipment. Policies must be followed by procedures. A technical staff, such as a clinical engineering department or variation thereof, is needed to write and implement equipment performance verification, safety, and calibration procedures. The same group must work closely with the clinical staff, both nursing and medical, in developing safe and effective operating procedures.

The Scheduled Service Procedure shown in Appendix B is an example of a protocol used by the technical staff at specified intervals to assure that the equipment is both safe and effective when properly used. This kind of procedure is written and implemented before the equipment is ever placed into clinical service. Hence, it serves as the major portion of Metro Hospital's acceptance test for the equipment. The balance of an acceptance test protocol includes inspection for shipping damage, assurance of complete shipment, and other routine and less technical matters. Note that forms for full documentation are included with this procedure.

Availability of the Clinical Engineering Staff

Metro Hospital has clustered most of its special care units and operating rooms on a single horizontal plane. Support services, such as radiology and respiratory therapy, either have satellite facilities within this cluster, or they serve the entire hospital from this area. The clinical engineering department is also located within the cluster. This author finds this rare in the hospital community, but extremely useful to the critical care function. Technicians are immediately available for problem-solving and they have developed excellent rapport with the various nursing staffs. While they do not participate in direct patient care, they certainly enhance it by their immediate availability to the bedside nurse.

Reducing the Communications Barrier

Safety and effectiveness in the application of high-technology equipment to patient care is less than optimal when the clinical and technical staffs are unable to understand each other's language. The clinical staff must have at least some rudimentary appreciation of the principles which operate sophisticated equipment, and the technical staff must understand something of the clinical aspects of equipment application. Without this mutual understanding, neither group can fully appreciate the hazards associated with the patient/equipment interface.

Each group benefits by both formal and practical education in the other's field of specialization. At Metro, BMETs are encouraged to attend weekly in-service education classes sponsored by each of the special care units. Here they learn something of the nature of disease, its diagnosis, and treatment. Some of the classes are devoted entirely to equipment safety and are taught by a member of the clinical engineering staff. One of the most effective of these classes addresses safe use of a defibrillator. The sequence described below was presented several years ago when Metro used grounded defibrillators, i.e., one paddle was electrically bonded to power line ground through the power cord. The user was taught to make sure that he or she never contacted the metal plates of either paddle during use, whether directly or through excess conductive gel applied prior to discharge. The demonstration was particularly effective because it illustrated the hazard to the operator in very unambiguous terms.

In the demonstration, a desk top gooseneck lamp with a 50 W incandescent bulb was "doctored up" to simulate a nurse using a defibrillator (see Figure 1). Two wires of the power cord, simulating the nurse's arms, were terminated with alligator clips. One clip was attached to a water pipe (simulating the nurse inadvertently touching ground), and the other to one of the defibrillator paddles. When the defibrillator discharged, the extremely bright flash of light which occurred just before the bulb filament disintegrated convincingly argued the potency of the defibrillator. Visible energy — not meters, nor a slide show, nor a lecture — convinced the audience that the defibrillator is powerful indeed. The communication barrier can drop to remarkable lows with this kind of presentation.

INFECTION CONTROL

The topic of infection control is fully discussed in another section of this handbook and the reader is referred there for an understanding of the principles of infection development, transmission, and prevention. The problem of infection control in the special care unit is really a much magnified version of the problem in general patient care areas. There are two primary reasons for this.

First, patients in these units are subjected to the largest number of invasive procedures, and the opportunity for infection is increased with each invasion. Multiple i.v. lines, endotracheal tubes, suction tubes, arterial pressure lines, arterial stick sites, cen-

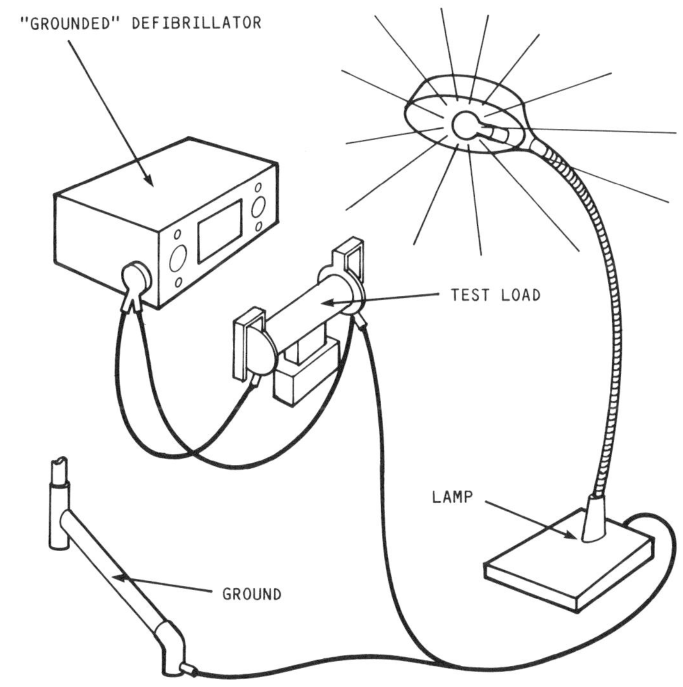

FIGURE 1. Setup to demonstrate defibrillator potency.

tral venous pressure lines, cardiac output and right heart pressure catheters, abdominal and thoracic drainage tubes, and nasogastric tubes each contribute to the likelihood of infection. To reduce attendant infection risks, special sterile or clean procedures must be followed for both insertion and maintenance of these lines.

Second, even without invasion, patients in special care units are the most susceptible to infection, either due to directly impaired immune systems or their generally weakened condition. Age, too, strongly influences the patients' ability to resist infection; newborns and the elderly are most susceptible.

Compounding the problem of the patients' condition, the staff sometimes tends to cut corners in the intensive care environment, particularly as crises develop.

Proper facilities design and thorough indoctrination of the staff to infection control protocols can act to enhance a low infection rate. The following environmental factors need to be considered in the design of any special care unit, regardless of specific function.

Environmental Factors

Handwashing facilities — There is virtually universal agreement that handwashing is the single most important procedural factor in preventing the spread of infection. Every special care patient room and work area must have a sink with hot and cold water and soap, which can be used immediately after contamination with any unclean material.

Traffic control — As discussed earlier, facilities design and administrative procedures should discourage unnecessary movement through the special care unit. People spread airborne infection simply by moving about; they also spread infection as asymptomatic carriers. Obviously, persons with clinical symptoms of infection (other than resident patients) must be prohibited from the special care unit.

Separation of functions — Each special care unit should have separate areas for clean and dirty functions. Dirty linens, for instance, should not accumulate or be removed through the clean linen supply area. Good facilities design should support administrative procedures prohibiting staff members from contacting clean supplies immediately after contact with contaminated material. This is accomplished by convenient location of handwashing facilities.

Ventilation — The pressure relationships, filtration characteristics, and air exchange rates in Tables 1 to 3 are all designed to minimize the spread of airborne contaminants. Ventilation systems serving patients extraordinarily susceptible to infection should be served by high efficiency filters.

Isolation rooms — Each special care unit should have an isolation room separated from the main corridor by an anteroom. The isolation room should have handwashing, bathing, and toilet facilities. The ventilation system serving the isolated patient should prevent the mixing of isolation room air with air in the rest of the facility. To this end, the anteroom should be designed to serve as an airlock. The anteroom must have storage space for gowns and masks, and it must have a handwashing sink for staff use.

General Procedures

Most infection control protocols are diagnosis or procedure specific. There are, however, general rules to be written and enforced which apply to the care of patients in all categories, and to all medical procedures as well.

General procedural guidelines for infection control in the special care unit include the following:

1. Effective handwashing must be done between handling of different patients, after handling the patients' excretions or secretions, before contacting the patients' face and mouth, before eating, after using the toilet, and when hands are otherwise known to be soiled.
2. Tubing and i.v. bottles should be changed at least every 24 hr and the change should be documented.
3. Nursing personnel must wear clean uniforms every day; sweaters should not be permitted.
4. When handling large amounts of patients' drainage or secretions, a gown should be worn during the process, and then discarded.
5. Patient and staff contact with visitors should be minimized, and consistent with reasonable short visiting privileges.
6. Excess linen, equipment, and other supplies should not be kept in the patient room.
7. Equipment used with patients in isolation should remain in the isolation room until the patient leaves, at which time the room and equipment should be disinfected.
8. Used hypodermic needles should be safely discarded in a nonglass container, and then incinerated.
9. The housekeeping staff should keep all areas of the special care unit clean and disinfected. Special precautions must be taken in cleaning rooms after use by patients with communicable diseases. Walls, floors, and equipment in these rooms must be disinfected by the housekeeping department immediately after use.

ELECTRICAL SAFETY SURVEY - SPECIAL AREAS

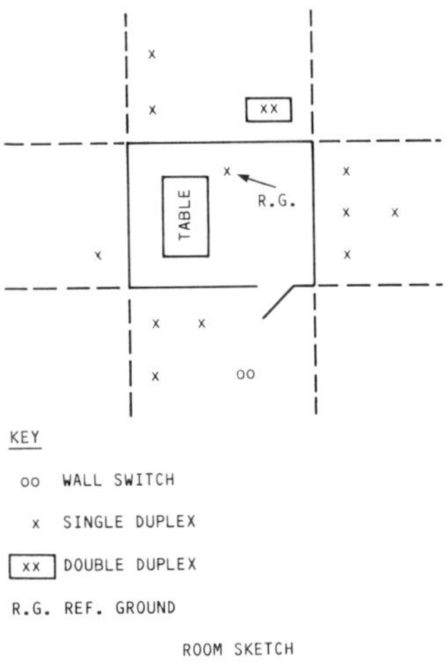

1. Room Sketch - Show outlets, switches and reference ground location on room sketch. Observe physical condition of each.
2. Light Switches - verify that light switches are working.
3. Receptable Tension - Minimum acceptable tension on all three terminals is 8 oz.
4. Receptacle Wiring - All receptacles must be wired correctly.
5. Ground Potentials - Note location and magnitude of ground potentials greater than 5 mV.
6. Interground Resistance - Resistance from reference to other grounds should be 0.1 ohms or less.

COMMENTS:

DEFFECTIVE RECEPTACLES IDENTIFIED BY RED DOT

Building ______
Floor ______
Room No. ______
Function ______

Date ______
By ______

FIGURE 2. Electrical survey form.

APPENDIX A: SAMPLE PROCEDURES FOR SURVEYING THE ELECTRICAL ENVIRONMENT IN SPECIAL CARE AREAS

Metro Hospital Electrical Safety Survey Procedures for Areas Processing Patients Susceptible to Microshock Hazards

1.0 General

Any area processing patients susceptible to microshock hazards requires periodic surveys to assure that it remains a safe electrical environment. Operating rooms, catheterization labs, and intensive care units are examples of such areas. Patients in these areas are subjected to devices and procedures which may produce a direct electrical path to or through the heart. Unintentional currents flowing through the heart must be kept to a minimum.

For convenience, and because it presents a logical approach to the analysis of such areas, the survey will be split into two parts. First, the power in the room, including receptacles and switches, will be considered. Then, the individual devices which use that power will be reviewed.

2.0 Survey of Area Power Facility

The survey first considers the area exclusive of any devices normally plugged into 117 VAC power. Therefore, all devices used in the area should be unplugged so that all receptacles are available. Then, using an electrical safety survey form (see Figure 2), proceed as indicated in paragraphs 2.1 through 2.6.

2.1 Room Sketch

Make a rough outline of the room. The outline must be suitable for showing the location of each receptacle in the room and for indicating where faulty conditions exist in the room. The diagram should be clear and well-labeled so that it may be easily used in the future. See the sample electrical safety survey form. Identify the room further by noting its location, number, and function in the upper right hand corner of the form.

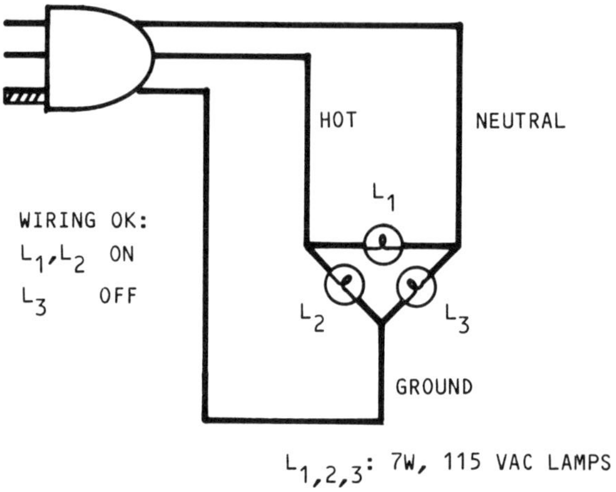

FIGURE 3. Receptacle wiring tester.

2.2 Light and Power Switches

See that all light and power switches are in good operating order. Listen and watch for signs of arcing or mechanical disorders. Note the location of defective switches on the room sketch.

2.3 Receptacle Tension

Evaluate each receptacle terminal for plug-gripping tension using an Instrutek RC-2 or equivalent. The minimum acceptable tension level is 8 oz. Use the room outline to locate defective receptacles.

2.4 Receptacle Wiring

Using a three-lamp polarity checker, see that receptacles are wired correctly. Figure 3 is a diagram of such a checker using incandescent lamps. Indicate improperly wired receptacles on the room sketch.

The incandescent lamp checker is preferred over the neon type because it gives an indication of the quality of wiring, as well as correctness. For example, a 60K Ω ground termination might indicate "ok" on a neon tester, but a tester using 7-W incandescent bulbs would indicate poor wiring for a ground termination of more than about 500 Ω.

2.5 Ground Potentials (See Measurement Technique at End of Procedure)

It is important that any two exposed conductive surfaces be equipotential. The maximum acceptable potential difference between such surfaces is 5 mV, from DC-1000 Hz.*

The first step in looking for potential differences between various surfaces is to select a single receptacle-ground terminal in the room from which to reference all voltage measurements. This point is appropriately termed "reference ground" (R.G.). R.G. is most conveniently located in the center of the room, from which point measurements

* The National Electrical Code claims that the maximum safe and allowable potential is 100 mV. While 100 mV is probably physiologically safe, it does represent a potential hazard in an apparently well-grounded room. Simply stated, it takes 1 A to generate 100 mV across 0.1 Ω. Should the ground resistance increase for any reason, the 100 mV could possibly increase to the full line potential. In fact, a 5-mV maximum is easy to achieve in most clinical environments, and anyone observing a higher potential should look for the source and correct the problem.

can be made with minimum length meter leads. Select R.G. and indicate its location on the room sketch.

After selecting R.G., measure the voltage from the reference to all exposed conductive surfaces that might be connected to the electrical system. These include water pipes, radiators, and window frames, but not such things as paper towel dispensers and coat hooks. Specifically include the ground terminal of each receptacle in the room. (All devices normally used in the room have been unplugged.) Remember, as soon as an instrument with a metal cabinet is plugged into the receptacle, the ground terminal becomes an exposed conductive surface. Making voltage measurements with clinical instruments unplugged precludes high ground currents in these instruments from contributing to high potentials in the room. These effects will be identified later in the survey.

Care must be taken when measuring potentials to chassis of instruments wired directly to the power mains (no plug). Chassis-potential measurements must be made with the device power switch in both the on and off position. If possible, set operating controls to maximize the chassis potential.

2.6 Interground Resistance

Interground resistance is the resistance between R.G. and all conductors allegedly connected to ground.

Resistance from R.G. to any other ground terminal in the room must be $\leqslant 0.1\ \Omega$. This measurement should be made at 60 Hz using the highest possible test current (up to 20 A), from a current source which cannot induce more than 5 V across its terminals. Due to the possible hazard associated with the use of high currents, this test is generally restricted to new or renovated areas.

3.0 Survey of Devices Used in Area

The second major portion of the electrical safety survey consists of a review of individual devices using 117 VAC within the room. A CED inspection form (Figure 4) will be used to record results for each device.

3.1 Device Identification

It is necessary to keep a separate record for each device that contains as much detail as possible about the instrument from the safety point of view. Identification data should include

1. Device description
2. Manufacturer
3. Model number
4. Serial number
5. High technology equipment number
6. Date
7. Tester's name

3.2 Preliminary Inspection

Before making measurements, observe and note the condition of the power cord, power and signal cable strain reliefs, power plug, fuses and fuse holders, controls, meters, and lamps. Evaluation of these items often involves sight, sound, and touch. For instance, a power switch failure may often be anticipated by feeling its mechanical action and listening to the contact closures. Use the CED inspection form to record results.

CED INSPECTION, ELECTRO-MEDICAL DEVICES

PRELIMINARY INSPECTION	IDENTIFICATION
1. Power Cord_____	Device_____
2. Strain Reliefs_____	Maun._____
3. Power Plug_____	M/N_____
4. Fuse (Holders)_____	S/N_____
5. Controls_____	HTE_____
6. Meters_____	Date_____
7. Lamps_____	By_____

GROUNDING RESISTANCE

Case-to-Power Plug Ground:_____ohms.

LEAKAGE CURRENT

	Normal Polarity	Reverse Polarity
Power On*	uA	uA
Power Off		

*Controls set for maximum leakage.

ISOLATION CURRENT**

Normal Polarity_____uA

Reverse Polarity_____uA

**Subtract leakage current measured above from total ground current measured with 110 VAC applied to patient leads.

FIGURE 4. CED inspection form.

3.3 Grounding Resistance

Any electrically operated device which is housed in an exposed metal cabinet or chassis should have that metal surface connected to power mains ground through the grounding terminal of the power plug. Case-plug grounding resistance $\leqslant 0.1\ \Omega$ is considered acceptable.

Case grounding serves two purposes. First, it is a safety measure allowing internal fault and leakage currents to be carried to ground through the case and power plug. If a short circuit should develop from a hot power line to the device case, and the case is not returned to ground through the power plug, then a person touching the case and ground simultaneously would provide the ground return path. This is obviously a hazardous condition which should not be encouraged by such infamous devices as 3-2 wire adapters or removal of the plug grounding prong.

The example concerning a direct short from the hot power line to chassis is an extreme case demonstrating how an operator can inadvertently be placed directly across 117 VAC. Note that two faults (power line short and open ground) have to exist for this to occur. It is not always necessary to have a double fault for a hazard to exist. Patients in the locations surveyed here are subject to electrocution from the microcurrents associated with normal leakage. These currents can be routed through an individual when only a single fault (open ground) occurs.

The second justification for grounding metal cases is to prevent radiation of unde-

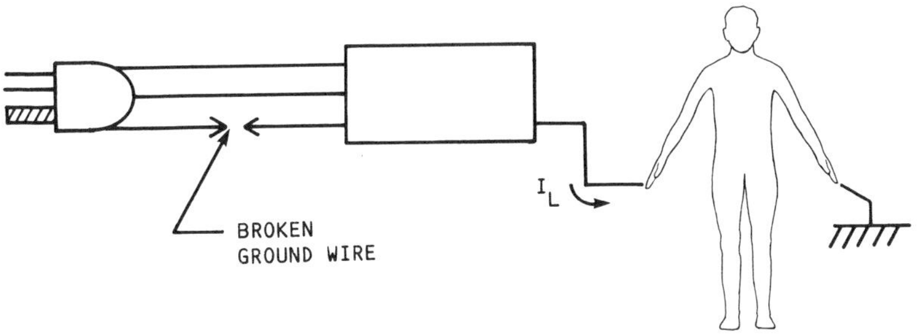

FIGURE 5. Patient provides path for leakage current (I_L) when ground wire is broken.

sirable electromagnetic interference. For instance, when an electric bed motor case loses its ground, the resulting radiation from the motor compartment may cause gross interference on the patient's ECG. The power line-related interference disappears when ground is restored to the motor frame. Thus, the grounded case serves as a radiation shield.

It is clear from the above examples that it is important to maintain a low resistance path from a device case to its power plug ground terminal.

When measuring case-plug grounding resistance, be sure to check each metal chassis subassembly. Sometimes these are joined in a mechanically secure, but electrically discontinuous manner. Beware of a dependence on bearing surfaces for electrical continuity. These paths tend to be intermittent, and, therefore, electrically unreliable. Another source of intermittent contact is in chassis-mounted male power receptacles on instruments where the power cord can be removed.

3.4 Leakage Current

Leakage currents are measured with an Instrutek LR-200, or equivalent. Current is noted with the equipment on and off, and with normal and reverse polarity applied.

The purpose of these measurements is to know how much current would flow in a line (connected from chassis to ground through an inadvertent path) in the event the power cord grounding connection is lost. Figure 5 illustrates this condition. The power cord ground connection is broken and a patient (or anyone else for that matter) contacts both the instrument chassis and earth ground. The device leakage current, I_L, which normally flows through the power cord and plug to ground, now flows through the patient to ground.

Instruments designed to measure these leakage currents generally do so by interrupting the device grounding conductor with a fixed resistance (500 or 1000 Ω) and responding to the current passing through that resistance. Provision is made to measure leakage currents for either correct or reverse polarity of the hot and neutral power lines.

Expected values of leakage current vary with several factors. However, some leakage current will always be present, even if it is very small. Power cords generally contribute about 1.3 μa/ft. Therefore, if a device has a 6-ft power cord and a meter of the type described above indicates 0-μa leakage, then it is reasonable to suspect that either the power plug grounding connection is broken or a shunt (redundant) ground path is being provided. If a continuity check reveals case-plug integrity, then redundant grounds may be assumed to exist. These shunt paths must be eliminated in order to measure leakage current.

There are various contributors to leakage currents. First, every electrically operated device will have a leakage current component due primarily to the capacitive coupling between the hot power line and ground. This occurs along the line cord as discussed above and from chassis to various components connected to the hot line, such as transformers, fuses, and power switches.

Typical leakage currents contributed by these factors range from 5 to 50 μA. As an instrument gets older, an increasing proportion of leakage current is from resistive sources since insulation qualities of certain materials degrade with age, and leakage paths develop due to dirt and moisture accumulation.

Second, devices having a DC motor will have low initial value of leakage current, such as are caused by factors discussed above. As usage continues, however, leakage currents will build up due to carbon brushes wearing out and forming a carbon powder conductive path from the windings to the motor case. Current can reach very high levels unless the motors are periodically cleaned. Respirators at MH reached leakage currents approaching 100 ma after several years of service.

Finally, any device that operates with water or in a humid environment should be regarded as a possible source of high leakage current. Moisture paths can build up around heating elements in humidifiers, suction motors in vacuum cleaners, etc. Heavy duty vacuum cleaners have been shown to have leakage up to 1 A. Such devices as submersible water heaters and vacuum cleaners should be subjected to regular and frequent inspection for high leakage current levels.

3.5 Patient Isolation

In this test, all patient leads are tied together and then subjected to 117 VAC (the hot side of the power line). As measured above, the increase in leakage current is attributable solely to the application of 117 VAC, and is, therefore, a measure of patient circuit isolation.

Care must be taken that the test is only performed on devices that are designed to withstand application of the full line potential to patient inputs. Even when so designed, a preliminary check with an ohmmeter is recommended before applying the 120 VAC. Connect the ohmmeter between the combined patient leads and chassis ground, and observe 1 to 50 mΩ.

Voltage Measurement Technique Using a Leakage Current Meter

Remember that a leakage current meter is an ammeter, and not a voltmeter. With proper precautions, however, it may be used to measure ground potentials up to several hundred millivolts. Simply multiply the current reading by the imput resistance of the meter. For example, if 50 μa is observed on a 500 Ω meter between two points in a ground circuit, the potential difference between the points is 25 mV. Note that if a 1000-Ω meter were being used for the same measurement, the reading would be 25 μa.

Be very careful in interpreting leakage current meter readings. It is crucial to know when the source is a voltage source and not a current source. Always assume a voltage source when looking across two points in the ground circuit; use an ohmmeter if in doubt. While the 25 or 50 μa used in the example above might seem innocuous enough at first glance, several amperes may be flowing in the ground circuit to produce these readings. Such current levels almost always indicate either a fault or an improper wiring technique.

APPENDIX B: SAMPLE SCHEDULED SERVICE PROCEDURE WITH DOCUMENTATION FORMS

Metro Hospital Scheduled Service Procedures

38.5 Thermotic Pump, Gomco Models 765 and 765A

I. Preventive Maintenance (after each use)

1. Thoroughly clean and dry all tubing, fittings, stoppers, and both bottles after each use.
2. Replace the 1-gal bottle stopper and interbottle connection tubing as required for a good vacuum seal.
3. Inspect the Aerovent overflow valve after each use and lightly lubricate the shaft to insure free operation.

II. Performance Verification (every 3 months) (see Figures 6 and 7)

Equipment Required

1. Leakage/Resistance Meter, Instrutek, LR-200A, or equal.
2. Vacuum manometer.

Procedures

1. Observe mechanical condition.
   a. Thoroughly inspect the entire pump to see that all screws, nuts, bolts, and other mechanical fasteners are tight.
   b. Observe that the casters are intact and operate freely.
   c. Note that other mechanical aspects are in good condition.
2. Note the condition of the power plug.
   a. The plug must be a nonmolded hospital-duty variety in visibly good condition.
   b. Observe that the strain relief is effective where the line cord enters the plug. If it is loose, the plug must be opened, inspected, and rewired, if necessary.
3. Observe the condition of the line cord.
   a. Check the line cord for breaks in insulation, signs of crushing, and other indications of excessive wear.
   b. Note the condition of the strain relief where the line cord enters the pump.
4. Verify ground wire-to-case continuity.
   a. Using the LR-200A, measure the resistance between the plug grounding pin and either front panel control nut.
   b. The resistance should be $\leqslant 0.1\ \Omega$.
   c. Values greater than this indicate poor electrical bonds. This can be due to oxidation or dirt deposits at various mechanical junctions of metal subchassis. Clean these places to insure a good bond.
5. Measure leakage current.
   a. For each position of either the power switch or the pressure range selector switch, leakage current should not be $<10\ \mu A$ or $>25\ \mu A$. This applies for either polarity of the applied line voltage.
   b. Leakage current below $10\ \mu A$ usually indicates a break in the grounding wire, either in the power cord or at the plug.
   c. Leakage currents $> 25\ \mu A$ may indicate insulation breakdown in the power cord, or the development of a conductive path within the device. This frequently occurs in devices that spend some portion of time in a liquid environment.
6. Measure suction pressure.
   a. Connect the mercury manometer to the patient tubing coming from the 1-gal bottle.
   b. Observe that at least 120 mmHg can be developed with the suction switch in the high position. Several minutes (about 5 min) may be required to develop this pressure.
   c. At least 90 mmHg should be developed with the suction switch in the low position.

PERFORMANCE VERIFICATION RECORD

TEST	TESTER & DATE											
1. Mechanical												
2. Power Plug												
3. Line Cord												
4. Continuity												
5. Leakage												
6. Suction Press												
7. Aerovent												
1. Mechanical												
2. Power Plug												
3. Line Cord												
4. Continuity												
5. Leakage												
6. Suction Press												
7. Aerovent												
1. Mechanical												
2. Power Plug												
3. Line Cord												
4. Continuity												
5. Leakage												
6. Suction Press												
7. Aerovent												

*CALIBRATION REQUIRED
**REPAIR MAINTENANCE REQUIRED

DEVICE: Thermotic Pump MODEL #: 765 I.D.#: ______
MANUFACTURER: Gomco SERIAL #: ______ C/C: ______ F/U: ______

FIGURE 6. Performance verification record.

SERVICE SUMMARY

Unscheduled Service

Item	Reported Trouble	Diagnosis	Action
0	Date By Loc	Date By	Date ______ By ______
1	Date By Loc	Date By	Date ______ By ______
2	Date By Loc	Date By	Date ______ By ______
3	Date By Loc	Date By	Date ______ By ______
4	Date By Loc	Date By	Date ______ By ______
5	Date By Loc	Date By	Date ______ By ______
6	Date By Loc	Date By	Date ______ By ______
7	Date By Loc	Date By	Date ______ By ______
8	Date By Loc	Date By	Date ______ By ______
9	Date By Loc	Date By	Date ______ By ______

Service Schedule

PM											
PT											

Initials & Date

Service History

RM											
PM											
PV											
C											
RM											
PM											
PV											
C											
RM											
PM											
PV											
C											

Identification

Device ______ Manu. ______
Model # ______ S/N ______
I. D. # ______ First Usage ______
C/C ______ F/U ______
Item No. ______

FIGURE 7. Service summary form.

7. Check operation of the aerovent overflow system.
   a. Allow the 1-gal collection bottle to collect water.
   b. Note that suction is interrupted when the liquid is within 2 to 3 in. of the top of the bottle.

REFERENCES

1. Safety Guide for Health Care Institutions, American Hospital Association and National Safety Council, Chicago, 1972.
2. Life Safety Code 1976, NFPA No. 101, National Fire Protection Association, Boston, 1976.
3. Memorandum on Use of Carpet in Hospitals, American Carpet Institute, New York, 1964.
4. Minimum Requirements of Construction and Equipment for Hospital and Medical Facilities, U.S. Department of Health, Education, and Welfare, Rockville, 1974.
5. Accreditation Manual for Hospitals, Joint Commission on Accreditation of Hospitals, Chicago, 1979.
6. National Electrical Code 1978, NFPA No. 70-1978, National Fire Protection Association, Boston, 1977.
7. Occupational Safety and Health Standards, *Federal Register,* Vol. 39(125), Part 1910, Washington, D.C., 1974.

MEDICINE-PHARMACY SAFETY

Warren Kramer and Bruce C. Carlstedt

INTRODUCTION

From the time that a drug enters the hospital (whether it is a raw product used in manufacturing or a finished product from a pharmaceutical manufacturer) until it is consumed by the patient, there are many opportunities for the drug to cause harm to someone. Failure in a "safe" system for the use or control of the drug or drug products is most often responsible. The two most important concerns are the safety of the patient and the safety of the hospital employee.

Patient — As a patient in the hospital, the individual needs to be assured that he will receive the right drug in the right strength, and in the right dosage form at the right time. Although the time of administration is important, the right dose is more critical in that toxicity or lack of response may occur from over- or underdosing, respectively. Of course, it is even more critical that the right drug be given. This should encompass assurances that the patient is not allergic and does not have a contraindication to the drug. Or, it might include more basic assurances that the drug is manufactured according to good manufacturing procedures, and that when one product is selected from multiple sources that product is active and will give the desired therapeutic response. As an out-patient, the patient must also be assured that he is receiving the right drug and that his safety (i.e., protection from further harm from his disease state) is incumbent upon his proper utilization of the drug. That is, the patient must comply with the prescribed drug therapy.

Employee — Various degrees of safety policies must be applied by the employees in the pharmacy in order to protect them from the medications (and resultant allergies) or mechanical devices used in the preparation of the drug products. Also, some drugs (e.g., ether) may be flammable or cause an explosion if handled improperly, therefore, adequate safety procedures must be developed and followed with the use of these drugs. Nurses handling medications must have some of the same concerns (due to cut fingers from opening glass ampules or hepatitis from contaminated needles used in administration of drugs, etc.) and appropriate policies must be instituted.

One could argue that additional safety measures need to be designed to protect visitors from pharmacy operations. However, because of the nature of its business, this department must be unavailable to visitors in the hospital. Safety features designed to protect the employees in the pharmacy should be sufficient to protect the occasional visitor observing the pharmacy. Control measures which provide assurances that drugs, especially "controlled" substances, are not diverted can be construed as protecting the public-at-large from the illegitimate use of all medications.

In the following sections, areas in the hospital are identified where good safety practices must be applied to the general concept of medicine use. We do not present hard and fast remedies to situations, but rather recommend that the topic or subject headings be used as a means to identify whether your hospital has policies and procedures which would prevent the safety problems as outlined here.

PROCUREMENT

Procurement of drugs and drug supplies is one of the functions of the pharmacy. Although there are many items which may be used in the pharmacy for preparation of patient-ready medications (e.g., alcohol swabs in preparation of i.v. solutions or injectible medications), drugs and the process of drug product selection are of particular importance.

Drug Product Selection

A drug is usually known by several names: a chemical name, a generic name adopted by U.S. Adopted Name (USAN) — usually the "common" name by which medications are called — and a brand or trade name (the name given and copyrighted by a manufacturer for a specific generic-named drug product). One problem that faces some pharmacists in certain states occurs when a prescriber orders a drug by a brand name, and the pharmacist *must* dispense that brand of the drug even though there may often be an equivalent (and less costly) product (generic equivalent) on the market. Many states are repealing these "anti-substitution" laws, thus making hospital drug product selection easier. Another method which is in effect now is the use of the formulary system. It is described in the next section. Rather than being required to carry many brand name products, the pharmacy need stock only one suitable drug product. The crux of the matter comes in the determination of what is suitable and what is not suitable. Here, the term "bioequivalence" denotes that the selection of the drug product must be made so that if one brand name product is ordered and another (generic) product is used, the effectiveness to the patient will be identical. The selection criteria for the safety of the patient is expressed in terms of an equivalent drug product. The Food and Drug Administration (FDA) has attempted to define those products which hold approved new drug applications and are manufactured under good manufacturing procedures therefore meeting the bioequivalence criteria. However, for some drugs, the amount of drug absorbed is dependent on the formulation of the dosage form, or there is a "window" between the blood levels needed for minimum effectiveness and those for toxicity. For these drugs, the possible differences in bioequivalence vs. possible cost savings must be weighed against patient safety and effectiveness of the selected drug product.

There are no rigid guidelines to tell which product is the one to be selected when a brand vs. generic decision must be made. Complicating this is the fact that many brand name pharmaceutical houses are now making available lines of "branded generics" which are not necessarily manufactured by that company, but are quality-controlled and often warranted by that company.

The basic question is how to make the decision to purchase either a brand name or a generic product. There are some comparisons of brand vs. generic products for bioavailability and these may help in the selection, however, they may not truly represent bioequivalence. Each drug product must be handled separately, and the decision must be made independently. It would seem that the pharmacist, with a background, training, and education in pharmaceutical formulations, could gather appropriate data from the literature and manufacturers. Armed with this information and in concert with the medical staff, these professionals should make an appropriate determination of the suitability of all drug product selections; they should first determine whether to buy generically or buy brand name, then determine which specific product to purchase.

Cost savings are certainly an important factor in the decision; cost containment is an important aspect of hospital management. However, it should never be the only parameter used. It may be that a manufacturer has the lowest price for a certain product, but is unable to guarantee that the product would be in sufficient supply at all times or that it would be manufactured using the same formulation which could affect the bioavailability of the desired drug.

Formulary System

The hospital formulary is a continually revised compilation of pharmaceuticals which reflects the current clinical judgment of the medical staff. It is a system whereby the medical staff of the hospital, working through the pharmacy and therapeutics committee, evaluates, appraises, and selects from numerous medicinal agents and dosage forms those that are considered most useful and beneficial to patient care. Generally, the pharmacy will stock only those items which are "on the formulary".

The system is more than a drug list; it is continually changing. Since it is changing, not all drug products are available within the hospital. Thus, mechanisms should be available to obtain nonformulary items for individual patients until they are presented for approval into the formulary.

An advantage of the formulary system is the elimination of duplicate brand name products which are generically identical. Implementation of this system should be accomplished as quickly as possible. However, resistance by the medical staff may be encountered due to: (1) elimination of their prerogative to prescribe a favorite brand name or (2) a perceived inability to obtain drugs which are not contained in the formulary.

Each of these concerns can be significantly diminished with development of pharmacy policies. A concern of not being able to prescribe brand name products is also easily eliminated. Formulary guidelines should include the statement that a particular brand of product will be obtained if the name of the drug is checked, underlined, or circled, or the brand name necessary is written in the prescription. If one of these mechanisms is used by the prescriber, the pharmacist has the option of calling the physician and asking if the particular product which is maintained in the pharmacy would be acceptable; if not, the brand name product prescribed could be obtained. One will find that insistence of a particular brand is almost never required. This mechanism should eliminate concern that the formulary will decrease prescribing prerogative.

The development of pharmacy policies which include a mechanism to obtain nonformulary items within 24 to 48 hr after an order has been written will eliminate the concern of not being able to obtain drugs. This is a reasonable length of time and can usually be met even if the order is written on Saturday.

Receiving Drugs

The pharmacy should mainly be concerned with two aspects of drug safety associated with the delivery of drugs before arrival at the pharmacy. These include

1. Safe transportation of drugs as they were shipped from the supplier to the hospital
2. Safe delivery of drugs from the loading dock of the hospital to the pharmacy

Safety of drugs delivered to the hospital does rest in the hands of the delivering company. Probably, the major control the institution may have is in the selection of a carrier which provides good service relative to time and safety. The shipper is liable for the merchandise until it is received and signed for at the receiving dock. After the drugs are received by the hospital, they become the responsibility of the hospital, and accurate detailed records need to be maintained. The institution needs to identify and implement procedures which maintain records of the delivery of all drugs to the hospital, and precautions which decrease the potential for diversion within the institution. It is impossible to make specific recommendations of procedures, but some basic principles should be followed. If possible, the ordering should be the responsibility of one individual, and the receipt, storage, and issuance of merchandise should be under another person. Also, inventory should have periodic (monthly) spot checks.

Purchasing — This responsibility should be limited to the issuance of purchase orders and the determination of how much and what items should be purchased from a vendor at a particular time, although predetermined guidelines should be established and followed. That is, quantities to be ordered are generally predetermined by establishing EOQ's, but flexibility must be maintained in order to respond to increases and decreases in usage patterns and to take advantage of special offers. In addition, because of the high cost in processing a purchase order, all items from a common vendor should be reviewed whenever a purchase order is cut. This will necessitate good communication with the individual who maintains inventory. If computer services are available, a daily perpetual inventory would provide the most accurate feedback. Armed with this information, generating larger but fewer purchase orders becomes easier, and this results in a decrease of paperwork.

Receipt — The receipt of drugs should be placed in the hands of the pharmacy department. This can be accomplished by either having the goods delivered to the pharmacy department or having pharmacy personnel at the receiving dock receive pharmaceuticals. This may sound unreasonable, but Drug Enforcement Agency (DEA) regulations require that controlled substances be delivered from the shipper into the hands of a pharmacist. In the event that the merchandise does not match the packing slip or the purchase order (e.g., back-ordered merchandise) and there is no additional information the vendor must be contacted immediately to clarify the situation.

Storage — There are two factors to be considered under this topic. The first is to ascertain that the area has the appropriate physical conditions, e.g., temperature and humidity control. If the drugs require refrigeration, an appropriate refrigerator must be obtained. The temperature in such a unit should be monitored on a daily basis. The other factor is to maintain these drugs using a good inventory control: reduce the physical inventory as it is requisitioned and/or dispensed, conduct spot checks periodically, perform an entire physical inventory yearly, and maintain these items in an area which has controlled access. These two factors must be considered in any area where drugs are stored. It is complicated and the work is compounded in larger pharmacies where drugs are stored in an area separate from the main pharmacy. More specific details are considered next.

STORAGE OF DRUGS

Bulk Storage

The storage, maintenance, and handling of drugs and drug products is another primary function of the pharmacy department. In the department, bulk quantities of drugs, i.e., the large containers of drugs purchased from the manufacturer, are frequently divided into smaller quantities which can either be used more efficiently in the pharmacy or be used for direct dispensing to the patient. These smaller units of drugs may also be packaged in such a fashion so as to be sent to a nursing unit for direct distribution of single doses to a patient.

Expiration dates — On most drug products now supplied to a pharmacy, an expiration date is placed on the label. Emphasis should be placed on the fact that this date is well within the stability of the product and therefore is safe to use if maintained under proper storage conditions and used before the indicated expiration date. The date only refers to the sealed, unbroken storage container; once the seal is violated, the date is no longer applicable. Thus, the expiration date on a bottle must be closely watched by the pharmacy personnel so that newer stock is placed in the back and older stock with closer expiration dates is used first.

General standards — The U.S. Pharmacopoeia (U.S.P.) establishes standards for the purity and content of many, but not all, drug products.[2] In these standards, inclusion of temperature, light, and humidity requirements greatly aids the decision as to the storage conditions of many pharmaceutical products.

The bulk storage of pharmaceuticals must take into account many variables and conditions based on different types of drug products as identified below.

Alcohol — Bulk quantities of alcohol are often used in the hospital pharmacy. When it is used as a tax-free substance, the disposition must be carefully controlled through scrupulous record keeping. In addition, 95% alcohol is a flammable liquid; therefore, it must be maintained under special storage conditions. These include a special room or vault with an outside "blow-out" wall to take the force of an explosion should it occur; a ventilating fan to remove alcohol fumes; increased smoke- or fire-detection equipment in the immediate area of the storage site; quick access to fire fighting equipment (if necessary) and a rapid means of identification to firemen (responding to a call) as to the location of the large alcohol storage tanks; and special temperature regulating devices (e.g., air conditioning) in the room or area to maintain a cool temperature.

Flammable liquids — The pharmacy is often responsible for the bulk storage of many flammable or explosive drugs such as ether, acetone, or benzene, and these require the same storage conditions as outlined for alcohol.

External medications — The JCAH (Joint Commission on Accreditation of Hospitals) requires separate storage areas for drug products that are used externally and internally in order to avoid any possibility of using an external product internally.

Narcotics and controlled substances — The bulk storage of narcotics and controlled substances (i.e., those with a high probability for abuse and/or dependence) represents a most challenging area for the hospital and especially for the hospital pharmacist. From a safety standpoint, the importance is probably not as great in terms of safety to the patient, but rather to the pharmacy personnel in terms of potential robberies or burglaries. Bulk narcotics and controlled substances must be kept in a locked vault or safe with strict and stringent record keeping. Specific information is identified in state and federal laws. Access to the keys for the vault or combination to the safe should be closely controlled and limited to as few individuals within the pharmacy as possible.

Cleanliness — Of paramount importance anywhere in the hospital is cleanliness. This is also very important as a safety factor in the storage and dispensing areas of the pharmacy. Open bottles of drugs may become contaminated with dirt, spores, or microorganism; therefore, this practice is to be discouraged (ultimately, these drugs will be consumed by patients who are already ill). In addition, cleanliness leads to neatness and this provides an atmosphere in which fewer errors are made.

Temperature — As previously discussed, various temperature requirements are needed for storage of medications. These may range from normal room temperature (15 to 30°C) to a refrigerator (2 to 8°C) to a freezer (<0°C). The requirements for a drug are usually included in the labeling and must be followed to be certain of its potency. If not properly stored, drugs (especially biologicals) may rapidly deteriorate (within hours).

Light — Certain medications are affected by light and these must be protected in an unlit room or by amber storage containers or boxes.

LABELING

The correct labeling of a drug product is an important factor in safety to the patient and cannot be overemphasized. Discussion has already emphasized proper storage conditions and the need to place such information on the label. The minimum information which must appear on the label is identified in the examples on the following page.

Pharmacy-Manufactured Product*

Hospital Name, Address, and Phone Number	
Product Name and Strength	
Quantity or Amount	
Expiration Date	
Lot Number	Storage Condition

Unit-of-Use Container

Generic Name and Strength per Dosage Unit		
(Brand Name, if Applicable)		
Storage Conditions/Special Warnings		
Lot Number	Expiration Date	Stock Bottle

Hospital Name, Address, and Phone Number

Generic Name and Strength per Dosage Unit	
(Brand Name, if Applicable)	
Quantity or Amount	
Storage Conditions/Special Warnings	
Lot Number	Expiration Date

Prescription Bottles**

Hospital Name, Address, and Phone Number	
Prescription Number	Date of Dispensing
Patient Name	Prescribers Name
Directions for Use	
DEA Number and Prescribers DEA Number for Controlled Substances	
Generic Name (or Brand Name) Strength, and Quantity Dispensed	
Expiration date	Initials of Dispensing Pharmacist

I.V. Bottles

Patient	Room
Bottle #	
Contents	Amount
Rate of Infusion in ml. or Drops per Hour or Minute	
Expiration Time	
Storage Conditions	Initials of Pharmacist

In summary, the labeling associated with medications must be accurate, complete yet concise, and easy to read to assure the right drug to the right patient. Labels that are used for the same purpose should have the same format. In this way, these labels are less confusing and are therefore, less likely to be misread.

MANUFACTURING

In a hospital manufacturing operation, there are three areas of safety which must be considered: the machinery, the products themselves, and the record keeping.

* Additional information may include special warnings (e.g., external use, poison, etc.).

** Additional information may include storage conditions, special warnings and instructions, and state requirements.

Drug Product

If the product itself in the final manufactured container is considered the primary concern in the operation, the other two ingredients identified above will be maintained naturally. The products in the final container must conform to U.S.P. specifications as identified under the specific product monograph, as well as the general specifications for that particular type of dosage form. FDA specifications must also be met. Some of the U.S.P. definitions which are used in many but not all of the individual specifications for oral dosage forms follow.

Tight container — Protects the contents from contamination by extraneous liquids, solids, or vapors, from loss of the drug, and from efflorescence, deliquescence, or evaporation under the ordinary or customary conditions of handling, shipment, storage, and distribution, and capable of tight reclosure. Where specified, it may be replaced by a hermetic container for a single dose of a drug.

Well-closed container — Protects the contents from extraneous solids and from loss of the drug under the ordinary or customary conditions of handling, shipment, storage, and distribution.

Light-resistant container — Protects the contents from the effects of light by virtue of the specific properties of the material of which it is composed, including any coating applied to it. Alternatively, a clear and colorless or translucent container may be made light-resistant by means of an opaque covering, in which case the label of the container bears a statement that the opaque covering is needed until the contents have been used. Where directed to "protect from light" in an individual monograph, storage in a light-resistant container is intended.

Cool — Any temperature between 8 and 15°C (46 and 59°F).

Room temperature — Temperature prevailing in a working area, with controlled room temperature a temperature maintained thermostatically between 15 and 30°C (59 and 86°F).

Excessive heat — Any temperature above 40°C (104°F).

Other definitions less frequently used are also identified in the U.S.P.

Prepackaging — Probably the most used method of manufacturing is in the area of prepackaging. Although one may not consider this a manufacturing operation, by definition it is clearly a manufacturing operation. It is taking the contents of a manufactured item, breaking it down into smaller dispensing units, and having them available for use in the dispensing operation. There are only a few basics one needs to keep in mind in a prepackaging program: (1) maintaining identity of the product, (2) maintaining the manufacturer's lot number and expiration date, (3) transferring the contents in a clean atmosphere, (4) repackaging the item into a clean container, and (5) labeling appropriately as defined above. Safety can best be maintained by doing one prepackaging operation at a time, and all equipment should be cleaned before and after the operation to keep the possibility of cross contamination to a minimum. The specific detergents and disinfectants which one uses to clean the environment will depend upon the equipment which is being used and the surface on which the operation is to take place. Cleanliness is the watchword in an operation of this nature. In addition, paperwork associated with the prepackaging operation should be maintained as the operation is continued so that the identity of the product is maintained. It is imperative that all stock bottles and final containers be labeled at the time they are prepackaged. The specific information contained on the label will be identified under record keeping.

Unit-of-use packages — A unit-of-use package is one where one dose is prepared and individually packaged. This may consist of two 5-mg tablets if the dose is 10 mg, or it may consist of a 15-mℓ bottle if the dose is a tablespoonful, etc. This type of packaging is generally, but not exclusively, used in a unit dose drug distribution system. The same basic precautions associated with prepackaging is associated with unit-of-use packaging. That is, it is extremely important to clean the machinery prior to and after the packaging operation. It is important to: (1) package only one item at a time, (2) maintain appropriate paperwork which identifies the medication as well as the individual control number and expiration date, and (3) work in a clean environment. Labeling precautions are the same as with the prepackaging operation and are identified above.

Bulk compounding — All compounding involves an additional dimension in that one needs to use a standard formula in the manufacturing of all items which are prepared for bulk preparations and subsequent prepackaging into smaller dispensing units. As identified with both prepackaging and unit-of-use packaging, it is essential that all equipment is washed and cleaned thoroughly and the environment in which it is to be prepared is clean. The formula must be available throughout the manufacturing process. As each ingredient is added and prepared as identified in the procedure, the specific information associated with that ingredient (name of product, manufacturer, lot number, etc.) must be recorded on the packaging sheet (or worksheet) so that there is positive identification as the product is prepared. Once the product is completed, the final container must be clearly labeled. In the event that it is necessary to allow the product to sit overnight uncompleted, it is imperative that the container be clearly labeled with the ingredients which have thus far been added and the step in the procedure which has thus far been completed.

Sterile products — The basic methods in the manufacturing of sterile products within the pharmacy encompass all of the above needs for cleanliness, record keeping, etc. but has the added onus of sterility and/or pyrogen testing if the product is to be used parenterally.

UNIT-DOSE SYSTEM

The unit-dose system may be one of the most recent innovations which directly benefits the patient's safety through reduction in medication errors. Rather than attempt a definition of unit-dose, a brief description may be better. In the past, drug acquisition by the hospitalized patient in a traditional system, or especially in ward stock systems, was subject to many of the errors inherent in the systems themselves: improper storage conditions, wrong medication, incorrect strength of medication, wrong time, and no dose administered. These often resulted because the medications were sent to the patient care area in a bulk quantity and were counted out or "poured" from these containers.

With unit-dose, the dose of medication for a particular patient to be given at a special time is prepared by the pharmacy and delivered to the patient care area once or twice daily, with each patient having a separate compartment for his medications.

However, before any medication is delivered to the nursing station, each dose can be checked for allergies and drug interactions by utilizing the patient profile. With this profile the pharmacy maintains a complete listing of drugs that have been or are being administered to the patient (as new drugs are added to the patient's regimen), and the pharmacist can quickly ascertain if there is either a potential allergy to the medication or a drug interaction or disease state contraindication. This was not possible with traditional systems. In addition, these medications are accurately labeled (as discussed) and stored under proper storage conditions. A safety advantage here is that the nurse can take this single dose of medication to the patient's bedside, open the package there (after appropriate patient checks), and give the medication directly to the patient. This has the advantage that the medication is not poured into a "souffle" cup at the nurses station and carried down the hall where it might be mixed accidently with other medications. An additional advantage is that after giving the medication, the empty wrapper or container can be checked against the medication profile to verify accuracy of drug and dose. Another safety check occurs when the individual patient's trays or bins are returned to or checked by the pharmacy. If there are medications still in the bin, they were obviously not administered. The pharmacist can check to ascertain why it was not administered and corrective measures can be initiated.[8]

Another part of the safety in the unit-dose system occurs with the use of duplicate physician order forms, although this is not necessarily unique to the unit-dose concept. In the past, ward secretaries or clerks transcribed the medication orders onto the patient's chart and onto an order form for pharmacy use. Since the pharmacist did not interpret the physician's original orders, a chance for error was increased. Use of carbon paper or noncarbon duplicating papers has allowed for a direct copy of all the physician's orders to be sent to the pharmacy.

In summary, the primary advantage of unit-dose for the safety of the patient is the reduction of medication errors. There may be additional safety features for the patient in terms of improved nursing care since the reduction in the time to prepare the medications by nursing personnel can be applied to patient care.

INTRAVENOUS ADMIXTURE PROGRAMS

Safety associated with an intravenous admixture program includes all of the following activities:

1. Large volume parenterals — These are primary administered i.v. solutions which are usually in volumes of 1000 mℓ (never larger), but are also available in 500 mℓ (and even smaller).
2. Hyperalimentation solutions — These are nutritional fluids which are administered parenterally in order to sustain life for those patients who cannot either consume nutrition by the oral route or absorb food which is consumed.
3. Piggyback medication — These are sterile medications which are usually diluted in a common carrier and administered using an administration set which is already inserted intravenously and carrying a fluid. Controversy has existed as to whether the "piggyback" or in-line burette is the safest for the patient.[9]

As with a unit-dose drug distribution system, one of the first prerequisites for the implementation of a pharmacy-based i.v. additive program is to implement the use of a duplicate physician's order form. This is not only necessary and important for ease of providing the service, but is necessary for assurance that i.v. bottles and additives are prepared from a copy of the original order and not from an interpretation order which was transcribed on the nursing unit.

In addition to the basic safety considerations which are an integral part of all pharmacists, the one additional aspect which must be borne in mind is sterile technique. Although this concept is now being taught in our schools of pharmacy, it was sadly lacking in the recent past. Therefore, concentrated efforts must be spent to assure that personnel involved in the preparation of i.v. solutions are using sterile technique. Educational manuals and workshops are available to provide opportunities to learn these skills. It is also important to ascertain that these techniques continue to be used after the initial interest wains.

A continuous concern with an i.v. additive program is the final product that is dispensed. Not only must these solutions be sterile, but they must also be free of glass and rubber particles. The potential of contaminating the fluid with glass particles can be reduced by drawing up syringes from ampules without rubbing the neck of the ampule with the needle. Another measure which should be considered is to use a filtered needle when utilizing solutions from an ampule.

Reduction of rubber particles from vials can be achieved by entering these solutions at a slight angle with the bevel of the needle up. This technique does not eliminate "coring", but has been shown to reduce the amount of rubber material entering the final solution.

Even with these precautions, it is imperative that the final solution be checked before it is dispensed. This should be done using both a black and white background to check for particulate matter. Solutions containing "floaters" should be filtered or discarded.

A quality-assurance program for the i.v. admixture program should be implemented and maintained on an ongoing basis.[10]

MEDICATION ADMINISTRATION

Medication Errors

When considering the safety of the patients in the institutional setting, a frequently encountered subject is medication errors. In defining this problem, the common factor is that the patient did not receive the intended therapeutic measure. This may have occurred for any one of several reasons.

Wrong Drug

This may happen at any level of the drug distribution system. It is possible, but not probable that the pharmaceutical manufacturer placed the wrong medication in the bottle. The solution to this is difficult to control, but surely includes purchase of drugs from quality manufacturers with good quality-control programs. A second way a patient may receive the wrong drug is through the pharmacy dispensing the wrong drug to the patient care area or directly to the patient (e.g., in an outpatient prescription). The solution to these problems is to have a quality-assurance program whereby the pharmacist is spot checked or there is adequate means for double-checking the contents of the orders or prescriptions. Also, the nurse who administers the medication should serve as another check on the right drug for the right patient. This brings us to the third level where the wrong drug may be given to a patient — the patient care area. There may be three reasons why the patient received the wrong drug.

Transcription error — This error occurs when either the physician's order was written in the wrong patient's chart or the order was taken off the right chart, but transcribed onto the wrong patient's chart. The solution to this problem is adequate training of ward clerk and pharmacy personnel and careful attention to the chart as orders are written and transcribing is done.

Wrong medication — Here, the wrong tablet, capsule, injection, etc. is obtained through confusion of names. Because there are many which sound alike and confusion exists with brand and generic names, this is understandable, but not acceptable. These problems are more likely to occur with ward stock systems or with the taking of drugs from stock bottles. Probably the best solution to this problem is the use of a unit-dose drug distribution system where the pharmacy prepares well-labeled medications and places them into the individual patient bins as described.

Administering medication to the wrong patient — This occurs when the patient's identification is not checked carefully at the time medications are administered. Clear policies must be implemented and enforced to check the identification of each patient.

Wrong Time

It is important to administer some medications to the patient at a specific time during the day. Some may be best absorbed when given on an empty stomach, while others are best given after meals to decrease GI side effects, and others should be given on a strict around-the-clock schedule to assure adequate blood levels for therapeutic effectiveness. The solution to this problem is complex, requiring close cooperation between the pharmacy, nursing personnel, and medical staff to determine the best times for the administration of each drug. A unit-dose system which incorporates patient medication profiles (complete with times of administration) should ease those problems. In addition, this system identifies drugs which should not be given together and allows for adjustment of administration times.

Wrong Dose

The administration of the wrong dose to a patient can result in either overdosage potentially resulting in toxicity, or underdosage which can lead to a lack of therapeutic effect. Reasons that a wrong dose may be given follow.

Incorrect transcription — For example, if the order is for 50 mg but the transcription onto the medication profile reads 5.0 mg or the other way around, a dosage error can occur. The solution to this problem is the use of clear (approved by the medical staff) symbols for decimal points and careful transcription. Also, a unit-dose system where the pharmacy prepares the dose helps to alleviate the problem since the right dose (not the incorrectly transcribed dose) should be present in the patient's medication bin and serve as a double check on the transcription. Both pharmacy and nursing would interpret the order before it was administered.

Selection of the wrong dose for the patient — There are many factors which influence the correctness of a dose: age of the patient, diseases (e.g., liver or kidney which influence drug metabolism or excretion), and other drugs which may interact and alter the pharmacokinetic parameters (absorption, distribution, metabolism, or excretion) of the drug. The solution to this problem is constant education of the nursing and pharmacy staffs to ensure adequate knowledge of drug doses and factors which affect them. Armed with this knowledge, the physician can be approached to make a dosage adjustment if appropriate.

Wrong dosage strength in stock bottle — There are several possibilities that fall under this heading: (1) incorrect labeling (e.g., if the bottle is incorrectly labeled 500 mcg when it should read mg) and (2) difficult to read labeling which has occurred with some medications. For example, a drug was labeled

XXXXXXXXX
100 mg/mℓ
10 mℓ

and an order was written for the patient to receive 1 g. The individual preparing the drug misread the contents of the vial as each vial contained a total of 100 mg, not 100 mg/mℓ. As a result, a dose of 10 vials was given which is 10 times the prescribed amount. Also, some medications are available in suspension dosage forms and require vigorous and complete shaking to assure adequate mixing of the contents. If this is not done, an underdose may be administered from the first doses of the bottle and an overdose (where there is increased amounts of drug) may be administered from the last doses. In addition, errors in measurement can occur with any liquid (oral or injection), but is more likely with a device containing two scales on the measuring device. A good example that was a common problem in the past occurred with the use of

U- ^{40}/U- ^{80} combination syringes. This problem has now been virtually eliminated with the use of U- ^{100} insulins. The important point is to use devices with only one scale.

Drug Allergy

An important factor is to ascertain that a patient does not receive a drug to which he is allergic. This is not a medication error per se, but obviously it is not the intended effect of the medication. To maximize prevention of an allergic drug reaction, known drug allergies should be recorded in the patient's chart, nursing medication sheets, and pharmacy profiles. This cannot stop a patient from developing an allergy, but surely there is no justification for giving ampicillin to a patient with confirmed penicillin allergy (without desensitization).

Reporting of Medication Errors

All medication errors should be reported to the patient's physician for the therapeutic plan to be controlled. For example, if a patient does not receive a dose of a drug, the prescriber may increase the dose thinking there was a lack of response to the previous dose. A formal mechanism to identify repeated types of medication errors should be instituted so that appropriate solutions can be found. In addition, clear and complete documentation is important in the event that a suit is filed.

Charting of Medications

One of the most important mechanisms in preventing, assessing, and/or documenting a medication error is the complete charting of the administered medications. This should not be done at the end of a shift, but immediately *after* each dose is given. Of course, if the dose cannot be given for some reason (patient is at X-ray), alternative scheduling must be employed. Also, documentation must be made as to why the dose was not administered.

Oral Syringes

Inaccurate measurement of oral liquids have always been a problem, partially because of the lack of standardization of teaspoonfuls, tablespoonfuls, etc. Vague measurements such as these should be standardized through the medical staff. Oral syringes, which more accurately measure and deliver (especially to children) the correct dose, can help alleviate the inaccuracy of liquid measurement. Of course, one must *never* use syringes intended for parenteral use since inadvertant parenteral administration of an oral preparation could be catastrophic.

Contaminated Needles

The use of parenteral medications can present a safety hazard to medical personnel through accidental injection or even scratching the skin with a needle from an infectious patient. Although puncture scratch from any needle could be of concern for any organism, the organism generally of most concern is hepatitis Type B or serum hepatitis. Anyone "innoculated" with a needle from a patient having hepatitis Type B should report the incident immediately and be treated appropriately according to the guidelines of the hospital. Even though the more serious incidents involve nursing or blood-drawing personnel, the pharmacists or technicians that prepare i.v. medications should also be aware of the procedure to follow if they are stuck with a needle.

Bedside Medications

Certain patients have medications kept at their bedside due to either immediate need (sublingual nitroglycerin), many doses per day (antacids), or chronic therapy (eyedrops for glaucoma). Here, it is important that the patient have adequate access to these medications, that proper storage conditions be met, and adequate supply be available in case of need.

Medications Brought into the Hospital

An important factor in the assessment of the therapeutic response of the patient is a complete knowledge of *all* the medication the patient is taking. Many patients will bring their current medications to the hospital and keep them hidden in a drawer beside them. The safety factor involves an awareness of the outcomes of such a practice by the patient and appropriate procedures must be implementted to ensure that the patient does not take these medications.

In summary, medication administration can pose a serious threat to the safety of the patient, the nurse, and pharmacy personnel if adequate awareness and knowledge of possible consequences is not appreciated.

NARCOTICS AND CONTROLLED SUBSTANCES

State and federal regulations define controlled substances very clearly and specifically. Therefore, these will not be repeated. Suffice it to say that controlled substances are divided into Schedules I through V. Schedule I substances either have no medical use or are investigational drugs with a high potential for abuse; they are seldom used. For those few institutions that do have these substances, they are strictly controlled because of their abuse potential and detailed records are required.

Schedule II substances have approved Food and Drug Administration indications, but also have an extremely high potential for abuse and drug diversion. Because of this, scrupulous record keeping is imperative. A perpetual inventory should be maintained on each of these drugs as they are received and issued. In addition, a physical inventory should be taken on a monthly basis to ascertain that this count matches the theoretical one. If they do not, some explanation must be found. Past experience indicates that discrepancies usually mean an error with the record keeping. However, if the audit does not uncover a pharmacy error and there becomes a strong indication of drug diversion, the Drug Enforcement Administration should be notified.

In addition to this control, it is also imperative that pharmacy personnel have some assurance that these drugs are not being diverted at the nursing station. This is accomplished by having a clearly defined procedure which includes a check of all doses that are administered at the nursing stations.

Individual dose-administration records with a perpetual inventory are not required for substances in Schedules III, IV, and V. However, it is imperative that controls are instituted to discourage drug diversion. Usage rates should be monitored and changes in usage patterns should be viewed with some concern until these changes can be verified.

Other requirements are identified in federal and state laws and will not be repeated here.

INVESTIGATIONAL DRUGS

Prior to F.D.A. drug approval for the marketing and release of a drug by a pharmaceutical manufacturer, it must undergo several phases of testing, the last of which is clinical testing on patients for whom such a drug would be indicated. At this stage, drugs are commonly referred to as investigational and are often found in the hospital setting, especially in larger hospitals or teaching medical centers. Depending on hospital policy, the storage of the drugs may reside with either the principal investigator (who has total control over who can and who cannot receive these drugs) or the pharmacy department. The safest place for these drugs to be stored and dispensed (the JCAH recommendation) is in the pharmacy since a number of problems can be identified with alternate patterns of control and use.

Record Keeping

While the investigator may often have adequate controls, the pharmacy should be the central facility in the hospital for storage and control through record keeping of all investigational drugs. This solution may help to eliminate several potential problems.

Storage — Generally, the pharmacy should have all necessary types of storage requirements whether freezer, refrigeration, light protection, etc. Expiration dating will more likely be observed.

Dispensing — An accurate record of all patients and amounts received, whether inpatient or outpatient, can be maintained.

Reordering — Pharmacies are oriented to inventory control and should ensure adequate replacement through appropriate reordering, thus protecting the patient from a lack of adequate drug supply and having to stop therapy.

Information

One of the major deficiencies either a patient who is taking an investigational drug or a nurse who is administering such a drug may have is inadequate information regarding that drug. For example, should the patient require medical care at another institution, it would be necessary to know what that drug is, its side effects, adverse reactions, etc. The principal investigator should be contacted, but when this is not possible, the patient could suffer severe consequences. By having the pharmacy act as a central clearing house for all investigational drugs, information on these drugs would be available to necessary medical personnel whether from an outside institution or within the same hospital.[11]

SAMPLE DRUGS

Although drug sampling by pharmaceutical companies is decreasing, the practice still continues. Therefore, the pharmacy and therapeutics committee should approve all drugs which are to be used in the hospital. Placing patients on sample drugs can cause problems because adequate supplies may not be available for continuous therapy, and personnel handling these medications may not be familiar with the essential information associated with their use. It would, therefore, be prudent to have a policy regarding sample drugs which identifies the following:

1. Where they will be stored (preferably in the pharmacy)
2. Who will order them for patients (very limited)
3. Who will reorder them to maintain the hospital supply
4. Adequate safeguards to ensure that supplies of these drugs have limited availability

In summary, while the threat to patient safety from sample medications may be small, it is nevertheless a topic for which policies should be developed and enforced.

PERSONNEL

People are our most valuable asset; at the same time, they can be our greatest liability. Because of these extremes, it is obvious that the institution must support supervisory personnel in providing orientation, training, and development of all individuals within any department. Although this section of the handbook addresses safety practices within the pharmacy, many of the concepts that are identified here can be easily practiced in other departments of the hospital.

An individual cannot function at peak efficiency unless that person is familiar with the environment in which he is working. The first step in accomplishing this is to provide a good orientation program. This will probably take several days to complete, especially within a large institution, but should begin on the first day. Topics which should be included, but certainly not limited to, are

1. Importance of the individual's job
2. Introduction to the other employees
3. Organization chart of the department and hospital
4. Rest rooms
5. Coat racks
6. Dress code and/or uniform
7. Cafeteria (hours of operation)
8. Coffee breaks and lunch time
9. Work schedule
10. Policies and procedures (department and hospital)
11. Job description
12. Vacation requests
13. Tour of the hospital
14. Location and use of time clock
15. Use and care of equipment
16. Authorized individuals within the department

As the new employee is being oriented, he is receiving training in the new environment. However, it is important to extend this training beyond the initial orientation. As new programs and systems are planned and implemented, all personnel must be oriented and trained. This becomes easier and more productive if department personnel are included in the development and implementation of these programs.

Other training programs which should be a part of the pharmacy is in the area of continuing education. These are usually sponsored by professional organizations, but are also presented by individuals and companies.

An important element in assuring that safety practices are maintained is with the use of a policy and procedure manual. This book should not be focused on safety, but on elements for the smooth operation of the department. The subject is mentioned here as another element in the development of the department as it relates to safety.

One important job of the pharmacy is dissemination of information relative to drugs, drug use, and related subjects. This information is given not only to patients, but to physicians, other professionals, and many times the general public. It is better to give out no information than inaccurate responses; in fact, this is critical. Therefore, if the answer to a question is uncertain or not known, the answer should be delayed or not given until such information is positively confirmed.

DRUG RETRIEVAL

A mechanism should be available so that medication can be retrieved in the event of a drug recall (the product is defective, hazardous, or outdated).[12]

Drug Recalls

A drug recall occurs when the manufacturer has determined that one of their products does not meet specified standards. The recall can either be ordered by the FDA or be voluntary on the part of the manufacturer. This multiplicity of initiators of drug recalls may lead to confusion and cause some drugs which should have been recalled to still be available.[13] In any event, whenever such a recall is initiated, the pharmacy should be able to put a plan into effect to retrieve all medications that are affected by the lot being recalled.

Maintaining a record of all lot numbers for medications which come into the hospital is one place to start in implementing such a program. In this way, one can quickly determine if the institution ever purchased any of the medications bearing the lot of the affected recall.

Outdated Medications

Another area of concern relative to drug retrieval is outdated medications. In order to assure retrieval of any outdated products, some system should be implemented to eliminate having these items within the hospital. Two methods which have had success follow.

1. Specific individuals within the pharmacy are responsible to check certain sections of the pharmacy on a monthly basis and remove all products which have expired or are due to expire, during the following month.
2. Another system is to establish a card file that is separated according to month and year. As drugs arrive at the pharmacy, the name is recorded on the card which corresponds to the month it will be expiring. Then, on the first day of the month, the respective card is removed and the drugs which are recorded on the card are checked to determine if any of the drugs on hand will become outdated.

In addition to maintaining the controls mentioned above, one must also be concerned with the medications on the nursing units. Regardless of the drug distribution system in effect, there is always some medication on the nursing units. Outdated and expired medications are easily checked at the time the monthly nursing inspections are made. Since these inspections are required by the JCAH, implementation of this check is easily made.

PATIENT COMPLIANCE

In a very broad sense, one must consider the role the patient plays in achieving or maintaining a state of well-being as a factor in patient safety. Again, defined in broad terms, patient safety concerns those factors which protect the individual from harm. One could argue that the patient who is noncompliant (i.e., does not take his medications according to the way they were prescribed) is being harmed either through an overdosing or, more likely, an underdosing of medication. Studies too numerous to document have demonstrated that one half to two thirds of all patients do not take medications in the manner in which they were intended. There are several reasons this occurs:

1. Asymptomatic patient: the patient does not feel sick (e.g., in hypertension) and therefore, does not take the medication even though it is necessary to control the disease state.
2. Taste: some medications taste bad and the patient may avoid this displeasure by not taking it. (Sometimes this can be overcome by cooling the liquid medicines.)
3. Frequency of administration: if medications are given too frequently (e.g., antacid every hour) or the patient is taking too many different medications, the patient may be noncompliant simply because there are too many to "monitor" properly.

4. Duration of therapy: patients on long-term chronic medications tend to be more noncompliant.
5. Side effects or adverse reactions: the patient is not likely to be too compliant in taking a medication which makes him feel worse or nauseous.
6. Fear of medications: the patient may fear drugs, either because of past experiences or becoming "addicted" and, as a result, may not take them.

Solutions to the problem of noncompliance in a patient are complex. Careful and complete education of the patient is probably the maximum that can be accomplished. For each medication, the patient should understand (at the minimum) the following:

1. Name of the medication
2. Purpose for which it is being taken
3. How it is to be taken, including route and special instructions (e.g., with food)
4. Amount or number of dosage units to be taken as a single dose
5. Maximum amount to be taken in a day (or at a dose) and what to do if one, two, three, etc. doses are missed
6. Length of time to use the medication
7. Possible side effects or adverse reactions, with an appreciation of their significance and what to do if they occur
8. How to store the medication properly

Although it is abundant, it is generally felt that knowledge and understanding of this information for each medication the patient is taking will help to improve compliance and achieve safer and more efficacious drug utilization, along with better patient participation in his health care.

REFERENCES

1. Holders of Approved New Drug Applications for Drugs Presenting Actual or Potential Bioequivalence Problems, U.S. Department of Health, Education, and Welfare, Food and Drug Administration, Rockville, 1976.
2. The United States Pharmacopeia, U.S. Pharmacopeial Convention, Inc., Rockville, 1975.
3. **Wolfert, R. R. and Cox, R. M.,** Room temperature stability of drug products labeled for refrigerated storage, *Am. J. Hosp. Pharm.,* 32, 585, 1975.
4. **Pray, S.,** Quality assurance of manufacturer-supplied unit-dose packages, *Hosp. Pharm.,* 14, 6c, 1979.
5. **Jeffrey, L. P., Temkin, L. A., and Krugman, M. E.,** Assuring the quality of medications stored in patient care areas, *Am. J. Hosp. Pharm.,* 32, 283, 1975.
6. **D'Arco, J. A. and Williams, R. L.,** The poison prevention packaging act and resistant containers, *J. Am. Pharm. Assoc.,* NS12, 380, 1972.
7. **Barbieri, J.,** The new prescription drug labeling requirement, *U.S. Pharm.,* 4, 19, 1979.
8. **Jarosinski, P. F.,** The importance of pharmacist surveillance in a unit-dose distribution system, *Hosp. Pharm.,* 13, 491, 1978.
9. **McAllister, J. C., Buchman, E. C., and Skolaut, M. W.,** A comparison of the safety and efficiency of three intermittent intravenous therapy systems — the minibottle, the minibag, and the inline burette, *Am. J. Hosp. Pharm.,* 31, 961, 1974.
10. **Turco, S.,** Quality assurance in i.v. admixture programs, *Hosp. Pharm.,* 14, 307, 1979.
11. **Archambault, G. F.,** Investigational drugs — legal implications of their use, *Hosp. Form. Mgmt.,* 9, 36, 1974.
12. **Morrison, M.,** How defective products are recalled, *Hosp. Formul. Manage.,* 9, 36, 1974.
13. **Gumbhir, A. K. and Jamison, M. L.,** Assessing the effectiveness of drug recalls in pharmacies, *Drug. Cosmet. Ind.,* p. 40, 1975.

SAFETY IN THE HOSPITAL LABORATORY

James D. Barger

INTRODUCTION

The safety program of the hospital laboratory is a product of an overall safety program for hospitals. The laboratory is unique when compared to the rest of the hospital in that here the hazards also present in the hospital environment are concentrated to a greater degree, and there are hazards peculiar to the laboratory itself.

Until recently, safety programs in hospital laboratories were neglected to a great extent. The presence of noxious fumes from such agents as dioxane in tissue processing was not fully appreciated. Fire extinguishers may have been present, but often were not of the right type and frequently were not checked regularly to see that they were in operating condition. Smoking was allowed throughout the laboratory. Biohazards, especially hepatitis, were not fully appreciated. With this lack of attention to various hazards, it has been fortunate that accidents in hospital laboratories have not been more numerous. Very little attention was paid to this aspect of laboratory operations and many of the accidents probably were not reported.

Accidents do happen and not always to "somebody else". For these reasons, a growing appreciation of safety programs has developed in recent years. Changes have been brought about not only by awareness of the safety problem, but also by various OSHA review programs and legal restrictions. The Occupational Safety and Health Act of 1970 and subsequent state safety acts have focused attention on safety. Insurance carriers for workman's compensation have also insisted that the working conditions be improved because of their financial interest in accident prevention. These pressures will continue to increase, and with increased vigilance will come a safer work environment. Continuing technical developments and an appreciation for safety already have made for marked improvements in these aspects of laboratory operation when compared to just a few years ago.

It is most important that management realize the importance of safety. Laboratory personnel are a highly trained and valuable resource and waste of this resource due to a needless accident is an unnecessary economic burden. Laboratory personnel must be educated by in-house programs. Installing and maintaining a laboratory safety program is not an easy task. It must be sold to all persons involved from top management to those with the lowest positions in the organization. This selling is not easy as there are many who may not want to be "saved" and will resist such education vigorously. Additionally, safety programs cost money. These costs are in capital expenditures and personnel time. The cost effectiveness of such a program is difficult to determine, but is actually irrelevant when all factors are considered. The objectives of the safety program are to provide a safe environment in which to work, with safe tools for performing the work. There are no absolutes in these programs. All risks cannot be completely eliminated, but significant risks can be reduced to an acceptable minimum.

THE SAFETY PROGRAM

The essence of safety is the prevention of accidents, most of which are due to human error and only a few to mechanical failure. This emphasizes the need for more vigilance of all people while at work. Prevention of accidents is brought about by careful planning of the work and elimination of such existing hazards as may be present before the work is started.

An important part of any safety program is the training of personnel to deal with accidents. Even in the best work environment, the possibility exists that accidents may occur. Prompt action in dealing with any accident may be of great importance in preventing more serious complications as a result of such an accident. This training should be given to all personnel, and the knowledge and skills necessary for treatment of various types of accidents should be continually emphasized so that proper responses will be carried out no matter what the situation.

In a recent monograph on safety, the Dow Chemical Company has given the following definition of safe: "A situation is 'safe' if it can be handled by a careful and prudent man using sound procedures and rules working with properly designed and maintained equipment." This definition contains three key phrases that delineate the responsibility of management in providing a safe work environment. These are proper employee selection for training and motivation of this employee in regard to safety, development of sound procedures and rules by management, and the provision of adequate equipment. Not only is it good management to provide a safe working environment, but is now a legal requirement. The Occupational Safety and Health Act of 1970 (PL 91-596) applies to any employer with one or more employees in a business effecting interstate commerce. This has been interpreted rather broadly and certainly applies to hospitals and hospital laboratories. The objective of this act is to reduce the number of work-related accidents, illnesses, and fatalities and "insure so far as possible safe and healthful working conditions for every American worker". The act authorizes the OSHA to set mandatory safety and health standards to carry out an effective program of enforcement. Additionally, the Federal Occupational Safety and Health Act provides that "any state which at any time desires to assume responsibility for development and enforcement therein of occupational safety and health standards relating to any occupational safety or health issue with respect to which the federal standard has been promulgated...shall submit a state plan for the development of such standards and their enforcement" and further "that the secretary shall approve the plan...if such plan in his judgment...will be at least as effective" as the federal plan. At the present writing, 21 states have such plans.

The details of the standards promulgated by the OSHA are to be found in the Federal Register of June 27, 1974. Standards that would affect operations of hospital laboratories are found in several sections of the Federal Register and refer to lighting, ventilation, safety equipment, general housekeeping, personal protection, equipment, signs, labels, fire extinguishers, gas cylinders, toilet facilities, drinking water, etc. These regulations have been summarized in several monographs. A laboratory safety checklist has been prepared by the Lab Safety Supply Company in Janesville, Wis. which details many of these requirements and gives their OSHA section number for reference.

Voluntary accrediting bodies have also given increased attention to adequate provision of a safe environment in hospital laboratories. The Joint Commission on Accreditation of Hospitals has new standards for hospital laboratories that became effective January 1, 1979. These are much more detailed concerning safey procedures than previous standards. The College of American Pathologists' inspection and accreditation program has also devoted a great deal of attention to the provision of a safe environment in the hospital laboratory. Many of the questions on the check list used for inspections are devoted to evaluation of safety programs. Lack of attention to the safety procedures leads to "Phase II" deficiencies that must be corrected within 30 days for the institution to be accredited. It is expected that all accrediting and licensing organizations, both private and governmental, will continue to devote close attention to safety procedures and precautions.

Provision of a safe environment and operation of the hospital laboratory requires a thoroughly planned safety program that is diligently applied at all times. This safety program consists of two parts, the first of which is the provision of proper environment. This requires a thorough inventory, including the evaluation of fire extinguishers according to availability and adequacy, the inspection of electrical equipment according to proper grounding, storage of flammables, proper ventilation, lighting, etc. throughout the entire laboratory. This inventory should be performed with meticulous detail, and repeated on a periodic basis to insure that the laboratory continues to be a safe environment.

The second part of the safety program is the teaching of safety. In this connection, we may use the paraphrase "safety is everybody's business and if safety is not everybody's business it may be no ones business". The teaching of safety requires a program of regular safety meetings beginning with the start of employment. Safety standards for the laboratory should be written and provided as a manual for each employee. The employee is required to be thoroughly familiar with these safety standards. Meetings must be held on a periodic basis to assure that everyone has an adequate knowledge of these standards. It is especially important to begin this safety indoctrination with the start of employment. The experience of Dow Chemical shows that 25% of accidents in the laboratory happen in the first 6 months, and 42% in the first year of employment. Furthermore, 19% of the employees in these laboratories are in the 20 to 29-year age group, and these persons accounted for 35% of the accidents. Safety is the price of eternal vigilance beginning at the start of employment.

SAFETY ORGANIZATION

There must be a person(s) assigned definite responsibility for the safety program. Depending on the size of the laboratory, this may be the laboratory manager, chief technologist, a supervisor who is designated as safety officer, or a committee of various persons from both management and the technical work force. The definite assignment of this responsibility to a specific person(s) is necessary for the continuity of the laboratory safety program. Without such continuity, there is a definite tendency to overlook or miss unsafe practices that may develop. A safety survey should be performed by a safety officer at least once a year. This person is also responsible for the investigation of all accidents in the laboratory. It is most important that investigation of any accident be carried on not as a punitive measure, but as an educational measure aimed at correction of unsafe procedures and prevention of future accidents. If such investigations are punitive, they will effectively destroy much of the safety program.

There are times when, in spite of safety programs, education and counseling, an employee will persist in unsafe practices in the laboratory. If this cannot be corrected, such an employee must be separated from the job not only for his own protection, but for the protection of other workers.

GENERAL GUIDELINES

Certain general guidelines are common to all laboratory safety programs. The most important of these, and one not peculiar to the laboratory, is the proper handling of specimens for analysis. All specimens must be considered infectious and must be in a proper container with a proper label identifying the specimen. Careful and judicious handling of these specimens must be impressed upon all persons having any contact with them, including the nursing service. No specimen with organic matter on the outside of the container should be accepted by the laboratory, and labels or requisition slips stained with blood or other material should be recopied and the original destroyed. Specimens from patients in isolation require special handling. They should be transported in paper or plastic bags, and opened in the laboratory in biohazard type hoods.

Handwashing is a necessity to prevent contamination between patients and employees. It is especially important for technicians to wash their hands with soap and water between each patient when drawing blood. Probably the most important safety precaution for employees of the laboratory is handwashing, an aspect of safety often not sufficiently stressed in laboratory safety programs. The Center for Disease Control (CDC) conducted a study on the importance of handwashing in the hospital. Results of this study show that for most hospital personnel, handwashing with plain soap and water is sufficient, but in certain critical areas (one of these is the laboratory), an antiseptic agent should be used with the soap. Often, laboratory personnel will use hand lotion after washing. It has been shown that hand lotion can be contaminated with gram-negative bacteria, especially pseudomonas, and these organisms may account for some disease. Hand lotion, therefore, should not be used in the laboratory.

There must be a prohibition of smoking in the laboratory. This ban serves several purposes. The smoking material may become contaminated and serve to introduce infectious or toxic material into the mouth of the smoker. It must also be prohibited where flammables or solvents are used because of fire hazards.

Eating and drinking are also prohibited in the work areas because of the possibility of contamination. The storage of food is not permitted in laboratory refrigerators.

SAFETY MANUAL

The safety manual will vary as to its length and sophistication, depending upon the size and complexity of the laboratory and the depth of the subject matter that needs to be considered in light of the technical knowledge and expertise of intended users of the manual. It must be decided whether this is to be a comprehensive text on safety procedures or a set of guidelines that will be augmented by written specific instructions for each section of the laboratory. In larger institutions, a common practice is to provide a comprehensive manual covering all aspects of the laboratory service, and then provide sections of this comprehensive manual showing general guidelines and specific details for each section of the laboratory. The organization of such a manual determined by the complexity of the laboratory services should be such that it is readily available and useful to all laboratory personnel.

Suggestions for organization of the laboratory manual have been outlined by the Analytical Division of the Chemical Society of Great Britian, and can be found in the Proceedings of the Analytical Division of Chemical Society, December 1977. This provides a rather complete outline for a safety manual for a chemical laboratory and should be readily adaptable for hospital laboratories.

THE SAFETY PROGRAM DETAILS

Laboratory Fire

Fires in any hospital area may be disastrous. The materials present in the laboratory to fuel such fires make the potential for disaster very great. The laboratory ranks fifth amongst hospital areas with the highest number of fires. Patient rooms, employee quarters, the power plant, and store rooms are the only areas where fires occur more commonly. According to the National Fire Protection Association (NFPA), fires in the laboratory area are the result of carelessness, inattention, lack of knowledge, an unsafe environment, unattended operations, and smoking. All laboratory fires are preventable. Prevention is the primary object of any laboratory safety program.

Some basic considerations are readily apparent for fire prevention. These are specific requirements for all accrediting and inspecting agencies, as well as OSHA. The first of these is good housekeeping. Laboratories are not noted for good housekeeping. Many are overcrowded and lack adequate work space. For these reasons, halls may be cluttered with equipment or used for storage of supplies. Often, because of shortage of space, areas are serviced for laboratory use even though they were not originally designed for these purposes. The explosive growth of laboratory technology and instrumentation has greatly magnified this problem in older laboratories.

The general impression given an inspector on first viewing the laboratory often depends on the housekeeping. A sloppy, carelessly kept laboratory with materials stored in halls and sometimes blocking exits, often indicates that there may be many violations of the safety requirements. Often, hospital management or laboratory directors may not be fully aware of deficiencies in housekeeping because of their constant contact with the situation. Appraisal of an inspector unfamiliar with the environment is most helpful in pointing out to management defects in housekeeping that usually are easily corrected.

As previously stated, smoking may be a hazard not only to the individual worker, but to his colleagues as well. The College of American Pathologists' fire regulations for laboratories specified "no smoking" areas as follows:

1. Within 25 ft of gasoline tank, oil, solvents, liquid, petroleum gases, or other storage flammables in use
2. Where "no smoking" signs are displayed
3. By employees whose clothing is contaminated by explosive dust or inflammable liquids, or who handle these materials
4. In areas where there is reason to doubt the safety, even though this area may not be posted
5. In all elevators
6. In all hazardous locations where "smoking areas" have been established by the chief fire marshall and plainly marked (operating personnel will be responsible for strict adherence to this regulation)
7. In all other such places as may be directed by the chief fire marshall

Laboratories may differ significantly from one another in many ways, but in the working areas, smoking should be entirely prohibited.

Smoking may be permitted in the employee lounge area, hospital dining room, or some other area not directly involved in laboratory operations. The restricted areas should include outpatient waiting rooms as well as other areas.

Waste receptacles used in the laboratory should be designed to self-extinguish accidental fires. Metal receptacles with removable dome rim tops are effective in extinguishing accidental fires. Plastic waste receptacles should not be used in the laboratory area.

Electrical

Electrical hazards probably constitute the greatest number of safety violations in the laboratory setting. Strict application of tighter safety standards for electrical equipment by accrediting agencies have markedly decreased the violations. Most violations are seen in expanding laboratories, and consist mainly of improper grounding of electrical outlets, improper extension cords, and overloading of circuits.

All electrical installations, repairs, replacements, and modifications must be made in accordance with requirements of the National Electrical Code (NFPA No. 70). It is the responsibility of the laboratory director or the hospital engineer to be sure that this code is observed in the laboratory.

All electrical appliances should have three-prong plugs with adequate grounding and be approved by UL. No items should be allowed in the laboratory that do not meet electrical standards. Extension cords should only be used when there is no alternative. Only one outlet is permissible on the end of such cords. They should be UL-approved. Old frayed plugs and cords should be replaced, and electrical circuits should not be overloaded. Electrical outlets for fume hoods should be placed on the outside of the hoods.

Any shock, including minor tingling, should be reported immediately as this is an indication of instrument malfunction. Shut off the current and unplug the instrument. Do not continue to use such an instrument; not only is it potentially dangerous, but any results from this instrument would be suspect.

Repair of any instrument should be undertaken only by those persons using proper precautions and familiar with electrical and electronic circuits. Repairs of the electrical system of the building are to be performed only by the building maintenance personnel.

Short circuits may occur causing overload of electrical circuits. In most instruments, circuits are protected from overload by fuses or circuit breakers. However, short circuits may generate enough heat to cause fires. If such an event occurs, the equipment should be disconnected, and the fire extinguished with a carbon dioxide, dry chemical, or liquified gas extinguisher. Water should not be used on these fires.

CHEMICAL

Hospital laboratories have a wide range of chemicals in storage. These include toxic and explosive compounds oxidizing agents, and corrosive chemicals. A current inventory should be maintained for all these materials. This inventory should identify the location of the material, the amount present, and its potential safety hazards. It is not necessary to store these compounds in an alphabetical manner since this could result in the storage of incompatible chemicals with one another. Should fire occur in these storage areas, fire fighters must be alerted to the presence of possible toxic compounds. The toxicity of all compounds must be known by responsible persons in the laboratory. A system must be used for the ready identification of any potentially dangerous compound.

Many of the routine procedures in a clinical laboratory employ reagents that are caustic, corrosive, poisonous, and flammable. These reagents must be properly labeled as to their hazard, and appropriate precautions must be taken. The introduction of automated testing equipment has reduced these hazards somewhat by prepackaging reagents, but there are still many such reagents that are not obtained in this manner.

Dangerous chemicals may be grouped into the following classifications:

1. Caustic or corrosive
2. Poisons
3. Explosives (oxidizers)
4. Carcinogens

Caustic or corrosive substances are those acids or alkalies that may cause burns of the skin or mucous membranes of the mouth, eyes, or respiratory passages. They may also damage equipment and even the storage area. Such material should be stored near the floor to prevent its falling from shelves. All storage of chemicals should be on shelves with retaining "shock" cords to prevent such accidents. Further, organic acids (acetic acid and acetic anhydride) should be stored separately from oxidizing agents such as nitric, sulfuric, and perchloric acids to prevent interaction of fumes, and subsequent corrosion of storage cabinets. Acid bottle carriers must be used for containers over 1 ℓ in size.

When quantities of acids and alkalies are being used, a shield or barrier should be present; eye-protection devices are essential. With highly corrosive materials, aprons and gloves are required. These materials should never be pipetted by mouth or tested by smell. Great care should be used in mixing these substances. Acid should always be added to water and not vice versa. Additions to the mixture should be made slowly and the mixtures should not be allowed to over heat.

In the event of breaks or spills, prompt action is needed. For skin, eye, or mouth contact, wash immediately with copious amounts of water. Clothing should be removed immediately to prevent skin contact. For large spills on the body, the subject should be placed under a drenching shower immediately. At times, this has been life saving. Such showers should be tested periodically to make certain they operate properly. Spills should be contained with sand and absorbent materials which are then placed in a sealed can and marked "CHEMICAL WASTE — HAZARDOUS". Wash the area thoroughly. Liquids may be flushed down the drain by using large amounts of water.

Mercury vapors are extremely poisonous. Fortunately, newer analytic techniques have minimized the amounts of metallic mercury present in the laboratory environment. If at all possible, spills of metallic mercury should be avoided. Any spills should be cleaned up as soon as possible and the area thoroughly ventilated to remove mercury vapors. Metallic mercury should never be placed in drains since it will remain in the traps and become a dangerous source of toxic mercury vapor. Mercury is also present in other reagents, such as Nessler's reagent and Zenker's solution, and it is wise to use alternative methods that do not require these reagents.

The danger from cyanide used in hemoglobinometry is somewhat exaggerated. The amount of cyanide present in these reagents is small and below toxic levels. However, the wastes from hemoglobinometry should not be mixed with acids because of the possibility of generating hydrogen cyanide gas even in small amounts.

Some of the reagents used in the clinical laboratories are carcinogens. OSHA has established regulations for the proper handling of these compounds. Although there are only a few of these compounds in routine use in the laboratory, and then in dilute solutions, these precautions must be followed and an inventory of such materials must be maintained.

Substances considered by OSHA to be carcinogenic and subject to regulation are the following:

- 4 Nitro biphenyl
- 4,4′ Methylene bio (2 chloraniline)
- Methylchloromethyl ether
- Beta Naphthylamine
- 4 Aminodiphenyl
- Beta Propiolactone
- 4 Dimethylaminoazobenzene
- Alpha Naphthylamine
- 3,3′ Dichlorobenzidine and its salts
- Bischloromethyl ether
- Benzidine and its salts
- Ethylenimine
- 2 Acetyl aminoflourene
- N Nitrosodimethylamine

Regulations for the possession and use of these compounds include the following:

1. Specific work areas and their restricted areas must be designated.
2. Personnel authorized to work in the area must be listed.
3. Inventory of the types and quantities of compounds on hand must be made. (The extent of this requirement is not clear and may not apply to nonfederal laboratories.)
4. Personnel must be specifically trained in safety procedures.
5. Records of exposure must be maintained.

6. Procedures for monitoring, storage, decontamination, disposal, and emergencies must be established.
7. Medical surveillance of personnel will include a preassignment examination, followed by periodic examinations with complete medical records.
8. Protective clothing must be provided and cleaned daily. Gloves must be provided if necessary.
9. Eating, drinking, smoking, and mouth pipetting is prohibited in the work area, and handwashing is required immediately after handling carcinogenic compounds.
10. Work areas must have clearly marked limited access. The work surfaces must be impervious, and procedures performed in a hood or closed system to control aerosols.
11. Facilities for changing clothes (with showers) must be available to personnel.

For the most part, these compounds have been eliminated from clinical laboratories by changes in methodology. Furthermore, it would be very difficult, if not impossible, for most hospital laboratories to comply with the requirements of these regulations. When satisfactory substitute methods not using these compounds cannot be found, a minimal program for use of the compounds should be instituted. This is best done using a glove box or safety cabinet to provide safe storage and limited access. The other inventory and personnel safety requirements must be met in this minimal program.

Oxidizing agents are chemicals with supply oxygen in any chemical reaction. Compounds such as peroxides, dichromates, perchlorates, and nitrates are commonly found in hospital laboratories, and should not be stored with flammables, organic chemicals, dehydrating, or reducing agents. These compounds should be kept only in small quantities. The methods for identification and storage of these potentially dangerous compounds should be thoroughly understood. Oxidizers are classified into four types depending on their relative reactivity. The general definition and some of the more common compounds in each class follows.

Class I — Oxidizing material that may increase the burning rate of the combustible material with which it comes into contact:

- Barium chlorate
- Calcium nitrate
- Hydrogen peroxide solutions (more than 8%, less than 27.5% W/V)
- Nitric acid (70% or less)
- Perchloric acid (less than 60% w/v)
- Potassium dichromate
- Silver nitrate
- Sodium chlorate
- Sodium nitrate
- Sodium perborate
- Zinc peroxide

Class 2 — Oxidizing material that can cause spontaneous ignition when in contact with combustible materials:

- Calcium hypochloride (50% or less w/v)
- Chromium trioxide (chromic acid)
- Hydrogen peroxide (27.5 to 52% w/v)
- Nitric acid (more than 70% concentration)
- Potassium permanganate

Class 3 — Oxidizing material that can undergo vigorous, self-sustained decomposition when catalyzed or exposed to heat:

- Hydrogen peroxide (52 to 91% w/v)
- Calcium hypochlorite (<50% w/v)
- Perchloric acid solutions (60 to 72.5% w/v)

Class 4 — Oxidizing material that can undergo an explosive reaction when catalyzed or exposed to heat, shock, or friction:

- Ammonium perchlorate
- Ammonium permanganate
- Guanidine nitrate
- Hydrogen peroxide solutions (<91% w/v)
- Perchloric acid solutions (>72.5% w/v)
- Potassium superoxide

The potential danger of these compounds is readily discernible. If possible, alternate analytical methods should be sought to eliminate the use of these compounds, as well as other incompatible compounds.

A short list of some of the incompatible chemicals that may be present in the laboratory is given here with those chemicals with which they may react:

Chemical	Incompatible chemicals
Acetic acid	Chromic acid, nitric acid, hydroxyl-continuing compounds, ethylene, glycol, perchloric acid, peroxides, and permanganate
Acetone	Concentrated sulfuric and nitric acids
Acetylene	Copper, halogens, silver, mercury, and their compounds
Chromic acid	Acetic acid, naphthalene, camphor, alcohol, glycemine, turpentine, and other flammable liquids
Hydrogen peroxide	Copper, chromium, iron, most metal and their salts, flammable liquids, and other combustible materials
Iodine	Acetylene, ammonium
Mercury	Acetylene, fulminic acid, ammonia
Oxalic acid	Silver, mercury
Potassium permanganate	Glycerine, ethylene glycol, benzaldehyde, sulfuric acid
Sulfuric acid	Chlorates, perchlorates, permanganates

This list is by no means exhaustive, but it does illustrate the need to identify the potential hazards of any chemical stored and used in the laboratory, and to inform all laboratory personnel of these hazards and the means of avoiding potentially dangerous situations.

Probably the most hazardous materials found in the laboratory are flammable and combustible liquids. These materials are easily ignited, burn with great rapidity, and the fires are difficult to extinguish. They must be handled with great care, and all personnel must have a thorough understanding of their hazardous properties.

Certain definitions are essential to this knowledge. The "flash point" means the minimum temperature at which a liquid will give off vapors in a test vessel at sufficient concentration to form an ignitable mixture with air near the surface of the liquid. A "flammable liquid" is any liquid having a flash point below 37.8°C (100°F), or any mixture with components having flash points at 37.8°C or higher in which the components constitute 99% or more of the total volume. "Combustible liquids" are those with flash points above 37.8°C. Flammable liquids are further divided into three classes depending on the flash point and the boiling point of the liquid. Combustible liquids are further divided into two classes depending on their flash points.

The flash points and ignition temperatures of some commonly used flammable liquids are as follows:

Liquid	Flash point (°C)	Ignition temp (°C)
Acetic acid	39.4	529
Acetone	−20	538
Benzene	−16.7	562
Ethyl alcohol	12.8	423
Ethyl ether	−45	180
Formalin (with methanol)	50	430
Isopropyl alcohol	−27.8	399
Lubricating oil	150—230	260—370
Toluene	4.4	536

The amounts of flammable liquids that can be stored in the laboratory are limited by the size of containers as outlined in OSHA regulations. Table 1 gives the maximum allowable size of containers for these types of liquids.

All flammable liquids should be stored in "safety cans". These are metal containers having a spring-loaded closing lid and spout cover that will safely relieve internal pressure when exposed to fire. They should be painted red and clearly labeled as to contents and the hazard of those contents. These containers should not have more than a 5-gal capacity.

Those liquids requiring refrigeration must be stored in an approved explosion-proof refrigerator or freezer. Ordinary household refrigerators must not be used for the storage of any of these solvents. Such storage can result in very dangerous and destructive explosions and fire. All refrigerators must have appropriate signs indicating whether they are explosion-proof and suitable for storage of flammable liquids. Storage of such liquids in proper refrigerators must be in safety cans. Appropriate preventive maintenance of these refrigerators is also necessary.

When not in use, flammable and combustible liquids should be stored in a protected storage area such as an approved safety cabinet. These cabinets must be labeled "FLAMMABLE—KEEP FIRE AWAY—NO SMOKING". Only minimal amounts of these liquids (consistent with efficient operations) should be stored in the laboratory.

For the efficient and economical operation of a hospital laboratory, it is often desirable to purchase supplies in quantities that may be unsafe for storage in the laboratory. For such storage, it is desirable and necessary to have a separate storage room. These storage rooms must be constructed in accordance with local building codes, NFPA recommendations, and OSHA regulations.

Inside storage rooms must meet certain minimal standards such as 1-hr fire-resistant construction between the room and other parts of the building. UL- or FM-labeled Class B fire doors and a 4 in. sill or ramp, or trenched drain to prevent liquids from escaping from the room. Explosion-proof electrical equipment is required. There should be adequate fire fighting equipment. These rooms are often equipped with ceiling sprinklers. Storage in these rooms must be orderly, neat, and free of clutter, with provisions not to store incompatible chemicals in proximity to one another.

Some procedures now use liquid nitrogen. This can cause serious injury due to extreme cold, and should be stored in a suitable container (Dewar flask) with precautions to prevent accidental spills.

Compressed Gases

Compressed gases present several safety hazards. Any gas cylinder with a broken

Table 1
CONTAINER SIZES FOR COMBUSTIBLE MATERIALS

Container type	Class 1A Flash point 16°C Boiling point 38°C	Class 1B Flash point 23°C Boiling point 38°C	Class 1C Flash point 23°C and 38°C	Class II Flash point 38°C and 60°C	Class III Combustible liquids
Glass	1 pt	1 qt	1 gal	1 gal	1 gal
Approved with density polyethlene or metal	1 gal	5 gal	5 gal	5 gal	5 gal
Safety cans	2 gal	5 gal	5 gal	5 gal	5 gal
Metal drums 1 cc. specification (storage vaults only)	60 gal	60 gal	60 gal	60 gal	60 gal
Examples	Ethyl ether Propylene oxide Pentane	Benzol Methyl alcohol Gasoline Ethyl alcohol Acetone Xylene Toluene	Ethyl mercaptan Turpentine Methyl alcohol (30% in H_2O)	Methylamyl acetate Kerosene	Stoddard solvent Amyl alcohol Fuel oil

valve head becomes a missile capable of penetrating walls and causing great structural damage, as well as endangering lives. Some gases may be toxic or flammable, and heating of the gas cylinder may result in an explosion.

Gas cylinders must be secured at all times to prevent any possibility of falling. Valve safety covers should remain on the cylinders until pressure regulators are attached. Hand trucks or dollies must be used for moving cylinders. They should never be rolled or dragged. The contents of the cylinders must be clearly marked. The use of oil, grease, or lubricant on the valve regulators or other fittings is prohibited. Do not attempt to repair damaged cylinders or force fully open frozen cylinder valves.

Special care must be used with flammable gases in confined spaces. Cylinder size for these gases is limited to 200 ft^3. Stand-by cylinders, whether full or empty, must not be stored in the laboratory. No more than two cylinders should be manifolded together, however, several instruments or outlets may be derived from a single cylinder. Valves on all flammable gas cylinders must be shut off when the laboratory is unattended.

Cylinders of compressed gas not in actual use should not be stored in the laboratory. Empty cylinders should be marked. All empty or unused cylinders should be promptly returned to the supplier.

Biohazards

Hazards from biological sources are concentrated in the laboratory environment because it is here that biological specimens are received for processing from all areas of the hospital. Fortunately, laboratory workers are (or should be) more aware of the potential hazards inherent in these patient specimens.

The greatest danger for laboratory workers and others lies in the improper handling of such specimens. Criteria must be derived for proper handling of all specimens. These criteria must be reasonable, clearly written, and understood by anyone who will handle biological specimens in any way. The importance of all persons in this chain observing safety rules cannot be overemphasized.

As a general rule, specimens that are improperly handled according to the accepted criteria should not be accepted. It is realized that there may be exceptions to this rule, but these exceptions should only be made at the supervisor level or higher. Most specimens sent for microbiological examination are known to be potentially hazardous and are handled well. However, this may not be the case with specimens for cytology, chemistry, or hematology examination.

At the present time, the most frequently encountered hazard for laboratory personnel is hepatitis B (serum hepatitis). Exposure of laboratory personnel to hepatitis B ranks with that of the personnel of the renal dialysis unit. Hepatitis A (infectious hepatitis) does not present the hazard of hospital-acquired infection as does hepatitis B. Hepatitis nonA-nonB, or hepatitis C, has been transmitted by transfusions and, experimentally, to monkeys. The possible hazards of transmissions to medical personnel from usual patient care of this disease is presently not known.

Hepatitis B is an ever-present danger. The dose of virus containing blood is estimated at 0.0004 mℓ. The usual means of transmission is by accidental needle puncture, although other possibilities exist. These are aerosol that may result from breakage of a tube of blood in a centrifuge, by oral route from handling contaminated specimens, and through minor breaks in the skin while handling such specimens.

The prevention of hepatitis B is of paramount importance. The immune status of all laboratory personnel with regard to hepatitis B should be determined by testing for hepatitis B surface antigen (HB_sAg) and hepatitis B surface antibody (HB_sAb). This testing should be repeated on a periodic basis, probably every 6 months. Studies are being carried on to determine the efficacy of immune serum globulin given periodically for prevention of clinical hepatitis B. The results of these studies are inconclusive.

In the event of an accidental needle puncture or other similar accident, the following precautions are recommended:

1. Test the patient for HB_sAg.
2. If the patient is positive for HB_sAg, give hyperimmune hepatitis B globulin according to recommended schedule. This should be done with some urgency (at least within 48 hr of the accident).
3. If the patient is not positive, immune serum globulin may be given as a precautionary measure, at the discretion of the attending physician.
4. If the laboratory worker is known to have had hepatitis B, or has hepatitis B antibody, the case should be evaluated by a physician to determine whether precautionary measures are necessary.

Of course, hepatitis B can be transmitted by other than parenteral routes and materials other than blood. For these reasons, all patient specimens must be considered contaminated and handled accordingly. Specimen containers should be supplied for the disposal of specimens such as blood, urine, etc. and for other disposables such as syringes, needles, pipettes, etc. There must also be an absolute ban on mouth pipetting throughout the laboratory. Smoking and eating in the laboratory should also be banned.

Since aerosols are also a potential source of contamination, they may be avoided by forbidding such practices as "popping corks" from blood tubes, and properly using the safety locks on centrifuges.

The laboratory environment must be kept scrupulously clean. Blood spills should be wiped up immediately. Surfaces are best cleaned by using 1% hypochlorite (bleach) solution or 2% Amphyl® solution. There is some recent evidence that 1 to 2% hypochlorite in 50 to 70% methanol may be more effective. For sterilization of material contaminated by HBV, it is recommended that the material be autoclaved for 30 min at 132°C.

There has been a decrease in tuberculosis in the past 20 yr that lowered the suspicion of the possibility of tuberculous infection. Because of this, patients with tuberculosis may go unsuspected without proper isolation precautions. This presents an extreme health hazard for all hospital personnel. Periodic X-ray or tuberculosis skin testing should be available for all personnel on a regular basis.

Other organisms, especially fungal organisms, are potentially very dangerous. The diphasic fungi, such as *Coccidioides immitis,* are especially hazardous. These organisms, as well as mycobacteria, should only be handled in a bacteriological safety hood for protection of the environment.

The collection of specimens from patients in isolation should conform with established isolation procedures of the hospital. All such specimens must be transported to the laboratory in closed containers such as plastic bags.

The personnel of the microbiology laboratory must maintain strict cleanliness of the work area. The sterilization of needles and loops for bacteriological inoculations should not be done with open flames because of the possibility of spattering contagious material. Frequent handwashing is recommended. All patient specimens and culture materials must be sterilized by autoclaving or dry heat prior to disposal. After sterilization, they are placed in double plastic bags for further trash disposal.

Anatomic Pathology

Safety precautions for anatomic pathology are often taken lightly. There are three areas that must be controlled: the hospital morgue, the surgical pathology-examination room, and the tissue-preparation laboratory.

Safety problems of the hospital morgue are chiefly microbiological hazards encountered at autopsy. These hazards may be minimized by careful dissection techniques and by scrupulous cleanliness of all surfaces in the morgue. In many communities, bodies are arterially embalmed before an autopsy is performed. However, embalming fluids will not kill many organisms that may be encountered. Such organisms as myobacteria and fungi, as well as other pathogenic bacteria, may be cultured from embalmed bodies. Thus, embalming should not be considered as materially lessening the microbiological hazards of the autopsy.

Surfaces of the furniture in the morgue should be inpervious to water, and periodically cleaned with antiseptic solutions. Water lines must be provided with vacuum breakers to prevent any possibility of contamination of the water supply system by hazardous material.

The surgical pathology gross examination room is very similar in that, here, too, the greatest hazards are biological. The examination of lesions of unknown etiology, or those with potentially infective organisms, should be done in the surgical pathology examination room rather than the operating room in order to confine such hazards to the smallest area possible with exposure of the smallest numbers of people. Here, too, surfaces should be impervious to water and kept scrupulously clean. It is recommended that all surfaces be wiped down with dilute hypochlorite solution each day and that the dissecting instruments be sterilized using hypochlorite or formalin solutions at least daily.

The freezing microtome is a potential source of contamination and should be regularly defrosted, and the surfaces cleaned with an antiseptic solution.

The most frequently used fixative for tissue specimens is formaldehyde. The fumes of formaldehyde are especially irritating to the mucous membranes of the eyes and respiratory tract, and some persons will have allergic reactions (especially skin sensitivity) to very small concentrations of this substance. These effects are reversible upon discontinuance of the exposure. There is a very limited amount of toxicologic data concerning the effects of prolonged or chronic exposure to this substance, however, none suggest that it produces delayed types of toxicity. For the comfort of the workers, it is recommended that environmental concentrations of this substance be kept below that which can be detected by odor.

Of all the sites of anatomic pathology activity, the tissue-preparation laboratory has the greatest potential hazards. The various processing and staining methods use many different solutions, most of which are highly flammable and toxic. Automatic tissue processors use a combination of flammable toxic liquids with melted paraffin in their processing cycles. These machines should be fitted with an exhaust hood, if possible. Malfunctions of the machines have resulted in serious electrical fires.

Flammable liquids should be stored in the laboratory in minimal amounts, and safety cans provided for any such storage.

Thin section techniques using plastic as an embedding medium are becoming more routine. These techniques use highly toxic materials in the process, and it is recommended that the entire procedure of plastic embedding be carried out using a hood for protection of laboratory personnel.

Radioisotopes

There has been an increasing use of radioactive materials for various diagnostic laboratory procedures. The exposure levels to radiation from the amounts used in these procedures is usually well below limits that have been established by federal or state regulations requiring specific safety precautions. There is a broad structure of agencies with a body of laws and regulations by which both federal and state authorities act to insure the safe use of radioisotopes. These policies and regulations should not be a burden to the hospital laboratory since the analytic methods involve relatively low levels of beta and gamma radiations from a limited number of radionuclides. Even so, clinical laboratory personnel should be acquainted with rules and regulations governing the use of this material.

The most common isotopes for in vivo and in vitro testing are the following:

Hydrogen (tritium)	^{3}H
Carbon	^{14}C
Cobalt	^{57}Co
Iron	^{59}Fe
Iodine	^{125}I, ^{131}I

Regardless of the small amounts of radioactive material for diagnostic use, strict safety precautions should be observed to minimize exposure to even these small amounts of radiation. Appropriate monitoring equipment should be available and used on a periodic basis. Appropriate signs and warnings must be posted. The standard radiation warning symbol is a magenta trefoil on a yellow background. All rooms where radioactive materials are stored or used must be posted with signs stating "CAUTION RADIATION MATERIAL". Similar appropriate labels must be used on containers of radionuclides, including preparations made in the laboratory.

Complete records must be kept for all radionuclides. These records will include the date received, a description of the material and its radioactivity, the supplier, the condition of the package on receipt, and the use and disposal of the material. For amounts of radionuclides covered by legal rules and regulations, there is a prescribed manner for the keeping of records.

Not only is the amount and kind of isotopes a laboratory can possess regulated, but the manner of disposal is also regulated. Wastes from patients such as urine, blood samples, and fecal specimens may be disposed of into the sanitary sewer system and flushed with large amounts of water. Radioactive material disposed of in this manner is negligible in amount. Effluents from in vitro diagnostic tests may also be flushed into the sink with copious amounts of water. Amounts of radioactivity disposed of in this manner should not exceed 20 μCi/day. Larger amounts of radioactivity should be trapped in waste containers and allowed to decay to safe levels before disposal. Any unused isotopes are either allowed to decay in storage or be returned to the supplier for recycling of containers. No radioactive materials should be incinerated or buried.

The rules for handling of radionuclides are much the same as for any hazardous materials. They are not pipetted or handled directly, but are removed from vials using a syringe and needle or an automatic pipetting device. The vials are handled within lead containers and are not removed from these containers. Tubes are covered with caps, and caution is exercised to prevent spills. Protective clothing should be worn when using these materials.

The work, storage, and specimen-receipt areas, as well as the instrument areas, should be monitored daily. The following tolerance limits should be observed: surface areas not to exceed 200 mrem/hr and 3 ft distances not to exceed 10 mrem/hr. All personnel should have film badges available to them even though the levels of radiation are at such a low level that the badges rarely show any significant exposure.

The radiation safety program should be a part of the hospital safety program, and the hospital radiation safety officer should be intimately involved in the supervision of the laboratory program for compliance with legal rules and regulations for use of this material.

CONCLUSION

Safety programs for hospital laboratories require a systematic approach for their evolution and continuance. This starts with an inventory of the potential hazards existing in the laboratory. Physical features of the plant that do not meet standards must be corrected. From this inventory, a safety plan is developed to meet all rules and regulations and eliminate any real or potential hazards. This plan is committed to writing, and the staff familiarized with all aspects of the safety plan. This familiarization is continued on a permanent basis for all old and new employees. A method for following and recording compliance with the plan is developed. The entire plan is monitored and reviewed at regular intervals to eliminate any hazardous practice that may develop, and to improve safety conditions in the work place. Safety must become a way of life for all personnel for it is truly "everybody's business".

REFERENCES

1. **Flury, P. A. and Deluca, K.,** *Environmental Health and Safety in the Hospital Laboratory,* Charles C Thomas, Springfield, Ill., 1978.
2. **Henry, R. J., et al.,** *Safety in the Clinical Laboratory,* Bioscience Enterprises, Van Nuys, Calif., 1976.
3. **Pieters, H. A. J.,** *Safety in the Chemical Laboratory,* Butterworths, London, 1951.
4. **Steere, N. V., Ed.,** *Handbook of Laboratory Safety,* 2nd ed., Chemical Rubber Co., Cleveland, 1971.
5. NIH Biohazards Safety Guide, U.S. Department of Health, Education, and Welfare, Washington, D.C., 1974.
6. **Carlson, D. J.,** Guidelines for Laboratory Safety for Medical Technologists, Policies and Procedures, *College American Pathologists,* Skokie, Ill., 1976.
7. Laboratory Safety at the Center for Disease Control, DHEW Publ. No. CDC76-811, U.S. Government Printing Office, Washington, D.C., August 1975.
8. Laboratory Waste Disposal Manual, Manufacturing Chemists Association, Washington, D.C., 1973.
9. Public Law 91-596, Occupational Safety and Health Act of 1970.
10. U.S. Department of Labor and Occupational Safety and Health Administration, Occupational safety and health standards, *Fed. Regist.,* 39(125), III, June 27, 1974; 39(20) 11, January 29, 1974.
11. U.S. Department of Labor, Organizing a Safety Committee, OSHA Bull. 2231, Occupational Safety and Health Administration, June 1975.
12. **Dwyer, M. J. and Brindley, H.,** Commitment — another word for safety, *Lab World,* 30, 28, 1979.
13. Fisher Safety Manual, Fisher Scientific Co., Pittsburgh, 1974.
14. Fisher Scientific Co., Safety Wall Chart, Fisher Scientific Co., Pittsburgh, 1976.
15. **Bond, R. and DeRoos, G.,** *Environmental Health and Safety in Health Care Institutions,* Macmillan, Philadelphia, 1972.
16. **Anon.,** Sense and safety in laboratories: editorial, *J. Clin. Pathol.,* 32, 417, 1979.
17. **McCarthy, K.,** Safety of laboratory workers, *Lancet,* 1, 52, 1977.
18. **Thirkell, D.,** Safety in the laboratory, *Top. Biochem. Sci.,* p. N260, November 1978.
19. Safety in analytical laboratories: the contents of a laboratory safety manual, *Proc. Anal. Div. Chem. Soc. (England),* 14, 360, 1977.
20. **Straub, C. P., Ed.,** Safety, 4.1 patient and personnel safety, in *Handbook of Environmental Control,* Vol. 5, CRC Press, Boca Raton, Fla., 1975, 299.
21. **Straub, C. P., Ed.,** Safety, 4.2 laboratory safety, in *Handbook of Environmental Control,* Vol. 5, CRC Press, Boca Raton, Fla., 1975, 320.
22. **Straub, C. P., Ed.,** Safety, 4.3 fire safety, in *Handbook of Environmental Control,* Vol. 5, CRC Press, Boca Raton, Fla., 1975, 320.
23. Fire Resistance Index, Underwriters Laboratories, Inc., Northbrook, Ill., 1975.
24. Fire Regulations for Laboratories, College of American Pathologists, Skokie, Ill., 1974.
25. Laboratories in Health-Related Institutions, NFPA No. 56C, National Fire Protection Association, Boston, 1973.
26. Safe Handling of Compressed Gases, Pamphlet P-1, Compressed Gas Association, New York, 1974.
27. Characteristics and Safe Handling of Medical Gases, Pamphlet P-2, Compressed Gas Association, New York, 1974.

28. Fire Hazard Properties of Flammables, Liquids, Gases, Volatile, Solids, NFPA 325M, National Fire Protection Association, Boston, 1969.
29. Hazard Identification System, NFPA 704, National Fire Protection Association, Boston, 1975.
30. Signs, Labels, and Safety Equipment, OSHA Memo, American Hospital Association, Chicago, 1973.
31. Explosive Azide Hazard, DHEW Publ. No. CDC 76-8017, U.S. Department of Health, Education, and Welfare, Washington, D.C.
32. Classification of Etiologic Agents on the Basis of Hazard, U.S. Department HEW, 1976, Center for Disease Control, U.S. Department of Health, Education, and Welfare, Atlanta, 1976.
33. **Seidenberger, J. W. and Blum, F. M.,** New concept in laboratory safety: the chemical spill clean-up kit, *Am. Lab.,* June 1975.
34. **Duckworth, J.,**Hepatitis Precautions, 1975, Methodist Hospital, Memphis, 1975.
35. Hepatitis Surveillance, DHEW Rep. No. 38, Center for Disease Control, U.S. Department of Health, Education, and Welfare, Atlanta, 1976.
36. Hepatitis Surveillance, Rep. No. 39, Center for Disease Control, U.S. Department of Health, Education, and Welfare, Atlanta, 1977.
37. **Kobayashi, M., et al.,** Sterilization of hepatitis B surface antigen — contaminated material, *Med. Instrum.,* 12, 171, 1978.
38. **Pike, R. M.,** Past and present hazards of working with infectious agents, *Arch. Pathol. Lab. Med.,* 102, 333, 1978.
39. Carcinogens, Job Health Hazard Series, No. 2204, U.S. Department of Health, Education, and Welfare, Washington, D.C., January 1975.
40. **Loomis, T. A.,** *Formaldehyde toxicity, Arch. Pathol. Lab. Med.,* 103, 321, 1979.
41. Carcinogens — Working Carcinogens, DHEW Publ. No. (NIOSH) 77-206, U.S. Department of Health, Education, and Welfare Washington, D.C.
42. Eye Protection, Manual Guide-Safety Management, DHEW Publ. No. CDC-21, Center for Disease Control, U.S. Department of Health, Education, and Welfare, Atlanta, 1975.
43. **Halbert, M. D., Vesley, D., and Vick, N.,** Pipetting Aids and Other Safety Devices for the Biomedical Laboratory, NIH-NCI-CP-43285 University of Minnesota School of Public Health, Minneapolis, 1974.
44. **Kaye, S.,** What to do with those laboratory disposables!, *Lab. Manage.,* p. 37, June 1978.
45. **Graham, J. D.,** Troubleshooting laboratory fume hoods, *Ind. Res. Dev.,* p. 129, June 1979.

HOSPITAL RADIATION SAFETY

Paul L. Ziemer and Alan L. Orvis

SOURCES OF RADIATION IN HOSPITALS

A surprising variety of radiation sources may be found in hospitals. The size and shape of these sources may range from minute objects such as needles containing radioactive materials, to huge machines such as the accelerators used in radiation therapy. Some familiar devices might emit radiation unexpectedly, e.g., a microwave oven with dirty or worn seals in the door. Although radiation sources are most frequently located in radiology and nuclear medicine departments, they are also found in virtually any place in the hospital. This is true not only because of the wide use of portable X-ray machines and portable nuclear medicine cameras, but because patients who have recently received diagnostic or therapeutic doses of most radionuclides are, for a time, themselves sources of radiation.

The users of radiation sources must comply with regulations promulgated by several governmental agencies. Most states exercise some degree of control in this matter, usually through state health departments or through state environmental safety divisions. State laws are likely to be comprehensive and cover all kinds of sources, but the degree of regulation varies from simple registration of sources in a few states to licensure and inspection in others. The Nuclear Regulatory Commission (NRC) exercises strict control over the safe use of byproduct material (radioactive substances produced in a nuclear reactor) either directly in some states or indirectly in "agreement" states. Radioactive materials not produced in a reactor, such as radium which occurs in nature, and others which are accelerator produced, are much less strictly regulated in the nonagreement states. However, the very broad safety regulations of the Occupational Safety and Health Administration (OSHA) include all radiation sources not controlled by other agencies.

Radiation hazards are often not easily recognized. Therefore, an important element of all radiation laws is a requirement for the presence of signs or other means of source identification. For instance, the hospital rooms of patients containing therapeutic radionuclides must be placarded. These signs usually list the name and telephone number of a person to be called in case of questions or emergencies. This person is frequently called the radiation protection officer, designated as such by the hospital administration.

Radiation sources may be categorized as being either "ionizing" or "nonionizing." The ways that these kinds of radiation physically interact with matter are basically different, as are the resulting biological effects. X-ray machines and radioactive materials emit ionizing radiations. Microwave, ultraviolet, laser, and ultrasound devices are sources of nonionizing radiations. The main emphasis of this chapter will be on sources of ionizing radiation.

X-Ray Machines and Accelerators

Every hospital has at least one X-ray machine and most hospitals have many. Radiotherapy accelerators also produce X-rays which have higher energy and are therefore more penetrating than diagnostic X-rays. X-ray rooms are typically shielded with millimeters of lead, whereas cost considerations require that radiotherapy installations be constructed with thick, solid concrete walls and ceilings. X-ray machines do not emit radiation when the beams are turned off. Irradiated patients are not made radioactive.

X-ray protection requires a consideration of both X-ray energy and beam intensity.

X-ray energy refers to the discrete energy of each individual constituent (the photons or the rays) of the beam. Higher tube voltages produce higher energy radiations. Beam intensity is a measure of the number of photons or rays in the beam. Higher intensities are obtained by increasing the tube current — the milliamperes. In radiotherapy, high energy is needed for the beam to reach deep-seated tumors and high intensity is needed to damage the tumor.

Radionuclide Sources

Radioactive materials are unique among the various kinds of radiation sources in that their emissions cannot be turned off. The decay of radionuclides is unaffected by external physical or chemical factors. Therefore, radiation safety requires constant attention to the details of shielding, isolation, distance, and time.

Radionuclides are used both diagnostically and therapeutically in hospitals. Diagnostic studies may be either in vitro or in vivo. In vitro tests are those in which patient material, such as blood, is withdrawn and caused to react with a radioactive substance in a laboratory, away from the patient. The patient receives no radioactive material. Relatively small amounts of radioactivity are used per test but many tests are performed. Radioimmunoassay is an example of a group of in vitro diagnostic tests which have become among the most used laboratory tests. The principal hazard from these wet-lab tests results from poor housekeeping and contamination.

Patients are administered doses of radioactive tracer substances for in vivo studies and therefore carry an internal body burden of the material until it has decayed away or has been excreted. In a sense, the patient becomes a walking source. However, diagnostic tests usually involve small activities and/or short half-life radionuclides so special precautions are generally not required.

Radionuclide therapy requires the use of larger quantities which may be solutions which are ingested/injected or which may be sealed sources that are temporarily inserted into tumorous regions. Special precautions are invariably required and must be set forth in nursing instructions. Hospitals licensed for radiotherapy must designate a qualified individual to be responsible for radiation protection.

Microwave Devices

The nonionizing radiation emitted by microwave devices produces biological effects mainly by heating the tissue wherein it is absorbed. However, the exact nature of all biological effects is not completely understood. Contrary to common impressions, far more is known about ionizing than is known about nonionizing radiation. It is known that the lens of the eye is sensitive to both kinds of radiation relative to the formation of cataracts.

Microwave ovens and blood warmers are essentially self-contained and of low power so that hazards from leakage will only occur in the vicinity of the device. Since strict standards apply to the manufacture of microwave ovens, there is little leakage when new. However, deterioration of the door seal may occur with time so routine measurements of leakage should be made to verify the integrity of the oven.

Microwave diathermy machines are used in physical therapy for localized tissue heating. Intense focused fields are produced proximal to the radiator but stray fields are unlikely to be a problem except for the patient and the operator.

Ultrasound and Other Radiation Sources

The role of ultrasound in physical therapy is similar to that of microwave diathermy. Whereas X-rays, microwaves, ultraviolet, and lasers are all forms of electromagnetic radiation, ultrasound must be transmitted by vibrating matter. It is almost totally reflected at tissue-air interfaces. Ultrasonic diagnostic systems are finding increasing applications in neurology, obstetrics, and cardiology departments. Ultrasonic cleaning tanks are also widely used and have enough power to cause pain in a hand that is carelessly or curiously immersed in the water. However, none of these devices produce hazardous radiation fields away from the coupling medium.

The hazards of ultraviolet sources that are used for dermatology treatments and of ultraviolet sterilizing lights are fairly well-understood and pertain, of course, to the eyes and skin.

Lasers are the least widely used source of radiation in a hospital but accidental viewing of the beam or its reflection could cause significant eye damage. A moderately powerful laser may be a hazard at considerable distance from the source because of the nondispersive nature of the beam. The lasers used for retinal tacking in ophthalmology have mechanical restraints for safety but are capable of damage if improperly used. The lasers used for patient positioning in radiation therapy are low powered but should not be viewed directly.

FUNDAMENTALS OF IONIZING RADIATION PROTECTION

Types of Radiation

It is appropriate at this point to define the types of ionizing radiation that might be encountered in a medical facility. The main types of radiation that will be considered are alpha and beta particles, gamma rays, X-rays, and neutrons. The first two, alpha and beta particles, are said to be directly ionizing particles in that direct interaction of the particle with atoms or molecules results in the formation of ion pairs along the path of the particle. Gamma rays, X-rays, and neutrons are indirectly ionizing in that they interact with atoms or molecules to produce secondary particles which, in turn, cause ionization.

Alpha Particles

Most often associated with the decay of heavy elements such as radium, the alpha particle is really a cluster of four particles — two protons and two neutrons — ejected from the nucleus during radioactive decay. The alpha particle is thus identical to the nucleus of a helium atom, having a positive charge of 2 electron charges (3.2×10^{-19} C) and a mass of 4 amu.

Alpha particles have a relatively short range in matter and cannot readily penetrate very far into tissue. Because of their low-penetrating power, alphas do not generally constitute an external hazard and are unable to penetrate even the outer layer of skin. If, however, an alpha emitting radioactive material is ingested or taken into the body and deposited in organs or tissues, alpha particles may deposit their energy directly in the tissues with which they are in close, intimate contact. Alpha particles have a high specific ionization. This means that the number of ions formed per unit path along the track of the particle is relatively large, and hence the amount of energy deposited per unit path is also large. Alpha particles are thus referred to as high LET particles, with LET being an acronym for linear energy transfer.

Beta Particles

Beta particles are actually high-velocity electrons emitted during the decay of certain radioactive atoms. Although we ordinarily think in terms of negative electrons (negatrons), the emission of positive electrons (positrons) is not uncommon. In either case, the beta particles are emitted with energies ranging from close to zero up to some maximum energy, E_{max} and an average energy, E_{ave} characteristic of the particular radionuclide in question. Usually, beta particle energies are listed according to the E_{max} value in charts and tables of radionuclides. The average energy in most cases is approximately one third of the E_{max} value.

Beta particles carry a negative charge of 1 electronic charge (1.6×10^{-19} C) and have a mass of 1/1836 of a proton. The specific ionization of beta is much lower than for an alpha of equal energy. Likewise, the LET for betas is relatively low.

Gamma Rays

Gamma rays are electromagnetic quanta or photons that have no mass and carry no electrical charge. Gammas are usually emitted in combination with alpha or beta decay and represent an energy readjustment in the nucleus following radioactive decay. Whereas alpha and beta particles interact by forming ion pairs along their paths, thus giving up energy over the path of the particle, gamma photons give up all or a large portion of their energy in single discrete events. Ion pairs are then produced in secondary processes.

X-Rays

X-rays are essentially the same as gamma rays (photons of electromagnetic radiation) and differ only in their origin. Whereas gamma rays result from energy transitions in the nuclei of atoms, X-rays result from energy transitions involving orbital electrons. In some cases, X-rays are emitted in conjunction with radioactive decay, as in the case of the decay of ^{125}I, a radionuclide commonly used in medical procedures. More frequently, however, X-rays are manmade by X-ray machines such as diagnostic medical X-ray devices. In X-ray-producing devices, X-rays are generated when high-velocity electrons are caused to strike a target material (e.g., tungsten). The resultant X-rays have a spectrum of energies ranging from close to zero energy up to the maximum energy of the incident electrons.

Neutrons

Neutrons are not widely used in medicine, but have found limited applications in therapy in recent years. Thus, they are included here as a type of radiation that might be found in a hospital. Neutrons are neutral (uncharged) particles having a mass approximately 1 amu. They may be produced by accelerators or emitted during the fission of certain heavy elements (e.g., californium-252). The special requirements for protection from neutrons are beyond the scope of this chapter.

Definitions and Terminology

Activity

The amount of radioactivity or the activity of a radionuclide is expressed by the number of atoms in a mass that decay or emit energy (as particles or photons) per unit time. The activity is defined as the number of such disintegrations per second (d/s).

Historically, a common reference scale has been radium, whose disintegration rate is 3.7×10^{10} d/s/g, or curie (Ci). Thus, a curie of radioactivity corresponds to any radioactive material decaying at the rate of 3.7×10^{10} d/s. A millicurie (mCi) is 3.7×10^{7} d/s and a microcurie (μCi) is 3.7×10^{4} d/s.

In recent years, a special name, the Bequerel, has been given to the unit d/s for use in the nuclear field. The Bequerel (Bq) corresponds to 1 d/s. Thus, 1 Ci = 3.7×10^{10} Bq.

Half-Life

The activity of a radioactive sample decreases exponentially with time. If the number of radioactive atoms present at time t_o is N_0, then the number, N, present at any subsequent time, t, is

$$N = N_0 e^{-\lambda t} \qquad (1)$$

where λ = the decay constant. The time for half of the atoms present to decay is called the half-life, $t_{1/2}$. Thus, for one half-life period, $N/N_0 = 0.5$ and $t_{1/2} = \ell n 0.5/\lambda = 0.693/\lambda$. Each radionuclide has its own characteristic decay constant and half-life.

Exposure

The intensity of a beam of X- or gamma rays may be expressed in terms of the amount of ionization produced in air. The quantity called exposure technically refers specifically to this situation, although the term exposure is often used in a more general sense. Intensity and energy are terms that are sometimes confused. Intensity is actually a function of both the number of rays passing through a volume and the energy of those rays.

Measurements of radiation fields may be accomplished by actually measuring ions with an electronic device such as an ionization chamber with an electrometer. The electrical charge (ionization) per unit mass of air, or exposure, is expressed in units of coulombs per kg. Historically, the special unit known as the roentgen (R) has been used for expressing exposure. The roentgen corresponds to 2.58×10^{-4} C of charge per kilogram of air. Most X-ray and gamma ray measuring instruments are calibrated to read out directly in roentgen units such as R/hr or mR/hr. It should be emphasized that by definition the quantity called exposure and the unit called the roentgen refer only to ionization in air due to X- or gamma rays.

Absorbed Dose

To determine hazards one must know not only about the quantities of radioactivity involved (i.e., the activity) and the exposure, but also about the type of radiation emitted (alpha, beta, or gamma) and the total amount of energy that is deposited by the radiation in the tissues or organs of interest. The basic quantity used to express the deposition of energy from ionizing radiation in body tissues (or any other medium) is the absorbed dose, which indicates the energy deposited per unit mass of any material.

The basic unit for absorbed dose is joules per kilogram (J/kg). This unit has been given a special name, the gray (Gy) for use in radiation-protection work. Another special unit for absorbed dose, the rad, has been used for many years. The rad corresponds to an absorbed dose of 0.01 J/kg (or 0.01 Gy). Absorbed-dose rates may be expressed in J/kg/hr, in Gy/hr, or in rad/hr. Likewise, one may express absorbed-dose rates in millirads per hour (mrad/hr), etc.

For air, an exposure of 1 R results in an absorbed dose in air of 0.869 rad. If a small mass of tissue is placed in a location where the exposure (in air) is 1 R, the absorbed dose in tissue will be about 0.95 rad. (The relation is not exact because "tissue" is not a well-defined medium). Thus, for many practical situations involving X- or gamma rays, the exposure measured in air in roentgen units is approximately equal numerically to the absorbed dose in rads for tissue. This has led to the common interchange of the quantities exposure and absorbed dose, and the units roentgens and rad for routine radiation-protection work.

Dose Equivalent

One other factor that must be considered in radiation protection is that certain types of radiation are more efficient in producing biological effects than others for a given amount of energy absorbed. To account for this effect, the absorbed dose is modified by an appropriate correction factor to take into account the relative biological effectiveness. The quantity obtained by this weighting of absorbed dose is termed the dose equivalent. That is

$$D.E. = D \times Q^{*}$$

where D = the absorbed dose in rads (or grays), Q = the weighing factor (called the quality factor), and D.E. = dose equivalent. Use of the dose equivalent puts all types of radiation on a common biological-effects scale with X- or gamma rays used as the basis of comparison. The quality factors generally used for various types of radiation are

Type radiation	Q
X or gamma	1
Beta	1
Slow neutron	3—5
Fast neutron	10
Alpha	20

The higher values of Q are associated with high LET particles (see previous section on alpha particles). Since Q is a dimensionless number and absorbed dose has the units J/kg, D.E. is also considered to have the units J/kg. Admittedly, this has led to some confusion in many cases since it does not always represent an actual amount of energy absorbed.

Historically, when the rad was the accepted special unit of absorbed dose, the dose equivalent was expressed in rems. Thus the dose equivalent, in rems, is the product of absorbed dose, in rads, multiplied by the quality factor. The rem remains in common usage in legal dose-limit values in the U.S. A new special unit, the Sievert (Sv), has been suggested for use with the dose equivalent in association with the use of the gray, but has yet to be widely accepted. A Sievert corresponds to a dose equivalent of 1 J/kg.

Biological Considerations

The knowledge that ionizing radiation could produce biological effects dates back to the period shortly after the discovery of X-rays when numerous reports of such effects began to appear in literature. Reports of skin erythema, epilation, and similar effects appeared early in 1896 and blood changes, tumor induction, and leukemia were reported in the early decades following the turn of the century.[1-5] A common factor among these early examples was that the radiation doses were quite high. Indeed, the effects of radiation at high doses are quite well known, and have been for many decades. However, it is at much lower doses and dose rates that most occupational exposures and population exposures occur today. The effects in this case are not quite so obvious, and in many cases can only be inferred by a careful evaluation of the incidence of effects in population groups.

Radiation may produce effects in living cells by directly hitting sensitive cell material, or indirectly by initiating toxic chemical reactions in the environment of the cell. In the case of the indirect effect, the radiation ionizes the water in the environment of the cell producing chemically reactive species (free radicals and other molecular products) that act as oxidizing or reducing agents. Depending on the type and amount of such products formed, damage to cells may be manifested. Cellular damage, whether by direct or indirect mechanisms, may take the form of morphological changes, alter-

* The International Commission on Radiological Units uses the symbols $H = D \cdot Q \cdot n$ where H is the dose equivalent, D and Q are the absorbed dose and quality factor, and n represents other modifying factors which may influence the biological effect.

ation of permeability, retardation or inhibition of cellular division, cell mutation, and denaturation of proteins. The extent of such cell damage may be a function of several factors, including (1) the total dose, (2) the dose rate (fractionation of dose), (3) the type of tissue (radiosensitivity of the tissue), (4) the extent of the body irradiated (number of cells at risk), (5) the type of radiation, and (6) the cell environment (oxygen content, for example).

Certain types of cells are known to be more radiosensitive (more easily damaged by radiation) than others. For example, the immature blood cells found in the bone marrow are generally considered to be the most radiosensitive cells in the body. Likewise, the cells that form the lining of certain organs are fairly radiosensitive. In general, the more rapidly proliferating cells in the body exhibit the greatest radiosensitivity. It is for this reason that the susceptibility of the human fetus to relatively low doses of radiation has been of concern in recent years. Such exposures may occur as a result of occupational exposure of the mother or in connection with diagnostic or therapeutical medical exposures of pregnant women.

To get some idea of the scope of the biological effects of ionizing radiation, let us consider two extremes. First, the greatest effect will be produced by a high dose to the total body, delivered in a short time period (e.g., a day or less). This situation may be referred to as acute exposure. Table 1 summarizes the observable effects of acute, whole-body exposure to X- or gamma rays as a function of dose. Once the lethal dose range is reached, increases in dose have the effect of decreasing the survival time. It should be noted that the doses delivered to patients in radiation therapy are typically in the acute dose range. However, such doses are generally to a restricted portion of the body rather than the whole body. Furthermore, therapeutic doses are often fractionated over a period of several days to several weeks. Thus, a dose which might otherwise be lethal if delivered to the whole body, may be limited in its effect by restricting the target organ(s) and fractionating the dose.

Recovering from the effects of sublethal acute exposures can and does occur. However, there may be long term or late effects that appear perhaps years after the exposure. Examples of this include the survivors of the nuclear weapons dropped on Hiroshima and Nagasaki as well as individuals who have received radiation therapy. Late effects included both somatic effects (cancer and leukemia) and genetic effects manifested in the offspring of exposed persons. Tables 2a and 2b summarize the risks of leukemia and cancer based on studies of several exposed population groups. Data concerning fetal exposures are of particular interest, especially in a hospital setting where pregnant women (female doctors, nurses, and other personnel) may be occupationally exposed, and where female patients may be exposed during diagnostic or therapeutic procedures. Studies have shown that the risk of leukemia in children increases if the mother is exposed to significant levels of radiation during pregnancy. A report of the National Academy of Sciences indicates that for children under 10 years of age in the U.S., the incidence of leukemia could rise from 3.7 cases in 10,000 children to 5.6 cases in 10,000 if the children each received a dose of 1 rem before birth.[6]

Stewart and Kneale have suggested that obstetric X-ray examinations of pregnant women will increase the risk of subsequent childhood leukemia and other malignancies.[7] These findings were generally confirmed by MacMahon as shown in Table 3.[8] It should be noted, however, that these findings are not completely conclusive and have been seriously challenged in more recent studies reported by Oppenheim.[9,10]

At the other end of the exposure scale we can consider chronic exposure — relatively low doses fractionated over extended periods of time. The chronic-exposure situation applies to both natural and man-made background radiation, individuals exposed to occupational radiation levels, or diagnostic medical exposures. Table 4 summarizes the population exposure levels involved.

Table 1
REPRESENTATIVE DOSE-EFFECT RELATIONSHIPS IN MAN FOR WHOLE-BODY IRRADIATION

Nature of effect	Representative absorbed dose of whole body X- or gamma radiation (rads)
Minimal dose detectable by chromosome analysis or other specialized analyses, but not hemogram	5—25
Minimal acute dose readily detectable in a specific individual (e.g., one who presents himself as a possible exposure case)	50—75
Minimal acute dose likely to produce vomiting in about 10% of people so exposed	75—125
Acute dose likely to produce transient disability and clear hematological changes in a majority of people so exposed	150—200
Median lethal dose for single short exposure	300

Note: The dose entries in this table should be taken as representative compromises only of a surprisingly variable range of values that would be offered by well-qualified observers asked to complete the right hand column. This comes about in part because whole-body irradiation is not a uniquely definable entity. Mid-line absorbed doses are used (see paragraph 139 of original source); the data are a mixed derivative of experience from radiation therapy (often associated with "free-air" exposure dosimetry) and a few nuclear industry accident cases (often with more up-to-date dosimetry). Also, the interpretation of such qualitative terms as "readily detectable" is a function of the conservatism of the reporter.

From Basic Radiation Protection Criteria, NCRP Rep. No. 39, U.S. National Council on Radiation Protection and Measurements, Washington, D.C., January 15, 1971. With permission.

The effects of natural background, if any, are not obvious, although it is commonly postulated that such effects do occur. Even population groups living in areas of elevated background (such as those which occur in certain areas of India and Brazil) show no clear-cut evidence of effects. The effects of chronic exposure for occupational groups has been well documented for cases where the doses were relatively high. In recent years, there have been studies suggesting observable effects in population groups working within the occupational dose limits that have been in force over the past couple of decades (typically in the range of 5 rem/year or less).[11-16] These studies are not considered definitive in that the statistical methodology and the conclusions are still undergoing widespread debate in the scientific literature. This, in itself, indicates one rather pragmatic conclusion: if effects do occur for individuals exposed in the 5 rem/year dose range, such effects occur with low probability and are difficult to discern from other normally occurring health effects.

As one goes to lower and lower doses, effects become difficult to observe. To differentiate from other environmental causes, one has to examine large population groups for statistical evidence of effects. These effects, if any, are too small or too infrequent

Table 2
RADIATION RISKS

A. Leukemia

	Percent increase in relative risk per rad	Excess cases per 10^6 person-year-rads
Exposure below age 10		
A-bomb survivors	8.0	2.6
Thymus X-ray	8.1	3.0
Tinea capitis X-ray[c]	11.0	3.4
Exposure at age 10 or more		
A-bomb survivors	3.1	1.5
Spondylitis patients	2.3	0.88

B. Cancer Excluding Leukemia

	Percent increase in relative risk per rad	Excess cases per 10^6 person-year-rads
Exposure at age 10 or more		
A-bomb survivors	0.15	4.7
Spondylitis patients	0.24—0.49	3.6—7.3

From Jablon, S., Health Physics in the Healing Arts, Proc. Health Phys. Soc. 7th Midyear Topical Symp., U.S. Department of Health, Education, and Welfare Publ. (FDA) 73-8029, U.S. Government Printing Office, Washington, D.C., 1973, 25.

Table 3
IRRADIATION DURING PREGNANCY: LEUKEMIA AND CHILDHOOD CANCER

Rate (per 10,000 live births)

				Irradiated	
	Unirradiated (U)	Irradiated (I)	Relative risk (I/U)	1 or 2 X-rays	X-ray pelvimetry
Leukemia					
First born	4.7	6.9	1.5	—	—
Others	3.6	4.6	1.3	—	—
All	4.0	6.1	1.5	3.8	6.9
CNS cancer	1.6	2.5	1.6	2.7	2.3
Other cancer	1.8	2.5	1.4	2.7	2.1

From Fabrikant, J. I., Health Physics in the Healing Arts, Proc. Health Phys. Soc. 7th Midyear Topical Symp., U.S. Department of Health, Education, and Welfare Publ. (FDA) 73-8029, U.S. Government Printing Office, Washington, D.C., 1973, 36. (Based on data from MacMahon.[8])

to observe easily. Being unable to conclusively detect any deleterious effects at very low levels has led to a dilemma for scientists because no one is willing to say there is

Table 4
TYPICAL POPULATION EXPOSURES FROM NATURAL AND MAN-MADE SOURCES OF RADIATION

Source	Exposure range[a]
Background in the U.S.	
At sea level, outdoors (varies with soil composition)	0.09—0.20 R/year
Average genetic dose equivalent	0.125 R/year
At 5000-ft altitude, outdoors (e.g., in Denver, Colorado)	0.11—0.22 R /year
In wooden houses	0.09—0.20 R/year
In brick or concrete buildings (varies with structural material)	0.11—0.50 R/year
Fallout, additional to natural background	0.01—0.02 R/year
^{40}K in the the human body	0.02 R/year
Man-made exposures	
Radioluminous wrist watches, TV, etc.	Up to 4 R/year
Average genetic dose equivalent	<0.005 R/year
Chest X-ray[b]	0.01—1.0 R/film
Dental X-ray[b]	0.2—1.0 R/film
Fluoroscopic examination[b] GI tract	5.0—50 R/exam
All diagnostic medical procedures, average genetic dose equivalent	0.055 R/year
Estimated per capita dose in the population from all sources	0.200 R/year

[a] In this table, the roentgen (R) is taken to be equal to the rad or rem. No distinction is made between these quantities because the error resulting from this simplifying assumption is very small in comparison with the accuracy of the numerals provided.

[b] Assumes normal good practice.

From Bond, R.G., et al., Eds., *Environmental Health and Safety in Health-Care Facilities*, Macmillan, New York, 1973, 156. With permission.

no effect. Thus, the scientific groups responsible for recommending dose limits assume or postulate the conservative positions that:

1. There is a linear dose-effect relationship for all effects from high range to zero.
2. There is no threshold below which effects do not occur.
3. All doses are additive no matter how low the dose rate.
4. There is no biological repair or recovery of effects at low dose.

Once these assumptions are made, one then is operating on the premise that any radiation dose, no matter how low, is potentially harmful. The question of establishing dose limits then revolves around a philosophical consideration: if all radiation is harmful, is there a level for which the risk is acceptable? Establishing dose limits or "maximum permissible doses" is really an attempt to answer this question.

Dose Limits and the Philosophy of Radiation Risks

In April 1899, just 3 years following the discovery of X-rays, a committee was established by the British Roentgen Society to collect evidence concerning X-ray hazards.[17] Although these efforts had little immediate impact, this was probably the first organized effort to evaluate radiation hazards with an intent for developing protection standards. At about the same time, in 1902, the first documented effort to determine a "safe" dose of radiation was made by William Rollins, a dentist who suggested a number of radiation protection procedures and recommended an exposure limit.[18,19] This limit was based on the observation that radiation would not be of harmful intensity if it did not cause fogging of a photographic plate in 7 min of exposure.

In 1924, the American physicist Arthur Mutscheller presented an important paper to the American Roentgen Ray Society entitled "Physical Standards of Protection Against X-ray Hazards."[20] Based on his observations and measurements at a number of X-ray facilities, he proposed a so-called "tolerance dose" of 0.01 of a skin erythema dose every 30 days (or about 0.1 skin erythema dose per year). This recommendation was widely used at the time and became the basis for the early official standards that were later adopted by standards-setting groups.

At the meeting of the first International Congress of Radiology (ICR) in 1925, the need for recommendations on radiation quantities and units was recognized. Therefore, the ICR established an important organization — the International Commission on Radiological Units and Measurements (ICRU). The commission (known at that time as the International X-ray Units Committee) considered the need for an acceptable quantity for measurement of radiation exposure. At the second International Congress in 1928, the ICRU adopted the roentgen as the unit of exposure, thus paving the way for setting quantitative exposure limits. At that time, the International Congress of Radiology established another important group, the International X-ray and Radium Protection Committee (which later became the International Commission on Radiological Protection or ICRP). The ICRP published the first international radiation protection standards at that time, patterned largely after those of the British X-ray and Radium Protection Committee.[21] By the time of the second meeting of the committee in 1931, consideration was being given to introducing tolerance-dose limits following the recommendations by Mutscheller. However, no specific recommendations on dose limits were made at that time due to the limited scientific evidence. Thus, the first recommendations of the committee were confined to specifying working-hour limitations, X-ray shielding, electrical precautions, general recommendations on lighting, ventilation for the removal of ozone, and radium protection. It was at its third meeting in 1934 that the committee issued its first recommendation on dose limits, namely a tolerance-dose limit of 0.2 R/day. This value turns out to be quite close to the Mutscheller recommendation when the erythema dose values are expressed in terms of roentgen units.[22]

Radiation dose limits have been revised constantly downward since the first limits were recommended in 1902. It is of interest to see why this has occurred and to examine the assumptions and the philosophies relating to these limits. The changes in the philosophy of radiation protection over the years are reflected not only in the numerical values of the dose limits, but also in the names used to describe these limits.

Going back to the early recommendations by Rollins, to the limits recommended by Mutscheller, and to the 1934 ICRP recommendations, we find that a basic assumption was that there was a threshold below which there would be no adverse biological effects. Naturally, this was based on the observation that no immediate discernible effects were observed for workers whose exposures were below certain amounts. The tolerance dose was simply a level set safely below the threshold value. Mutscheller's recommendation, for example, was based on keeping doses below levels which produced an observable effect — erythema. In order to use the Mutscheller recommendation, efforts were made to quantitate what was called by some the "skin unit dose." This was the amount of radiation that, for a short exposure time, produced a definite skin reaction (erythema or reddening). This effect, thought to be harmless, was the "threshold." Based on a poll of radiotherapists at that time, the average value for one skin unit dose for the therapeutic X-rays then in use was about 550 R. Taking Mutscheller's definition of tolerance dose as 0.01 of the skin unit (erythema) dose per month, the value of the tolerance dose was in the order of 5 to 6 R/month. Morgan indicates that Mutscheller's value corresponded to 1 R/week for 200 KV X-rays.[23] The ICRP recommendation in 1934 of a tolerance dose of 0.2 R/day corresponds closely to these values if we assume a five-day work week.

As evidence began to accumulate that there was no threshold for some effects, such as gene mutations and certain types of somatic effects, a shift in emphasis occurred. By the early 1940s the idea of tolerance dose meant a dose that could be expected to produce deleterious effects that were tolerable.[23] Then, as the idea of a threshold was discarded, the term tolerance dose began to be replaced in the mid 1940s by the term maximum permissible exposure (MPE) and eventually by maximum permissible dose (MPD).

Meanwhile, in the mid 1930s L. H. Gray had developed the basic principle that the important factor in understanding the interaction of radiation with biological systems was the energy deposition in the tissue. By the late 1940s, proposals had been made by at least two independent groups of scientists to introduce a quantity based on Gray's principle of the energy deposited in or imparted to matter. These proposals were presented to the ICRU at its first meeting after World War II in London in 1950, and the concept was adopted in 1953 when the quantity absorbed dose of ionizing radiation was defined with the unit rad.

The idea of permissible dose has been developed with the assumption that any exposure to radiation involves some degree of risk. The practical problem in utilizing radiation for beneficial purposes is to limit the dose to some value such that the risk is not unacceptable either to the individual exposed or to the general population. On this basis, the ICRP has stated that the permissible dose for an individual is defined as "that dose, accumulated over a long period of time or resulting from a single exposure, which, in the light of present knowledge, carries a negligible probability of severe somatic or genetic injuries; furthermore, it is such a dose that any effects that ensue more frequently are limited to those of a minor nature that would not be considered unacceptable by the exposed individual...."[24] Using this concept of permissible dose, the ICRP then established limits for occupational exposure referred to as MPD limits.

A similar definition for MPD was developed by the National Council on Radiation Protection and Measurements (NCRP) in the U.S.: "The maximum permissible dose is that dose of ionizing radiation that, in the light of present knowledge, is not expected to cause appreciable bodily injury to a person at any time during his lifetime." The NCRP also specified that "appreciable bodily injury" is "any bodily injury or effect that the average person would regard as being objectional and/or competent medical authorities would regard as being deleterious to the health and well being of the individual."[25]

The key points in these concepts of MPD are (1) any biological effects which occur are not appreciable or are of a minor nature; (2) the probability of effects occurring in an individual is very low, and (3) the possibility of effects to the individual or to future generations is not excluded. It should be realized that because of the low probability of effects and the fact that the effects, if any, are not expected to be major, one could only expect to detect such effects by statistical methods applied to large groups. The dose limits currently recommended by the NCRP are given in Table 5. The regulatory limits of the U.S. Nuclear Regulatory Commission are based largely on the NRC recommendations and are given in Table 6.

When defining MPD the ICRP also stated: "It is emphasized that the maximum doses recommended...are *maximum* values; the commission recommends that all doses be kept as low as practicable, and that any unnecessary exposure be avoided."[24] This

Table 5
DOSE-LIMITING RECOMMENDATIONS

Maximum permissible dose equivalent for occupational exposure	
Combined whole-body occupational exposure	
Prospective annual limit	5 rem in any 1 yr
Retrospective annual limit	10—15 rem in any 1 yr
Long-term accumulation to age *N* years	$(N-18) \times 5$ rem
Skin	15 rem in any 1 yr
Hands	75 rem in any 1 yr (25/quarter)
Forearms	30 rem in any 1 yr (10/quarter)
Other organs, tissues and organ systems	15 rem in any 1 yr (5/quarter)
Fertile women (with respect to fetus)	0.5 rem in gestation period
Dose limits for the public, or occasionally exposed individuals	
Individual or occasional	0.5 rem in any 1 yr
Students	0.1 rem in any 1 yr
Population dose limits	
Genetic	0.17 rem av/yr
Somatic	0.17 rem av/yr
Emergency dose limits — life saving	
Individual (older than 45 yr, if possible)	100 rem
Hands and forearms	200-rem addition (300-rem total)
Emergency dose limits — less urgent	
Individual	25 rem
Hands and forearms	100-rem total
Family of radioactive patients	
Individual (under age 45)	0.5 rem in any 1 yr
Individual (over age 45)	5 rem in any 1 yr

From Basic Radiation Protection Criteria, NCRP Rep. No. 39, National Council on Radiation Protection and Measurements, Washington, D.C., January 15, 1971. With permission.

Table 6
RADIATION DOSE STANDARDS FOR INDIVIDUALS IN RESTRICTED AREAS[a]

Portion of body	Rems per calendar quarter
Whole body, head, and trunk, active blood-forming organs, lens of eyes, or gonads	1 ¼
Hands, forearms, feet, and ankles	18 3/4
Skin of whole body	7 ½

[a] Applies specifically to U.S. Nuclear Regulatory Commission licensees.

From Standards for Protection Against Radiation, Title 10, Code of Federal Regulations, Part 20, June 15, 1979.

philosophy has led to a new approach, that of maintaining exposures "as low as practicable," or "as low as reasonably achievable" (ALARA).

This is a consequence of the philosophy suggested by the ICRP as early as 1955. The recommendations published by the commission at that time stated "Whilst the values proposed for maximum permissible dose are such as to involve a risk which is small compared to the other hazards of life, nevertheless...it is strongly recommended that every effort be made to reduce exposure to all types of ionizing radiation to the *lowest possible level.*"[26] (Emphasis added.) In ICRP Publication 1, the comparable statement read: "...the commission recommends that all doses be kept *as low as practicable,* and that any unnecessary exposure be avoided."[24] (Emphasis added.) In a later recommendation, the ICRP stated: "As any exposure may involve some degree of risk, the commission recommends that any unnecessary exposure be avoided, and that all doses be kept *as low as is reasonably achievable,* economic and social considerations being taken into account."[27] (Emphasis added.)

The implications of this philosophy include the fact that although the so-called MPD limits are still utilized, any dose which does not meet the ALARA criteria is unacceptable, even though it may be below the MPD value. There are certain practical difficulties in the use of the ALARA philosophy in establishing dose limits, the principle one being the lack of definite numerical values for use in legal codes and regulations. Nevertheless, the concept is a sound one and practical methods to achieve ALARA limits for health physics practice are being developed.

Administrative and Regulatory Aspects

The underlying philosophy for radiation protection in a hospital should be to maintain the exposures of the staff, the patient, and visitors as low as reasonably achievable while obtaining the optimum beneficial use of radiation in diagnosis and therapy. To achieve this goal, the top administration of the facility must have a clear commitment to suitable radiation protection practices. This commitment includes providing the necessary qualified staff, equipment, facilities, resources, and administrative backing for carrying out an adequate radiation protection program.

In any hospital, clinic, or medical laboratory where individuals may be occupationally exposed to radiation, there should be a qualified individual designated as the Radiation Safety Officer (RSO) (or a variety of titles, such as Radiation Protection Supervisor, Radiological Control Officer, Radiation Protection Officer, or Chief Health Physicist) who should be a person who has the knowledge and training to evaluate radiation safety procedures and techniques, measure ionizing radiation, and advise the staff and administration concerning radiation protection needs. In large institutions, the RSO is usually a full-time position whereas in smaller hospitals or laboratories, the individual may be employed on a part-time or consulting basis. The RSO is responsible for administering the radiation safety program for the institution and must have authority to communicate directly with whatever level of management is needed to take corrective action or enforce rules when needed. The RSO must also have the authority to suspend activities when necessary in an emergency to protect life or health. This authority should be exercised only when it will not interfere with life-saving medical procedures which normally would have priority.

The Radiation Safety Officer must also be familiar with applicable Federal and State regulations and with the basic principles of radiation protection. Such an individual must assume the following responsibilities:

1. Establish and oversee the radiation protection procedures used in the facility, and assure that such procedures conform to applicable regulations and standards
2. Instruct or arrange instruction for personnel in the required radiation protection practices and procedures
3. Conduct area radiation surveys, personnel monitoring, instrument calibration, leak tests, and other such procedures in order to assure that radiation protection standards and regulations are met
4. Maintain records of area surveys, personnel monitoring, and other procedures in order to document radiation protection activities

In order to carry out the stated responsibilities properly, the RSO must have appropriate education, training, and experience in health physics (radiation protection). Regulatory Guide 1.8 of the Nuclear Regulatory Commission suggests the qualifications that should be met by such an individual (referred to by the NRC as a Radiation Protection Manager)[28].

A Radiation Safety Committee (sometimes designated as the Radiological Control Committee, the Medical Isotopes Committee, or similar name) should be appointed by the governing board of the hospital to serve as a policy-making body relative to radiation safety matters. Such a committee is required for facilities working under NRC licenses and is highly recommended for any hospital using radioactivity or radiation-producing devices. Membership on the committee should normally include representatives from the areas of pathology, hematology, radiology, nursing, administration, nuclear medicine, and radiation safety. The responsibilities of the committee should include the following:

1. Review and grant approval or disapproval of the use of radioactive material or radiation-producing devices within the institution
2. Specify the conditions, facilities, procedures, and qualification for individuals to use radiation or radioactive material (e.g., areas of use, facility requirements, handling and disposal procedures)
3. Assure that an adequate radiation protection program is carried out under the supervision of a qualified radiation safety officer; such a program will include laboratory and area surveys, personnel monitoring, instrument calibration, record keeping, and other practices to assure the health and safety of personnel and the compliance with standards and regulations

There are a variety of possible administrative arrangements for establishing a radiation protection program in a clinical facility. It is generally accepted that an organizational arrangement where the RSO and the health physics staff of the facility are independent of any of the departments that use radiation and radioactive materials is best. That is, the RSO should answer to a top administrator or to a high-level radiation safety committee. In the broad context, the radiation safety program might logically be a component of a facility-wide safety program that includes electrical safety, fire safety, sanitation, drug and chemical safety, and the like. In addition, activities in the hospital involving the use of radiation and radioactive materials will be subject to regulatory authority of a number of Federal, State, or other agencies that mandate or otherwise stipulate certain standards of practice. Although it will usually be the task of the radiation protection or health physics staff to meet regulatory requirements, it is important that hospital administrators and certain other personnel such as clinical engineers be aware of the regulation aspects of radiation protection.

Some of the agencies whose regulations and standards may impact on the radiation safety program of a hospital follow:

Nuclear Regulatory Commission (NRC) — This agency regulates the use of byproduct material (reactor-produced radioactive material) under the provisions of the Atomic Energy Act. The NRC regulations are set forth in Title 10 of the Code of Federal Regulations. Regulation is achieved through a program of licensing and inspection. Certain "agreement" states have entered into formal agreements with the NRC whereby regulation of byproduct material is carried out by a specified state agency (such as the State Health Board) rather than by the NRC, provided that the state regulations are compatible with the federal regulations as set forth in Public Law 86-373.

Environmental Protection Agency (EPA) — The EPA is charged with protecting human health and the environment through promulgation and enforcement of standards and regulations. A number of its legislative mandates, such as the Federal Water Pollution Control Act and the Clean Air Act have radiological implications. However, since environmental emissions from hospitals are largely governed by NRC regulations (or the equivalent for agreement states), the EPA will not generally be an agency with which a hospital has direct interaction with respect to radiation safety.

Bureau of Radiological Health (BRH) — The BRH is a part of the U.S. Public Health Service. This bureau has jurisdiction over electronic product radiation and certain medical devices. Electronic product radiation includes X-ray devices, laser and microwave devices, ultrasound and ultraviolet devices, and accelerators. The regulations of the BRH pertain primarily to the manufacture of such devices, and radiation protection is achieved largely through specification of performance standards for the devices as manufactured and installed. The BRH regulations are found in its Regulations for the Administration and Enforcement of the Radiation Control for Health and Safety Act of 1968, and in Title 21 of the Code of Federal Regulations (CFR).

Occupational Safety and Health Administration (OSHA) — The OSHA regulations set forth in 29 CFR 1910 are virtually identical to the Standards for Protection Against Radiation in 10CFR20. In the case of byproduct material, the NRC has jurisdiction. For other types of radioactive materials and radiation-producing devices, the OSHA regulations would apply.

Department of Transportation (DOT) — The shipping or transport of radioactive material is subject to the regulations of the DOT as set forth in Title 49 of the Code of Federal Regulations. Basically, the DOT regulations specify the packaging, labeling, and transportation restrictions on radioactive material based on the type, amount, and form of material shipped. For packages shipped by air, the Federal Aviation Agency (FAA) has additional restrictions which must be followed. Likewise, the U.S. Post Office has regulations governing the transport of radioactive materials via the postal system.

State Health Department — Most states exercise some control over radioactive materials and radiation-producing devices through state health agencies. The degree of regulation ranges from full licensing and inspection programs in NRC agreement states to simple registration programs.

National Council on Radiation Protection and Measurements (NCRP) — The NCRP is a nonprofit corporation chartered by Congress to develop information and make recommendations on protection against radiation and measurement of radiation. The NCRP issues reports from time to time on various aspects of radiation protection, including many facets of hospital radiation safety. Although the recommendations of the council do not have the force of law, they do represent what might be referred to as "good practice."

Radiation Protection Principles

The basic principles of radiation protection are not unique to medical facilities, although the specific implementation of such principles in the hospital setting may differ from other facilities. Usually radiation protection is directed toward minimizing exposure to personnel while maximizing the potential benefits from the use of radiation. This may be accomplished through a combination of regulatory means, the use of trained personnel, the utilization of monitoring and surveillance programs, and the use of proper facility design.

Personnel exposure control is based on a consideration of scientific information concerning the physical fundamentals of radiation, the biological effects of radiation, and the associated risks, together with philosophical considerations as to what constitutes acceptable risks. These considerations must be coupled with the practical considerations of developing workable rules, regulations, and standards, and must be carried out within a framework of appropriately trained persons and suitable radiation-monitoring programs. Radiation protection of personnel is achieved by controlling external exposure (exposure from sources of radiation outside the body) and internal exposure (exposure from radioactive materials that have been ingested or otherwise taken into the body). Such control is accomplished through the careful use of proper facilities and procedures by appropriately trained personnel who protect both themselves and others while gaining the beneficial use of radiation.

External Protection

External exposure control is accomplished by limiting the exposure time and by reduction of exposure rates through the use of distance and shielding. These three variables, time, distance, and shielding, can be effectively used individually or in combination to restrict exposures to any desired level. The use of time as a method of control is straightforward. Assuming that exposure rates are known from making appropriate measurements, the total exposure can be controlled by limiting the exposure time.

Distance is often used to control exposure from X- or gamma rays, and sometimes for beta particles as well. In the case of X- or gamma rays, the intensity of the radiation varies inversely with the distance from the source. In the ideal case where the physical size of the source is a point source (or relatively small) and a scattering medium is not close by, the intensity varies inversely with the square of the distance from the source. That is, if a source has an intensity of I_0 at distance d_0, then the intensity at some other distance d is

$$I = I_o \left(\frac{d_o^2}{d^2}\right) \qquad (2)$$

In the case of beta emitters, intensity varies inversely with distance, but the relationship is not quite as simple as for photons. For distances less than the maximum range of the beta particle (in air), the relationship between intensity and distance may be approximated by the inverse square relation similar to the relation used for X- or gamma rays. The intensity of the radiation essentially drops to zero for locations beyond the range of the beta particle.

Where time and distance are insufficient to produce the required protection, shielding material is interposed between the radiation source and the individual(s) being protected. Beta particles are readily stopped (shielded) by relatively small masses of many materials. Figure 1 indicates the range of beta particles of various energies for different absorbing materials. The range in soft tissue is similar to that in water or lucite. It should be noted that although the higher atomic-number materials seem to be effective as beta shields, they do present one complicating factor. As beta particles interact with material (thereby being stopped), they generate secondary X-rays called bremsstrahlung (from the German for "braking radiation"). The amount of these secondary X-rays generated is a function of the atomic number of the shielding material, with high atomic-number materials giving rise to relatively large amounts of bremsstrahlung. Thus, it is more practical to use low atomic-number material (such as plastics or aluminum) to shield betas so as to minimize the X-ray production.

For X- and gamma rays, attenuation of a beam of radiation, in the simplest case, is an exponential function. For a well-collimated beam of monoenergetic photons, the attenuation through thin layers of absorbing material follows the relation:

$$I = I_o e^{-\mu x} \qquad (3)$$

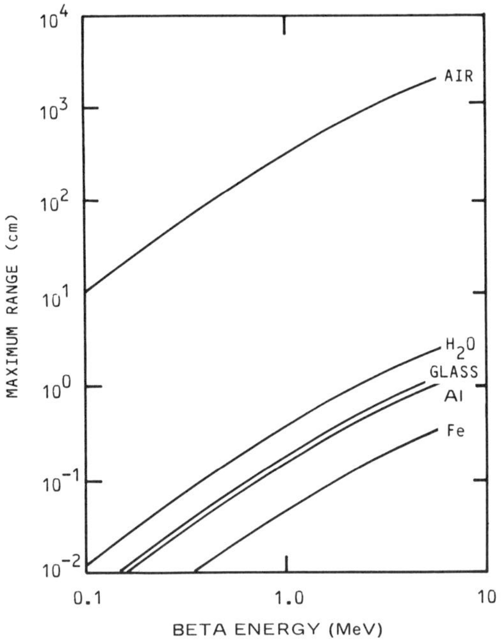

FIGURE 1. Penetration ability of beta radiation.

where I_0 is the initial intensity of the beam and I is the intensity after passage through an absorber of thickness x. The coefficient μ, called the attenuation coefficient, is dependent upon the energy of the photons and the atomic number of the absorber. In practical situations, where significant scattering of the beam occurs due to the geometrical size of the beam or the presence of relatively large thicknesses of shielding material, the ideal exponential relationship will not hold and one may have to rely on tables of shielding data. Likewise, when the radiation is not monoenergetic, as for most medical X-rays, shielding tables and graphs provide a practical way of determining shielding requirements. A convenient way of expressing shielding data is in terms of half-value layers. The half-value layer is the thickness of a specified material required to reduce the intensity of radiation by a factor of two. Referring to the shielding equation (Equation 3), the half-value layer $X_{1/2}$ is the thickness that causes I/I_0 to equal 0.5. Or,

$$e^{-\mu X_{1/2}} = 0.5 \tag{4}$$

This relation leads immediately to

$$X_{1/2} = \frac{\ln 0.5}{\mu} = 0.693/\mu \tag{5}$$

Examples of half-value layers for gamma-emitting nuclides are given in Table 7. Half-value layers for X-ray beams of various energies and the amount of shielding to reduce X-ray beams to 10% of initial intensity are listed in Table 8.

Internal Protection

Radioactive materials may enter the body by injection, inhalation, absorption (through the skin), or through openings in the skin (cuts, wounds). Once inside the

Table 7
HALF-VALUE LAYERS AND TENTH-VALUE LAYERS FOR SELECTED GAMMA-RAY SOURCES

				Half-value layer[a] (cm)			Tenth-value layer[a] (cm)			
Radionuclide	Atomic number	Half-life	Gamma energy (MeV)	Concrete	Steel	Lead	Concrete	Steel	Lead	Specific gamma-ray constant[b] Rcm²/mCi-hr
^{137}Cs	55	27 yr	0.66	4.8	1.6	0.65	15.7	5.3	2.1	3.2
^{60}Co	27	5.24 yr	1.17, 1.33	6.2	2.1	1.20	20.6	6.9	4.0	13
^{198}Au	79	2.7 days	0.41	4.1	—	0.33	13.5	—	1.1	2.32
^{192}Ir	77	74 days	0.13—1.06	4.3	1.3	0.60	14.7	4.3	2.0	5.0
^{226}Ra	88	1622 yr	0.047—2.4	6.9	2.2	1.66	23.4	7.4	5.5	8.25[c]

[a] Approximate values obtained with large attenuation.
[b] These values assume that gamma absorption in the source is negligible. Value in R/mCi-hr at 1 cm can be converted to R/Ci-hr at 1 m by multiplying the number in this column by 0.10.
[c] This value assumes that the source is sealed within a platinum capsule (0.5-mm wall thickness), with units of R/mg hr at 1 cm.

From Structural Shielding Design and Evaluation for Medical Use of X-rays and Gamma Rays of Energies up to 10 MeV, NCRP Rep. No. 49, U.S. National Council on Radiation Protection Publications, Washington, D.C., 1976. With permission.

Table 8
HALF-VALUE AND TENTH-VALUE LAYERS FOR X-RAYS[32]

	Attenuation material					
	Lead (mm)		Concrete (cm)		Iron (cm)	
Peak voltage (kV)	HVL	TVL	HVL	TVL	HVL	TVL
50	0.06	0.17	0.43	1.5		
70	0.17	0.52	0.84	2.8		
100	0.27	0.88	1.6	5.3		
125	0.28	0.93	2.0	6.6		
150	0.30	0.99	2.24	7.4		
200	0.52	1.7	2.5	8.4		
250	0.88	2.9	2.8	9.4		
300	1.47	4.8	3.1	10.4		
400	2.5	8.3	3.3	10.9		
500	3.6	11.9	3.6	11.7		
1,000	7.9	26	4.4	14.7		
2,000	12.5	42	6.4	21		
3,000	14.5	48.5	7.4	24.5		
4,000	16	53	8.8	29.2	2.7	9.1
6,000	16.9	56	10.4	34.5	3.0	9.9
8,000	16.9	56	11.4	37.8	3.1	10.3
10,000	16.6	55	11.9	39.6	3.2	10.5

Note: Approximate values obtained at high attenuation for the indicated peak voltage values under broad-beam conditions; with low attenuation these values will be significantly less.

From Structural Shielding Design and Evaluation for Medical Use of X-rays and Gamma Rays of Energies up to 10 MeV, NCRP Rep. No. 49, U.S. National Council on Radiation Protection Publications, Washington, D.C., 1976. With permission.

body, the material may deposit in one or more organs, depending on its chemical and physical form. When this occurs, the normal protective factors of time, distance, and shielding which were useful for sources outside the body no longer apply. Indeed, the material is in direct intimate contact with the tissue or cells, and may remain there for extended periods of time. Thus, the main defense or protection from internal radiation is to prevent entrance of the material into the body in the first place. Accordingly, those procedures, techniques, and equipment which serve to minimize the chance of intakes through the mouth, nose, or skin are important to stress whenever personnel are handling unsealed sources of radioactive material. Such simple precautions as using rubber or plastic gloves, using good housekeeping procedures, avoiding pipetting by mouth, etc. tend to minimize the probability of internal deposition of radioactive materials.

In situations where air or water may have become contaminated by radioactive materials, internal deposition may be controlled by controlling both the concentrations of radionuclides in the air and water to which workers are exposed and the time they are subjected to such concentrations. Tables of maximum permissible concentrations of various radionuclides in air and water are given by the ICRP and the NRC.[30,31] Representative values for nuclides frequently used in hospitals are given in Table 9.

Personnel Monitoring

External exposure for occupationally exposed personnel may be conveniently moni-

Table 9
MPC VALUES FOR OCCUPATIONAL AND NONOCCUPATIONAL EXPOSURE FOR SELECTED RADIONUCLIDES IN SOLUBLE FORM

Nuclides Most Frequently Used in Hospitals

	MPC in air (μCi/mℓ)		MPC in water (μCi/mℓ)	
Radionuclide	Occupational	Public	Occupational	Public
^{61}Cr	1×10^{-5}	4×10^{-7}	5×10^{-2}	2×10^{-3}
^{57}Co	3×10^{-6}	1×10^{-7}	2×10^{-2}	5×10^{-4}
^{68}Co	8×10^{-7}	3×10^{-8}	4×10^{-3}	1×10^{-4}
^{60}Co	3×10^{-7}	1×10^{-8}	1×10^{-3}	5×10^{-5}
^{198}Au	3×10^{-7}	1×10^{-8}	2×10^{-3}	5×10^{-5}
^{125}I	5×10^{-9}	8×10^{-11}	4×10^{-5}	2×10^{-7}
^{131}I	9×10^{-9}	1×10^{-10}	6×10^{-5}	3×10^{-7}
^{55}Fe	9×10^{-7}	3×10^{-8}	2×10^{-2}	8×10^{-4}
^{59}Fe	1×10^{-7}	5×10^{-9}	2×10^{-3}	6×10^{-5}
^{32}P	7×10^{-8}	2×10^{-9}	5×10^{-4}	2×10^{-5}
^{99m}Tc	4×10^{-5}	1×10^{-6}	2×10^{-1}	6×10^{-3}
^{113}Sn	4×10^{-7}	1×10^{-8}	2×10^{-3}	9×10^{-5}
^{133}Xe	1×10^{-5}	3×10^{-7}	—	—

From Straub, C. P., *CRC Handbook of Environmental Control*, Vol. 5, CRC Press, Cleveland, 1975, 275.

tored through the use of such devices as film badges, thermoluminescence dosimeter (TLD) badges, or pocket dosimeters. Generally, such devices are of the dose-integrating type. That is, they integrate the total dose received over a specified period of time (a day, week, month). The film badge has been the most widely used personnel monitoring device for many years, although TLDs have come into widespread use in recent years. Each type of personnel dosimeter has specific advantages and disadvantages and the type chosen is dictated by considerations of cost, convenience, reliability and accuracy for the particular application, and other factors.

The pocket dosimeter has the advantage of permitting the worker to check the total dose during and after working in an area of elevated radiation levels. Many pocket dosimeters are of the self-reading type, as shown in Figure 2, where the worker observes the reading by looking through a lens at a scale displayed. Frequently, the pocket dosimeter is simply used as a supplement to the film badge, with the badge providing the permanent dose record and the pocket dosimeter providing an immediate dose estimate.

Thermoluminesce dosimetry is based on the phenomenon that certain crystalline materials, such as the alkali halides, will (after irradiation) emit light when heated. TLDs are now available in a variety of physical configurations including rods, chips, and powders (Figure 3). These may be incorporated into badges or into tube-type pocket dosimeters. After use, the TLD materials must be evaluated by means of a reader which heats the phosphor and measures light emitted. This luminescence is, in turn, related to the dose received by the phosphor. Figure 4 is an example of a commercial TLD reader.

An additional method of personnel monitoring is the use of the pocket "chirpy," a pocket-size rate meter that provides an audible indication (chirp or beep) of radiation levels. Generally, this type of device fits into the pocket or clips on a belt. The frequency of the chirps is proportional to exposure rate, thus providing a convenient

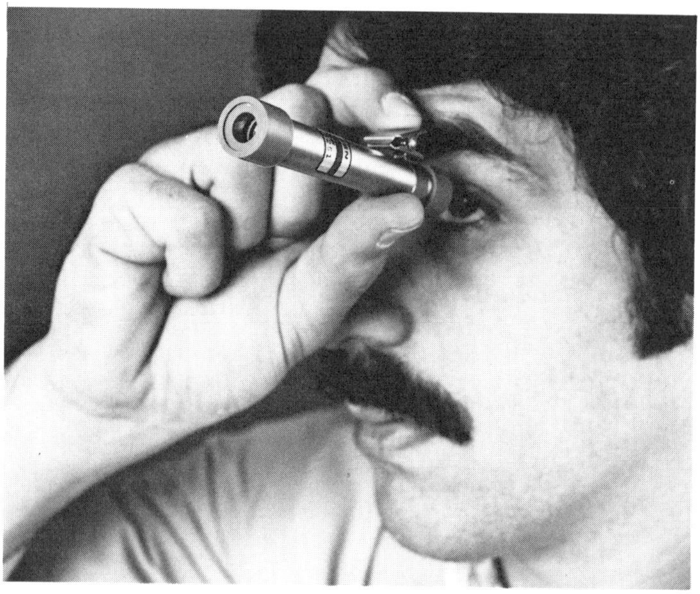

FIGURE 2. Radiation worker reading pocket dosimeter. (Courtesy of Victoreen Instrument Co.)

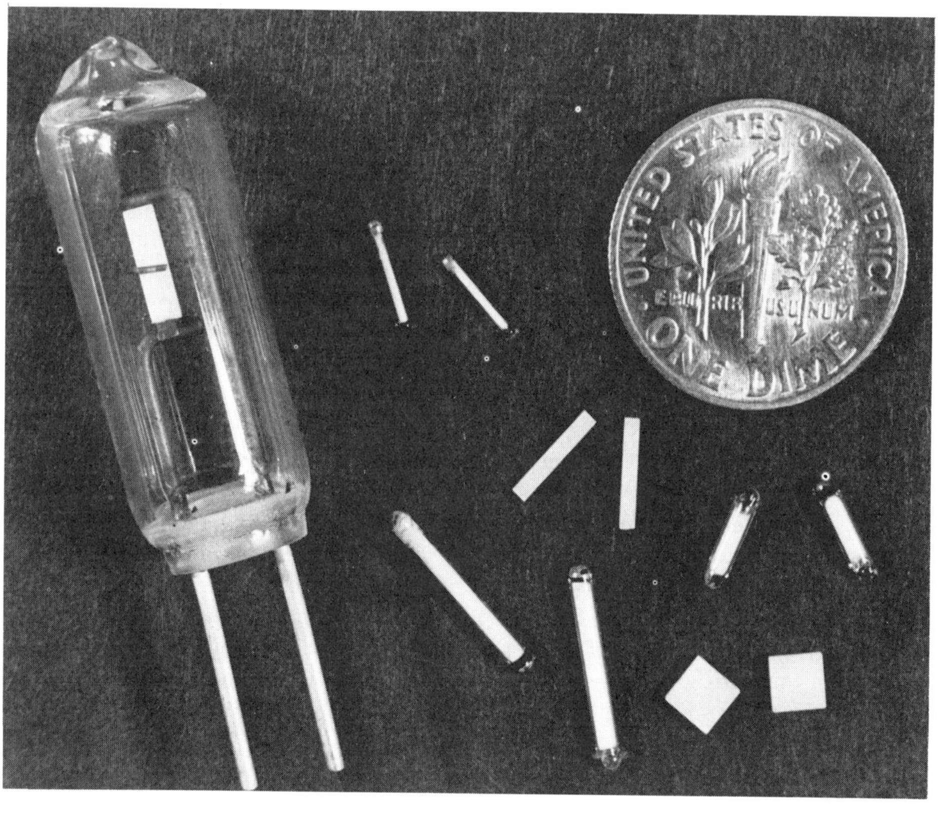

FIGURE 3. Examples of thermoluminescence dosimeter configurations: bulb type (far left); powder in glass tubes (upper and lower middle and middle right); extruded rods (middle); and extruded ribbons (lower right).

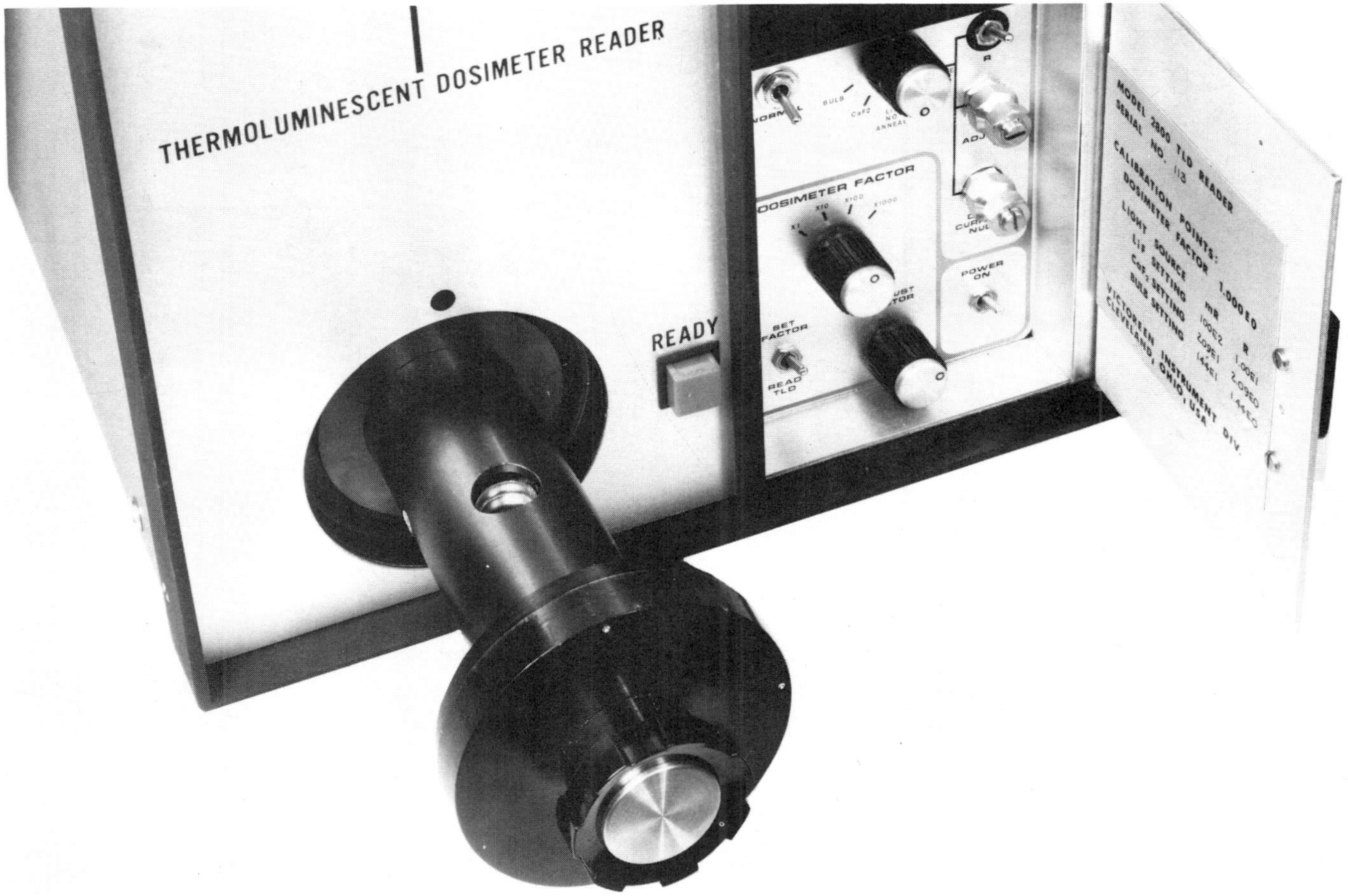

FIGURE 4. Example of TLD reader showing sample holder/heater in open position on left and operating controls on right. (Courtesy of Victoreen Instrument Co.)

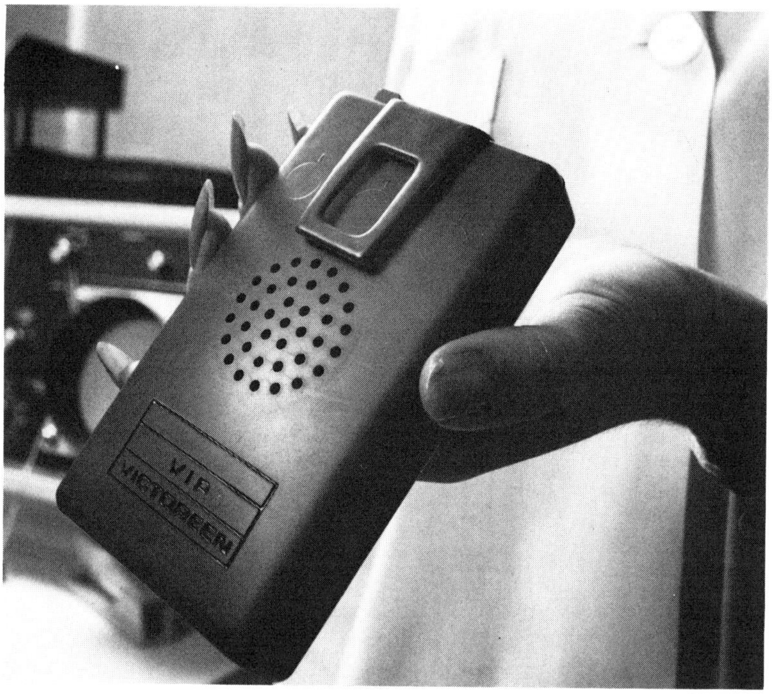

FIGURE 5. Pocket chirpy-type personal dosimeter. Unit is battery operated and has a small GM tube as a detector. Operating range is 0 to 999 mR and readout is a 3-digit LED display at upper end of dosimeter. (Courtesy of Victoreen Instrument Co.)

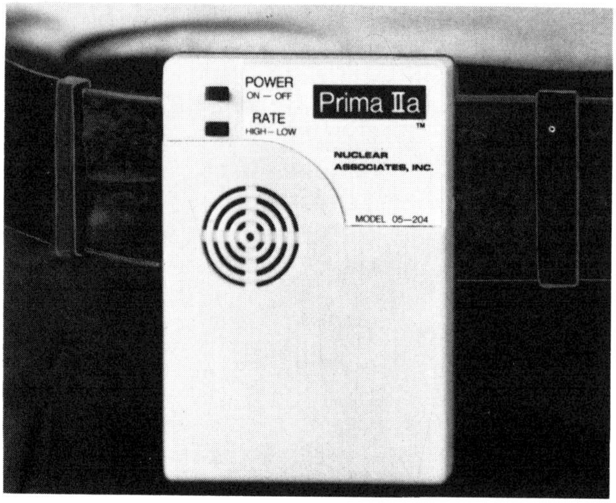

FIGURE 6. Personal monitor, battery operated, which serves mainly as a rate-meter type warning device. The unit emits a beep sound whose frequency varies with radiation intensity. Unit does not record total dose. (Courtesy of Nuclear Associates, Division of Victoreen, Inc.)

method of warning the wearer of the relative intensity or the exposure rate of the radiation. Figures 5 and 6 show examples of this type of personnel monitor.

Monitoring for internal exposures (ingestion or inhalation of radioactive materials) is accomplished through the use of bioassay procedures such as urine analysis, fecal analysis, breath analysis, external whole-body counting, or organ counting. The bioassay method selected depends on the particular nuclide taken in (or suspected of being ingested), the chemical and physical form of the material involved, and other conditions of the exposure. For example, bioassay for radioiodine deposition may be accomplished by external counting of the thyroid with a sensitive scintillation counter, whereas a suspected intake of tritium (hydrogen-3) would generally call for urine analysis. In the first instance, iodine would be expected to concentrate rapidly in the thyroid gland where it could be readily detected outside the body due to emission of gamma rays (for ^{131}I) or X-rays (for ^{125}I). In the other example, tritium, which emits only a weak beta, could not be detected by external detectors, but its presence in body water could be inferred by measuring concentrations in urine samples counted in an appropriate beta detector. Further details on personnel monitoring, including bioassay, will be provided in later sections of this chapter.

Facility Design

Proper facility design is an important component of radiation protection. In the case of radiation-producing devices (diagnostic and therapeutic X-rays, for example), consideration must be given to the amount of shielding needed, requirements for interlocks and warning devices, room layout and access, and even the use of adjacent areas. For facilities in which radioactive materials are used in unsealed forms (such as in nuclear medicine), attention must be given to the air flow and ventilation aquirements, the types of surface coverings on floors, walls, and laboratory equipment, the layout of the room, accessibility by personnel, and use of adjacent areas.

In most cases where shielded rooms are required, the services of a qualified expert should be sought to provide specifications on required shielding thickness and related design matters. Generally, the qualified expert will be a certified medical physicist or certified health physicist who has had experience and training in shielding design. Usually, the methods used in determining shielding needs for medical facilities are based on the recommendations of the NCRP given in NCRP Report 49.[32] This report also provides useful information on the proper installation of shielding materials so as to avoid loss of shielding integrity through cracks and voids in the shields.

Interlocks are frequently necessary in facilities where the potential for high exposures to medical personnel might occur. Generally, this is the case for therapy devices where outputs in the direct beam are substantial. There are a number of important points that should be considered in designing an interlock system:

1. Redundancy: when practical, use two interlocks at each location where an interlock is required.
2. Fail-safe: use interlocks which cause a safe condition to occur in case of failure of the interlock.
3. Multiple interlocks: utilize systems requiring more than one specified operating condition in order for system to function. (For example, door interlock must be activated, and keyed switch must be turned on, and timer must be set, and warning light must be turned on).

Systems in which interlock and warning components can fail without causing shutdown to a safe condition are generally unsatisfactory. As a simple example, if one were to rely only on a lighted warning sign to indicate that a therapy source was on without actually putting the light in series with the source control, a burnt-out bulb might go unnoticed and result in an individual entering the radiation area during an exposure. This still might not be a problem if the entry door was interlocked. However, if the door interlock were to stick in the closed position on such an occasion, someone might very well enter the area and be subjected to unnecessarily high exposure.

Some important lessons can be learned from the accidental exposure of a worker in a cobalt-60 irradiation facility as reported by Wade.[33] Although the situation did not involve a medical facility, the case does provide some interesting insights into the use of interlocks, warning systems, and the operational procedures associated with the use of such a facility. Engineers and physicists evaluating facility designs should give careful attention to the combinations of conditions that might lead to such an occurrence. The incident reported by Wade involved an irradiation facility containing 6 ^{60}Co sources totaling about 8000 Ci. The exposure rate at 1 m from such a source would be over 100 R/min. The facility included the following safety features:

1. TV camera with scan and zoom controls that provided viewing of the entire irradiation room from the control room.
2. Three radiation monitors in the irradiation room with meter outputs in the control room; when the sources were out of the shields in the irradiation room (high radiation conditions), a red light on the monitor, a warning light on the control panel, and three red flashing lights were all activated; the flashing lights were located in the irradiation room, at the entrance to the irradiation room, and at the entrance to the maze leading from the control to the irradiation room.
3. Limit switches located at the doors leading to the maze so that if the door was open, an irradiation could not be initiated; also, opening a door during an irradiation would cause the sources to return to their shield.

The system included several other safety features which will not be described here. In spite of the seemingly safe design of this facility, a research technician did enter the irradiation room when the sources were out, receiving a total body dose of about 260 rad. An investigation revealed the following.

Human errors — The facility operator did not follow established procedures and the technician did not observe the radiation meters, the red flashing warning lights, nor even the source itself raised out of its shield.

Equipment failures — Incomplete closing of the maze door resulted in the electric lock not preventing entry. In addition, the maze door limit switch did not cause the source to be lowered when the technician opened the door for entry.

Additional problems — The door limit switch had been bypassed by tying it closed a day or two before the incident. Also, the facility management had no formal procedures for training personnel who operated the facility.

This case illustrates that: (1) facilities must be properly designed, (2) the safety devices must be allowed to function and serve their intended purpose, and (3) personnel must be properly trained and must follow well-established safety procedures.

Personnel Training in Radiation Protection

Properly trained employees will be an asset to any facility in meeting the goal of minimizing radiation exposures. Such an individual is able to make informed judgment on more effective ways of using equipment and carrying out work assignments. Also, a properly trained worker will be aware of potential health risks and be better equipped to exercise sound judgment in an emergency.

The amount of radiation protection training needed for various categories of employees will depend on several factors such as the potential for radiation exposure and the complexity of the job or activity. Also, the level of responsibility and degree of supervision may dictate how much training is required. As a minimum, all employees involved in radiation work must learn the applicable radiation safety regulations governing their work (federal, state, or local); be informed of the risks associated with radiation exposure; use proper procedures for minimizing exposure; and know what actions and responses are to be taken in emergencies. The need for additional training will be dependent on the factors mentioned previously.

Persons in different job categories in a hospital, such as orderlies, nurses, and aides, have occasional duties with patients containing radioactive materials and are sometimes in and about the X-ray or nuclear medicine departments. Formal lectures on radiation safety or the use of videotape or cassette materials should be planned for all such groups. The rotation of assignments, particularly for nurses, presents special problems with respect to insuring that all persons are appropriately trained. The training requirements for the medical doctors who will use radiopharmaceuticals or other radioisotopes are specified in Appendix A of NRC Regulatory Guide 10.8.[34] Examples of instructions that should be provided for nurses may be found in Appendix K of NRC Regulatory Guide 10.8 and in Appendix 3 of Quimby's book.[34,35]

RADIATION SAFETY IN DIAGNOSTIC RADIOLOGY OR X-RAY DEPARTMENTS

Facility Design and Equipment

Several aspects of facility design have already been considered. For shielding of diagnostic X-ray facilities, the recommendations of NCRP Report 49 are suitable.[32] The tables and graphs in NCRP Report 49 are based on controlling doses to occupationally exposed workers (hospital personnel) to the equivalent of 100 mrem/week or 5 rem/year and for nonoccupationally exposed persons in the environment of the facility to 10 mrem/week or 0.5 rem/year. This is apart from the direct exposure of the patients. However, the NCRP also notes that when practical, in keeping with the ALARA philosophy, the doses to occupationally exposed persons should also be reduced to the 10-mrem/week level. Generally, this can be accomplished without substantial additional cost for shielding. Although the details of the report will not be considered here, it is useful to note the parameters upon which such shielding designs are based. They are

1. The energy of radiation
2. The work load (the amount of time the radiation producing device is on per week)
3. The exposure rate in the primary beam at unit distance for a given operational setting
4. The distance from the radiation source to the area of interest
5. The fraction of the on time that the beam is pointed in the direction of interest
6. The degree of occupancy of the area of interest (fraction of the time that it is occupied by personnel when the radiation unit is on)
7. The classification of the persons occupying the area of interest (general population or radiation workers)
8. Desired weekly exposure limit desired in the area of interest

Exposure to hospital personnel (radiologists, technologists, and others) can also be reduced through the use of proper diagnostic equipment. This is particularly true for fluoroscopy and special procedures equipment where the use of modern image-enhancement techniques can result in a reduction of the beam intensity required to obtain suitable diagnostic images.

Radiation Surveys and Monitoring Methods

The NCRP has recommended that area surveys be made in the following situations:[36]

1. Prior to initial use of a radiation installation or as soon as possible after radiation sources are brought into the area
2. Whenever changes in the equipment, shielding, sources, or procedures have occurred that may cause an increase in personnel exposure
3. Periodically, in order to detect long-term changes in equipment or other parameters that might effect personnel exposures
4. Whenever an accident has occurred or is suspected

For diagnostic X-ray facilities, the physical safeguards (facility design) and procedures suggested in NCRP Report Nos. 33 and 49 and in the federal standards for X-ray equipment generally provide the needed protection for personnel.[29,32,37] Radiation surveys then provide a means for confirming that the facility is continuing to meet the standards. These routine surveys are a necessary part of quality-assurance programs. Tests for compliance with the technical performance standards of the BRH (following installation of a facility) are set forth in detail elsewhere.[38] Thus, here we will only consider the radiation protection aspects of X-ray installations. The NCRP recommends that these measurements be made:[36]

Exposure rates in the useful beam — Because doses to both working personnel and patients will depend on the exposure produced by the X-ray tube operating at a specific peak kilovoltage (kvP), tube current (milliamps or mA), and timer setting (seconds), measurements of exposure rates should be made at a specified distance from the tube target for several kVP and mA settings.

Leakage radiation — Measurements of leakage radiation through the X-ray tube housing are usually only necessary if the housing specification is in doubt. A survey to locate inadvertent gaps in the shielding of the housing may be made during the initial survey following methods recommended in NCRP Report No. 33.[37] However, such measurements are not usually required on modern equipment and the manufacturer's certificate of compliance (with performance standards) is accepted.

X-ray transmission through primary and secondary barriers — Transmission measurements are needed for the beam orientations and field sizes used in practice that will give the greatest exposure rate at the point of measurement. For measurements in the direction of the useful beam, no phantom should be used whereas for measurements of scatter radiation, a phantom should be used to simulate the irradiated object.

In addition to the measurements indicated above, there are a number of items recommended in NCRP Report No. 33 as well as certain provisions of 21CFR1020.31 that should be tested for medical radiography installations. These include

1. Test collimators to confirm that the radiographic field cannot be adjusted to exceed the film sizes used
2. Test collimator alignment between the visual and X-ray fields
3. Check alignment of the axis of X-ray beam with the center of film
4. Determine the total beam filtration by measurement of the half-value layer
5. Confirm that the duration of the X-ray exposures agrees with the timer settings
6. Determine the exposure per milliampere second (R/mAs) for several of the current settings normally used; for a given tube kilovoltage and distance from the target, the R/mAs values should not differ by more than ±20%.
7. Confirm that the exposure switch can be operated only when the operator is in a shielded position; for mobile equipment, assure that the operator is both standing at least 6 ft from the patient, the tube, and the beam and is wearing a lead apron

8. Confirm that there is a positive indication that X-rays are being produced and that the operator can readily discern the indicator
9. Confirm that the operator can see the patient during exposure
10. For mobile equipment, confirm that the target-to-skin distance is not less than 30 cm

Likewise, flouroscopy installations must meet certain requirements of NCRP Report No. 33 and of 21CFR1020.32. Items that must be tested or checked are summarized in NCRP Report 57 and include the following:[36]

1. Determine that the entire cross section of the useful beam is intercepted by the primary protective barrier of the fluoroscopic image receptor
2. Determine that the exposure is automatically terminated when the image receptor is removed from the beam
3. Confirm that the dimensions of the X-ray beam cannot exceed the dimensions of the visible area of the image receptor (for fluoroscopes used only for fluoroscopy or recording of images through an image intensifier)
4. Determine that the center of the X-ray beam is aligned with the center of the image receptor
5. For fluoroscopes equipped with spot-film devices, determine whether the automatic field-size adjustment operates correctly and is properly aligned
6. Determine the source-to-skin distance, it should be not less than 30 cm; for stationary units, not less than 38 cm is preferred (and is required for newer units subject to the requirements of 21CFR1020.32)
7. Assure that a cumulative timing device is used to indicate the length of time of each procedure, to either interrupt operation or give a signal after a predetermined period of time (5 min)
8. Determine total tube filtration to confirm that it complies with values recommended in NCRP Report No. 33
9. Confirm that a cover for the film slot under the table and a shield (attached to the viewing device or table) to intercept scatter are provided
10. Evaluate the adequacy of provisions for both dark-adaption of eyes and exclusion of light from the room when nonimage-intensified fluoroscopes are used
11. Check protective devices such as aprons and gloves for shielding defects
12. Measure the table-top exposure rate in the center of the beam; exposure rate at the table top must not exceed the values specified in NCRP Report No. 33 (10 R/min, maximum; 5 R/min or less, preferred)
13. Measure the exposure rates 10 cm from any accessible surface of the fluoroscopic imaging assembly beyond the plane of the image receptacle and at areas by the fluoroscope commonly occupied; these measurements should be made with a phantom in the beam

Procedures for making diagnostic X-ray surveys vary among individuals and groups, and standardized protocols have not been completely developed. There are suggested protocols in the literature that are helpful in conducting surveys of X-ray installations. Hendee and Chaney have provided guidelines for survey procedures for fluoroscopic installations.[39] To assist individuals making radiation surveys of medical fluoroscopes, Dunlap has developed a survey form that provides for complete collection of facility information, equipment data, and radiation measurements.[40] Other examples of X-ray survey procedures and suggested survey forms include those of Collier at the Los Angeles County-University of Southern California Medical Center; Repacholi and Jack of the Radiation Protection Bureau of Canada; and the U.S. Public Health Service, Bureau of Radiological Health.[41-43]

Personnel Monitoring

Personnel monitoring would seem to be a straightforward procedure since film badges and TLD badges are in widespread use and have become well accepted and well established in medical institutions. Thus, it might be important here to discuss some of the problems associated with personnel monitoring in medical facilities.

Classification of Workers

The NCRP recommends that if a person may receive a dose exceeding one fourth of the MPD for radiation workers, that individual shall be classified as a radiation worker or occupationally exposed person and should wear a personnel monitor. Even though most X-ray technologists and other staff members who frequent the X-ray department (including some nurses, orderlies, or other aides) do not routinely receive exposures that are high, they are classified as radiation workers in the interest of good practice and the ALARA principle. Also, special attention should be given to the category of fertile or pregnant women working in the X-ray department. Personnel monitoring in this case should be directed toward assuring that the recommendations given in Table 5 are met.

Position of Personnel Monitoring Devices

There has been considerable debate in recent years over the location of film badges or dosimeters on the body. This has been particularly true for fluoroscopy where confusion has arisen as to whether dosimeters should be worn over or under lead aprons, at the waist, chest, or near the head (collar). Hendee and Chaney and Hendee et al. recommend that dosimeters or film badges used to estimate whole-body dose (trunk of body) should be worn at chest or waist level.[39,45] If protective garments such as lead aprons are used, the badge should be worn under the garment so as to reflect the actual dose to the wearer. If dose estimates are also required for other portions of the body not covered by protective apparel, the use of additional dosimeters is advised. For example, in fluoroscopy, one might also be concerned about the dose to the lens of the eyes of the radiologist. A badge positioned near the head (say on a shirt collar) may be useful in estimating dose to eyes.

The amount of exposure received by attending personnel in certain X-ray procedures is highly dependent upon the position of the individual in the room. This is because of the shielding provided by various pieces of equipment and because of nonhomogeneous scatter from the patient. Exposure of personnel can sometimes be reduced dramatically by small changes in their position in the room. Compact, audible radiation monitors such as the chirpy-type previously described, are helpful in locating regions of minimal exposure. Such devices are especially useful in fluoroscopy and in angiography rooms.

Procedures for Minimizing Dose to Patients

It is a well-established fact that the major contribution to population radiation exposure above normal background radiation is due to medical diagnostic X-rays. For example, the National Academy of Science-National Research Council (NAS-NRC) Committee on Biological Effects of Ionizing Radiation issued a report indicating that "medical diagnostic radiology accounts for at least 90% of the total man-made radiation dose to which the U.S. population is exposed."[6] This being the case, it is clear that efforts to minimize patient dose offer the potential of having substantial impact on reduction of long-term, low-level radiation effects in the population. The BRH has provided pertinent information on population exposures to X-ray and has made estimates of the mean gonad dose, the genetically significant dose (GSD), and the average dose to the blood-forming organs (mean marrow dose) for the U.S. population.[46,47] Tables 10a, 10b, and 11 summarize these data.

Table 10a
ESTIMATED MEAN GONAD DOSE PER EXAMINATION BY TYPE OF RADIOGRAPHIC EXAMINATION AND SEX, U.S., 1964 AND 1970[46]

	Millirads							
	Male				Female			
	1964		1970		1964		1970	
Type of examination	Mean	S.E.	Mean	S.E.	Mean	S.E.	Mean	S.E.
Skull	—	—	—	—	—	—	—	—
Cervical spine	—	—	—	—	—	—	—	—
Chest	1	—	—	—	5	1	1[a]	—
Radiographic								
Photofluorographic	—[b]	—	2[b]	2	5[b]	1	3[b]	—
Thoracic spine	46	55	3	3	17	8	11	2
Shoulder	—	—	—	—	—	—	—	—
Upper gastrointestinal series	22	11	1	1	128	19	171[a]	15
Barium enema	133	46	175	70	578	63	903[a]	111
Cholecystography or cholangiogram	—	—	—	—	72	15	78	17
Intravenous or retrograde pyelogram	537	172	207[a]	66	437	43	588[a]	47
Abdomen, KUB, flat plate	63	21	97	42	248	41	221	25
Lumbar spine	108	39	218	98	520	65	721[a]	50
Pelvis	444	101	364	76	130	19	210[a]	34
Hip	718	244	600	135	196	31	124[a]	15
Upper extremities	—	—	—	—	1	1	—	—
Lower extremities	38	11	15[a]	7	—	—	—	—
Other abdominal exams	331	178	857	332	256	48	524[a]	84
All other	1	1	—	—	4	2	6	4

Note: S.E. = standard error; — = less than 0.5 mrad.

[a] Change in mean gonad dose from 1964 to 1970 was statistically significant ($P < 0.10$).
[b] These figures are based upon assigned values of exposure, free-in-air at tabletop, because of the lack of specific exposure measurements.

One of the important questions that must be addressed is whether patient dose can be reduced without sacrificing diagnostic information and quality. Frequently, the answer is yes. By use of proper quality control procedures, trained operators, and proper X-ray techniques, unnecessary retakes, faulty films, and other problems leading to high patient exposure can often be eliminated. The NAS-NRC Committee has stated: "Medical radiation exposure can and should be reduced considerably by limiting its use to clinically indicated procedures utilizing efficient exposure techniques and optional operation of radiation equipment."[6]

Federal medical facilities are under a presidential mandate to follow this advice. In January 1978, President Carter approved Presidential Document No. 3195-01, "Radiation Protection Guidance to Federal Agencies for Diagnostic X-rays". It contains 12 recommendations for minimizing patient exposure. The recommendations are based on three broad principles:

1. Clinically unproductive examinations should be eliminated.
2. Optimal techniques should be used whenever X-ray examinations are performed.
3. Appropriate X-ray equipment should be employed.

Table 10b

ESTIMATED ANNUAL GENETICALLY SIGNIFICANT DOSE CONTRIBUTIONS BY TYPE OF RADIOGRAPHIC EXAMINATION AND SEX, U.S., 1964 AND 1970[46]

Millirads

Type of examination	Male 1964 N	Male 1964 GSD Cont.	Male 1964 S.E.	Male 1970 N	Male 1970 GSD Cont.	Male 1970 S.E.	Female 1964 N	Female 1964 GSD Cont.	Female 1964 S.E.	Female 1970 N	Female 1970 GSD Cont.	Female 1970 S.E.
Skull	39	—	—	112	—	—	39	—	—	88	—	—
Cervical spine	26	—	—	80	—	—	44	—	—	83	—	—
Chest	384	0.1	0.1	772	—	—	386	0.3	0.1	807	0.1	—
Radiographic												
Photofluorographic	226	—	—	118	0.1	0.1	260	0.2	0.1	155	—	—
Thoracic spine	17	0.3	0.7	38	—	—	16	—	0.1	46	—	—
Shoulder	17	—	—	48	—	—	26	—	—	56	—	—
Upper gastrointestinal series	71	0.1	0.1	142	—	—	77	0.4	0.4	170	0.4	0.2
Barium enema	32	0.4	0.7	76	0.3	1.4	46	2.2	1.4	98	1.7	1.4
Cholecystography or cholangiogram	29	—	—	65	—	—	50	0.1	0.2	118	0.6	0.5
Intravenous or retrograde pyelogram	46	1.3	4.0	93	1.0	0.9	37	1.4	1.4	99	2.2	1.0
Abdomen, KUB, flat plate	54	0.4	0.4	72	0.4	0.2	30	0.4	0.7	85	1.1	0.5
Lumbar spine	55	0.8	0.7	147	0.5	0.2	51	1.7	1.3	130	3.1	1.2
Pelvis	32	2.4	3.0	28	0.7	0.7	27	0.1	0.4	58	1.1	0.5
Hip	13	0.5	1.6	18	0.7	0.7	20	0.1	0.7	51	0.2	0.1
Upper extremities	114	—	—	231	—	—	77	—	—	205	—	—
Lower extremities	176	1.4	0.7	298	0.6	0.4	106	—	—	281	—	—
Other abdominal exams	13	0.7	1.6	29	0.8	1.2	16	0.4	0.8	59	3.0[a]	1.2
All other	46	—	—	114	—	—	36	—	—	100	—	—

Note: N = number of cases in sample; — = less than 0.05 mrad; S.E. = standard error; GSD Cont. = GSD contribution.

[a] Change in GSD contribution from 1964 to 1970 was statistically significant ($P < 0.10$).

Table 11
MEAN ACTIVE BONE MARROW DOSE TO THE ADULT POPULATION (1970)[47]

Examination	Mean active bone marrow dose per examination (mrad)	Annual per capita examination rate	Annual per capita dose (mrad ± S.E.)	
Head and neck				
Skull	78	0.020		1.6 ± 0.1
Cervical spine	52	0.022		1.2 ± 0.2
Other	—	—		0.6 ± 0.2
Thorax				
Chest-photofluorographic	44	0.073		3.2 ± 0.3
Chest-radiographic	10	0.306		3.2 ± 0.1
Thoracic spine	247	0.010		2.5 ± 0.4
Ribs	143	0.009		1.3 ± 0.2
Other	—	—		1.9 ± 0.4
Upper abdomen				
Upper GI series (total)	535			24.3 ± 4.7
Radiographic (subtotal)	294	0.046	13.5 ± 4.3	
Fluoroscopic (subtotal)	241	0.045	10.8 ± 1.9	
Scan	167			
Spot films	74			
Lumbar spine	347	0.023		8.1 ± 0.8
Gall bladder (total)	168			3.7 ± 0.4
Radiographic (subtotal)	129	0.027	3.5 ± 0.3	
Fluoroscopic (subtotal)	39	0.006	0.2 ± 0.3	
Scan	29			
Spot films	10			
Small bowel series	422	0.002		1.0 ± 0.3
Other				2.1 ± 1.0
Lower abdomen				
Barium enema (total)	875			21.2 ± 1.8
Radiographic (subtotal)	497	0.024	11.9 ± 1.0	
Fluoroscopic (subtotal)	378	0.024	9.3 ± 1.5	
Scan	268			
Spot films	110			
IVP	420	0.024		10.1 ± 0.6
Lumbosacral spine	450	0.013		5.7 ± 0.7
Abdomen KUB	147	0.020		2.9 ± 0.4
Other	—	—		0.4 ± 0.2
Pelvis				
Pelvimetry	595	0.002		1.4 ± 0.5
Pelvis	93	0.012		1.1 ± 0.2
Hip	72	0.009		0.7 ± 0.1
Other	—	—		1.2 ± 0.7
Extremities				
Femur	21	0.002		0.04 ± 0.02
Dental				
	9.4	0.312		2.9 ± 0.2
				Total 103 ± 5

Among the 12 recommendations are requirements for well-trained operators, equipment that meets the federal X-ray equipment performance standards and quality-assurance programs designed to provide satisfactory diagnostic requirements with minimal patient exposure.[38] The BRH is also seeking to promote voluntary adoption of these recommendations by nonfederal medical facilities.[48]

The quality-assurance aspects deserve further emphasis. Such programs involve equipment calibration, preventive maintenance, quality control of image processing, and procedures to reduce retakes. Koenig has discussed the close relation between radiation protection and quality in radiography.[49,50] Shaver et al. have indicated the need for such quality control based on the wide variations in patient dose throughout the country for essentially the same X-ray examinations.[51] They reported on pilot studies that were made to determine variations in organ doses delivered to a standard patient for a given X-ray examination. Large variations were observed in the techniques used for a specified exam from one facility to another and this resulted in an extremely wide range of patient doses for a specified diagnostic exam. For example, for a lumbosacral examination of a standard-size patient, the entrance radiation exposure varied from 100 to over 1500 mR, the mean ovarian dose from 11 to 660 mrad, and the testicular dose from less than 0.5 to over 1000 mrad.

Cameron and Bassano suggest that once the operating parameters of an X-ray unit are established at the time of installation, a competent radiological technologist can perform routine quality-assurance tests to detect changes and deterioration in the system.[52,53] These tests are basically:

1. A determination of the effective kV as a function of the kVP settings of the unit
2. Checking the performance of processing equipment with a standard exposed film
3. Determining the half-value layer and total filtration of the unit
4. Measuring beam output (in mR/mAs)
5. Determining effective focal-spot size

Hendee et al. provide details on quality-assurance programs in diagnostic radiology including film processors, film storage, dark rooms, X-ray generator variables, reproducibility of exposure, filtration checks, kilovoltage calibration, timer accuracy, milliampere accuracy, focal-spot size, beam restriction, target-to-film distance, film-screen contact, fluoroscopic beam alignment, fluoroscopic image intensifier, video system performance, and other variables.[45] Conducting an extensive quality-assurance program as described by Hendee et al. should be a goal of all hospitals and medical centers. Such a program requires cooperative efforts of the radiology staff including radiologists and technologists together with the medical physics or health physics staff, and clinical engineers. The immediate goal is, of course, improved diagnostic information, but the beneficial side products are reduced patient exposures and cost effectiveness.

RADIATION SAFETY IN NUCLEAR MEDICINE OR RADIOISOTOPE DEPARTMENTS

Many aspects of the safe handling of radioactive materials in hospitals have been reviewed elsewhere.[35,54] However, it is useful to both reiterate and expand some of the radiation safety concepts that have been developed in medical practice. Two other documents that should be consulted for guidance on the safe use of radionuclides in hospitals are NCR Guide 10.8 (Guide for the Preparation of Applications for Medical Programs) and their Guide on Maintaining Exposures in Medical Institutions as Low As Reasonably Achievable.[34,55]

Facility Planning

Radioactive materials may present both internal and external hazards. For this reason, they are most commonly used in laboratories that are specifically set aside for the purpose. In some cases, the amounts of radioactivity are so small that very little in the way of special facilities and precautions are needed. In other cases, high levels of activity may call for the use of completely remote handling facilities. Between these extremes, many laboratory designs are possible. There are no set rules as to what constitutes an adequate facility. Usually, one follows general guidelines such as the NCRP recommendations.[56] These give broad considerations both to the physical features of the facility and the degree of control exercised over the facility by the personnel involved.

In designing or setting up nuclear medicine laboratories, the main requirements are

1. Radiation exposures to personnel must be kept acceptably low (i.e., control direct radiation exposure using distance and shielding)
2. Prevent contamination of personnel
3. Prevent or minimize contamination of apparatus and equipment
4. Prevent spread of contamination to places and persons outside the lab

These requirements are not achieved by lab design only, but by good management and control by the workers in the lab as well. Hence, hazard control depends on both suitable facilities and good working practices.

Unsealed sources, in the form of liquids, solids, or gases that are not permanently sealed and are used in various nuclear medicine applications, present not only the possibility of external exposure, but also the possibility of internal hazards. Whenever radioactive materials are used as open sources, it is inevitable that some of the material will be transferred to apparatus (pipettes, bench tops, and even floors). Usually the worker is aware of this, especially in the case of apparatus that has come in contact with the radioactive material. However, small quantities may sometimes be transferred to benches and floors and then tracked out to uncontrolled areas. This is referred to as contamination. Once control of the material is lost, the probability of ingestion becomes quite high.

The importance of special design of radioisotope facilities lies in the control (or improved control) that results. A well-designed facility makes it easier for the worker to control the spread of contamination.

Facilities

Classification of Laboratories

Facilities for the use of radiopharmaceuticals or other radioactive materials must be designed to protect personnel from external and internal hazards and minimize interference by the radiation with diagnostic nuclear medicine measurements and radioassays. A number of general requirements can be set forth for radionuclide laboratories, but many of the specific requirements are dependent upon the following factors: (1) the radionuclide being used (type and energy of the radiation involved), (2) the level of activity being used, (3) the type of use or manipulation of the material, and (4) the chemical and physical form of the radioactive material. Using these factors (with perhaps some modification for unique features associated with a specific hospital), one can classify radionuclide laboratories in a reasonably objective manner and provide a rational basis for design requirements. The ICRP has recommended a laboratory classification scheme based largely on the four parameters listed above.[57] Basically, the various radionuclides are categorized into radiotoxicity classes based on type and energy of radiation emitted, half-life, and chemical and physical form as shown in Table 12. The term radiotoxicity is used to indicate the relative hazard of various radionuclides. This information is then coupled with the amount of activity used to give a laboratory-rating classification (Table 13). Finally, the laboratory classifications are modified according to the type of manipulations involved and the form of the material used (Table 13). Three convenient laboratory classifications are identified by this

Table 12
CLASSIFICATION OF ISOTOPES ACCORDING TO RELATIVE RADIOTOXICITY PER UNIT ACTIVITY

Group 1 (high toxicity)								
Pb-210	Po-210	Ra-223	Ra-226	Ra-228	Ac-227	Th-227	Th-228	Th-230
Pa-231	U-230	U-232	U-233	U-234	Np-237	Pu-238	Pu-239	Pu-240
Pu-241	Pu-242	Am-241	Am-243	Cm-242	Cm-243	Cm-244	Cm-245	Cm-246
Cf-249	Cf-250	Cf-252						
Group 2 (medium toxicity)								
Na-22	Cl-36	Ca-45	Sc-46	Mn-54	Co-56	Co-60	Sr-89	Sr-90
Y-91	Zr-95	Ru-106	Ag-110m	Cd-115m	In-114m	Sb-124	Sb-125	Te-127m
Te-129m	I-124	I-126	I-131	I-133	Cs-134	Cs-137	Ba-140	Ce-144
Eu-152 (13y)		Eu-154	Tb-160	Tm-170	Hf-181	Ta-182	Ir-192	Tl-204
Bi-207	Bi-210	At-211	Pb-212	Ra-224	Ac-228	Pa-230	Th-234	U-236
Bk-249								
Group 3 (low toxicity)								
Be-7	C-14	F-18	Na-24	Cl-38	Si-31	P-32	S-35	A-41
K-42	K-43	Ca-47	Sc-47	Sc-48	V-48	Cr-51	Mn-52	Mn-56
Fe-52	Fe-55	Fe-59	Co-57	Co-58	Ni-63	Ni-65	Cu-64	Zn-65
Zn-69m	Ga-72	As-73	As-74	As-76	As-77	Se-75	Br-82	Kr-85m
Kr-87	Rb-86	Sr-85	Sr-91	Y-90	Y-92	Y-93	Zr-97	Nb-93m
Nb-95	Mo-99	Tc-96	Tc-97m	Tc-97	Tc-99	Ru-97	Ru-103	Ru-105
Rh-105	Pd-103	Pd-109	Ag-105	Ag-111	Cd-109	Cd-115	In-115m	Sn-113
Sn-125	Sb-122	Te-125m	Te-127	Te-129	Te-131m	Te-132	I-130	I-132
I-134	I-135	Xe-135	Cs-131	Cs-136	Ba-131	La-140	Ce-141	Ce-143
Pr-142	Pr-143	Nd-147	Nd-149	Pm-147	Pm-149	Sm-151	Sm-153	Eu-152`
Eu-155	Gd-153	Gd-159	Dy-165	Dy-166	Ho-166	Er-169	Er-171	(9.2 hr)
Tm-171	Yb-175	Lu-177	W-181	W-185	W-187	Re-183	Re-186	Re-188
Os-185	Os-191	Os-193	Ir-190	Ir-194	Pt-191	Pt-193	Pt-197	Au-196
Au-198	Au-199	Hg-197	Hg-197m	Hg-203	Tl-200	Tl-201	Tl-202	Pb-203
Bi-206	Bi-212	Rn-220	Rn-222	Th-231	Pa-233	Np-239		

Group 4 (very low toxicity)

H-3	O-15	A-37	Co-58m	Ni-59	Zn-69	Ge-71	Kr-85	Sr-85m
Rb-87	Y-91m	Zr-93	Nb-97	Tc-96m	Tc-99m	Rh-103m	In-113m	I-129
Xe-131m	Xe-133	Cs-134m	Cs-135	Sm-147	Re-187	Os-191m	Pt-193m	Pt-197m
Th-232	Th-Nat	U-235	U-238	U-Nat				

From Report of Committee V on the Handling and Disposal of Radioactive Materials in Hospitals and Medical Research Establishments, International Commission on Radiological Protection Publ. No. 5, Pergamon Press, Elmsford, N.Y., 1964. With permission.

Table 13
CLASSIFICATION OF LABORATORIES FOR HANDLING RADIONUCLIDES

Group of radionuclide	Type of laboratory required for levels of activity specified below		
	Type 3	Type 2	Type 1
1	< 10 μCi	10 μCi—1 mCi	> 1 mCi
2	< 1 mCi	1 mCi—100 mCi	> 100 mCi
3	< 100 mCi	100 mCi—10 Ci	> 10 Ci
4	< 10 Ci	10 Ci—1000 Ci	> 1000 Ci

Modifying factors	Factors
Simple storage	× 100
Very simple wet operations (e.g., preparation of aliquots of stock solutions)	× 10
Normal chemical operations (e.g., analysis, simple chemical preparations)	× 1
Complex wet operations (e.g., multiple operations, or operations with complex glass apparatus)	× 0.1[a]
Simple dry operations (e.g., manipulation of powders) and work with volatile radioactive compounds	× 0.1[a]
Dry and dusty operations (e.g., grinding)	× 0.01[a]

[a] These factors could be increased by one or more orders of magnitude if the operations are carried out in closed boxes.

From Report of Committee V on the Handling and Disposal of Radioactive Materials in Hospitals and Medical Research Establishments, International Commission on Radiological Protection Publ. No. 5, Pergamon Press, Elmsford, N.Y., 1964. With permission.

method, ranging from a high level radionuclide laboratory (Type 1 lab) down to a low level laboratory (Type 3). An additional category, very low (Type 4) is added for convenience. The International Atomic Energy Agency uses this scheme for classifying working areas as shown in Table 14.

Laboratory Requirements

Laboratory requirements will be dependent upon the classification of the laboratory as previously discussed. General suggestions, recommendations, and guidance on design criteria were available from several sources.[34,58,59] Table 15 is such an example.

Surfaces

Generally, it is desirable to have smooth, nonporous floors for easy decontamination. Such floors are mandatory for Type 1, 2, and 3 labs, and desirable although not mandatory for Type 4 labs. Linoleum, vinyl, or asphalt tile (or similar smooth surfaces) fulfill this requirement. A coating of wax to seal cracks and seams is recommended.

Other surfaces (including walls) should be nonporous and readily washable, especially in locations near workbenches and sinks where contamination might be expected. Ceilings rarely cause problems with respect to contamination, although it is generally considered advisable to use nonporous materials for ceilings as well. Workbenches likewise should be of smooth impervious material. Stainless steel is frequently recommended in reference books on facility planning, but in fact is rarely necessary. Less

Table 14
CLASSIFICATION OF WORKING AREAS[59]

Area type	Definition	Control of access	Typical examples
4	Areas within the confines of a radiation facility where the external radiation levels are negligible and where radioactive contamination is also not present	Unrestricted	Administration block
3	Areas in which the average external radiation level is not greater than 0.1R/week; contamination is negligible and no special operating instructions are required	Access limited to radiation workers, no special clothing necessary	Working areas in the immediate vicinity of radiography operations, such as control rooms, etc.
2	Areas in which external radiation levels could exist and in which the possibility of contamination necessitates special operating instructions	Access limited to radiation workers in appropriate clothing and footwear	Luminizing factories and other equivalent installations
1	Areas in which the external radiation exposure levels and/or radioactive contamination levels could be high	Controlled access to radiation workers only, under strictly controlled working conditions and with appropriate clothing	Hot laboratories and similar facilities; highly contaminated areas

From Radiation Protection Procedures, IAEA Safety Ser. No. 38, International Atomic Energy Agency, Vienna, 1973. With permission.

costly materials are generally adequate and some of the newer workbench materials, such as epoxy resins, are excellent. Furthermore, even with an easily decontaminated laboratory bench, one should cover working surfaces with absorbent paper and use laboratory trays to hold materials and equipment.

Layout and Arrangement of Radioisotope Facilities

At minimum, a hospital with a nuclear medicine department will require a room for storage and dispensing of radioactive materials and another room for making uptake measurements or related radioassays. To some extent, grouping of such rooms may be advantageous, but consideration must be given to the fact that counting or radioassay rooms must be located so as to minimize interference by radiation levels in the dispensing area. Nuclear medicine facilities must, of course, be reasonably convenient and accessible to patients and other related supporting facilities and laboratories. At the same time, it is often economical to utilize basement locations to simplify shielding problems both with respect to providing natural wall shielding and floor loading requirements for storage shields or other local shields.

In all cases, the layout of the facilities should permit work to be segregated according to the levels of activity involved, ranging from low-level counting rooms to intermediate-level areas (including rooms for patients undergoing therapeutic treatment with radioactive materials), and to high-level storage and dispensing area(s). There is no

Table 15
FACILITIES AND INSTRUMENTS FOR WORKING PLACES

Type of laboratory	Facilities required	Instruments required: Essential	Instruments required: Optional	Remarks
Type 3	Those of a good chemical laboratory	Film badge	Wrist badge Ion chamber survey instrument, low range	
	Possibly fume hoods	Contamination monitor, fixed Contamination monitor, portable		
Type 2	All facilities to restrict radiation levels and avoid contamination	Film badge	Pocket dosimeter Wrist badge	Detailed operating instructions may be essential
	Fume hoods and glove boxes	Contamination monitor, fixed		Supplementary instruments for monitoring clothing, air monitoring, etc.
	Decontamination facilities	Contamination monitor, portable		
	Facilities for waste disposal	Ion chamber survey instrument, low range		
Type 1	All those for type 2 plus special structural features related to working surfaces, ventilation, etc.	Pocket dosimeter Film badge Wrist badge Contamination monitor, fixed Contamination monitor, portable	Portable gamma spectrometer Ionization chamber survey meter, high range	Siting and ultimate location to be carefully done
	Change room	Ion chamber survey instrument, low range	Portable wide-range survey meter	Strict compliance with detailed operating instructions essential
	Special decontamination facilities	Special hand and clothing monitors Air monitoring equipment	Permanently installed area monitors	Special instrumentation for measuring high-level radiation and for following up all operational phases from the radiation protection point of view

Sealed sources and radiation machines	Adequate shielding and clear demarcation of controlled areas Special facilities for mobile equipment	Film badge Contamination monitor, portable Ion Chamber survey instrument, low range X- and gamma-ray dosimeter with ionization chambers	Pocket dosimeter wrist badge TLD reader	Restricted access to controlled areas

From Radiation Protection Procedures, IAEA Safety Ser. No. 38, International Atomic Energy Agency, Vienna, 1973. With permission.

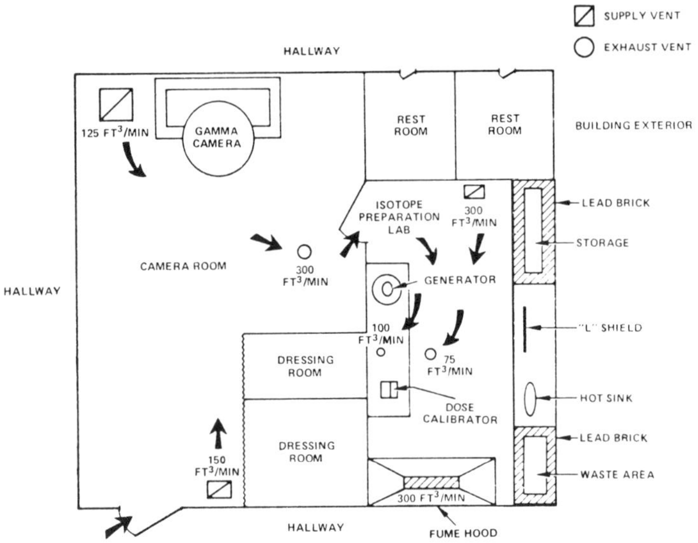

FIGURE 7. Nuclear medicine facility illustrating requirements and room layout. Scale: 1 in. = 4 ft. (Adapted from Regulatory Guide 10.8, U.S. Nuclear Regulatory Commission, Washington, D.C., 1979.)

single arrangement that is best. The layout chosen for a specific hospital will depend on the relative importance of the various factors mentioned and the relation of these factors to other aspects of the hospital program.

Ventilation

Although precautions should always be taken to avoid air contamination (from radioactive aerosols or radioactive vapors), as an added precaution it is wise to provide ventilation such that air flow is from low-level laboratories to higher-level laboratories, with high-level labs under a net negative pressure with respect to adjacent areas. The air from the high-level radioisotope laboratory should normally be exhausted via one or more radioisotope hoods. (See Figure 7)

Hoods provide containment for the handling of higher levels of materials, especially in cases where there is a potential of generating radioactive aerosols or vapors. In order for a hood to fulfill its intended use properly, there are several functional criteria that should be met.

Flow rate — The linear flow rate through the face of the hood should be 100 to 150 linear ft/sec (40 m/sec). This flow rate will generally prevent back-drafting of air out of the hood, yet not give an air current so strong as to disturb the materials in the hood. The face velocity can be altered in hoods with sliding sashes and may fall below the desired value when the sash is fully open. Thus, it is a good practice to clearly mark the position where the face velocity is adequate. Figure 8 is an example of a label used to mark radioisotope hoods.

Exhaust blowers — In order to maintain a net negative pressure in a hood duct, the blower should be located at the exit of the duct and not at the hood (see Figure 9). A negative pressure will assure that any leakage will be inward (into the duct) and that contaminated air does not escape the duct to other areas of the building. The exhaust point should be at the roof of the building so that proper dilution can occur (see Figure 10). The exhaust must also be located well away from building air intakes. If possible, the blower motor should be mounted outside the ducts to provide easy maintenance without potential contamination of maintenance personnel. It is also desirable to post

RADIOLOGICAL SERVICES

HOOD AIR FLOW CHECK

100 L.F.M.

WITH SASH AT MARK ⟶

DATE ______________

CHECKED BY ________________

FIGURE 8. Example of label to indicate sash location giving adequate flow rate.

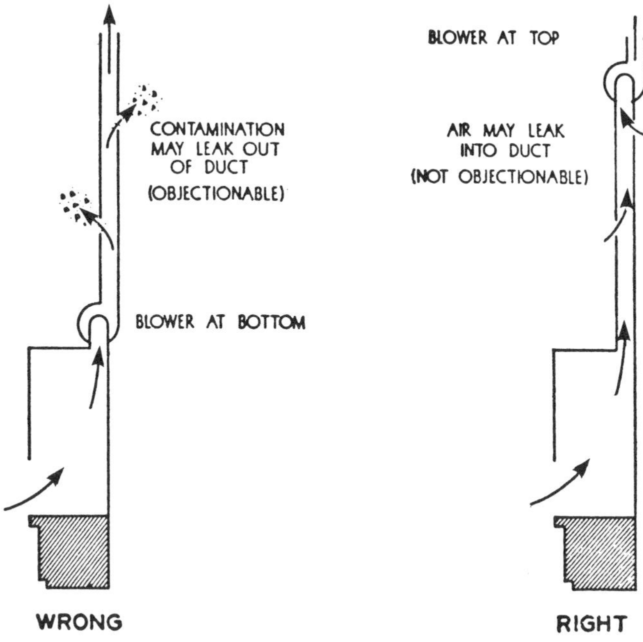

FIGURE 9. Wrong and right blower locations on hoods. (From Bradford, J. R., Ed., *Radioisotopes in Industry,* Reinhold, New York, 1953. With permission.)

exhaust ducts at the exit location to inform maintenance workers of a radioisotope hood (see Figure 11).

Hood controls — It is usually desirable to have controls for the hood (lights, blower) and hood services (water, gas) located on the outside of the hood. Such a placement serves to minimize hazards to the operator(s) by allowing adjustments to be made from outside.

Hood surfaces — The same guidelines already specified for lab benches should be followed, namely, provide smooth, easily decontaminated surfaces. Hoods made from epoxy resin materials that are easily decontaminated are now available. Other surfaces such as painted or coated metal are also acceptable.

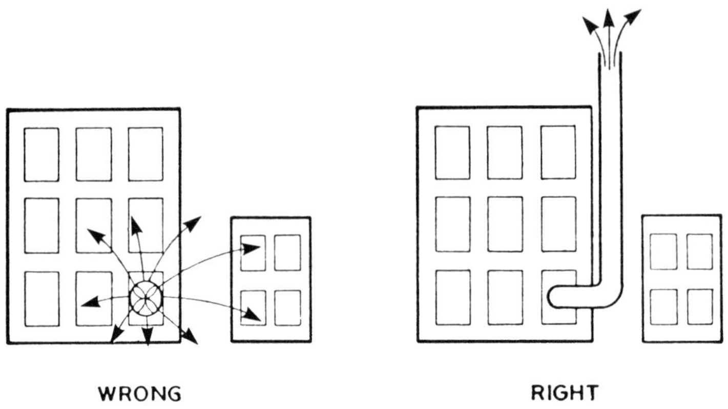

FIGURE 10. Wrong and right locations for discharging hood fumes. Discharge should be at top of the building. (From Bradford, J. R., Ed., *Radioisotopes in Industry*, Reinhold, New York, 1953. With permission.)

Hood location — In general, hoods should be located well away from traffic patterns and doors. A rapidly opening door or an individual walking rapidly past a hood can cause back-drafting and draw fumes or vapors out of the face of an operating hood (see Figure 12).

Filters — For hoods in which significant levels of nuclides in the high radiotoxicity category are used, filters are necessary. Normally, the filter system should include a prefilter (such as the standard fiberglass type) followed by a high efficiency particulate filter (HEPA filter). A HEPA filter is considered to be 99.97% efficient for removing particles down to 0.3 μm. If radioiodine is to be used in the hood, consider using an activated charcoal filter. If filters are used, a program of routine maintenance is necessary. If the filters become clogged, air flow may be greatly restricted and the flow rate may drop below the required level.

Storage and Shielding

Provisions must be made for storing radioactive materials in a secure area. For gamma emitters, shielding may also be required in the storage area. For radioisotope laboratories, it is necessary not only to protect those persons outside the room, but those working in the room routinely. For this reason, local shielding (as in Figure 13) around the sources is both more desirable and more economical than shielding the walls of the room as is done for X-ray facilities. In some cases, suitable shielding may be provided by constructing a barricade from lead bricks. More permanent storage shields or vaults may be constructed from lead or concrete. Although not always practical, such a vault is more convenient. Figure 14 illustrates several storage arrangements.

Portable shields and other temporary shields should be used as needed in laboratories where relatively high levels of gamma emitters are dispensed or used. Lead or steel bricks are convenient to use for this purpose. It should be recognized that such shields may weigh hundreds of pounds and should only be assembled on sturdy supporting structures.

Equipment

Several categories of equipment should be considered to adequately equip a nuclear medicine facility. The first, of course, are those instruments involved in assays and measurements for patient diagnosis. These will not be discussed here since our main

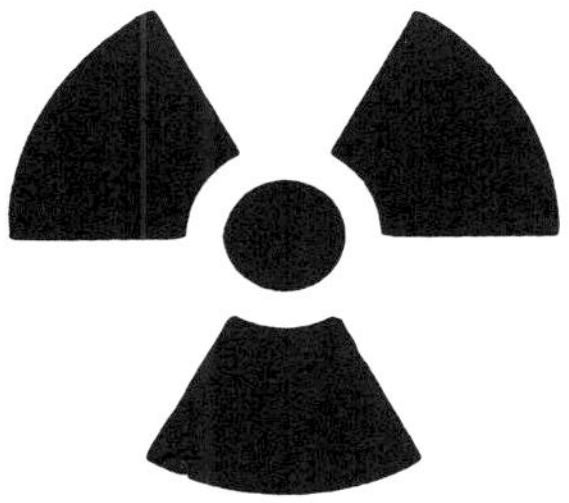

CAUTION:
RADIOACTIVE
MATERIALS

HAVE BEEN USED IN THE HOOD BELOW

BEFORE PERFORMING MAINTAINCE ON DUCTING OR BLOWER,

CALL ONE OF THE FOLLOWING IN THE ORDER LISTED

Name	Office Phone	Home Phone

FIGURE 11. Example of caution sign used near exit duct and blower to inform maintenance personnel of radioisotope hood.

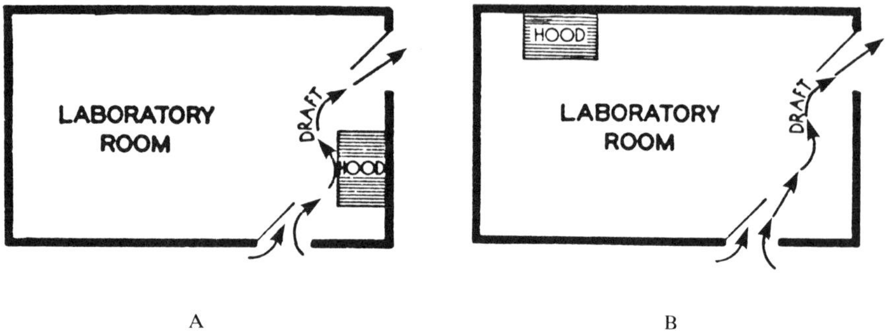

FIGURE 12. Illustration of the desirability of a draft-free hood location. (A) Poor hood location. (B) Good hood location. (From Bradford, J. R., Ed., *Radioisotopes in Industry,* Reinhold, New York, 1953. With permission.)

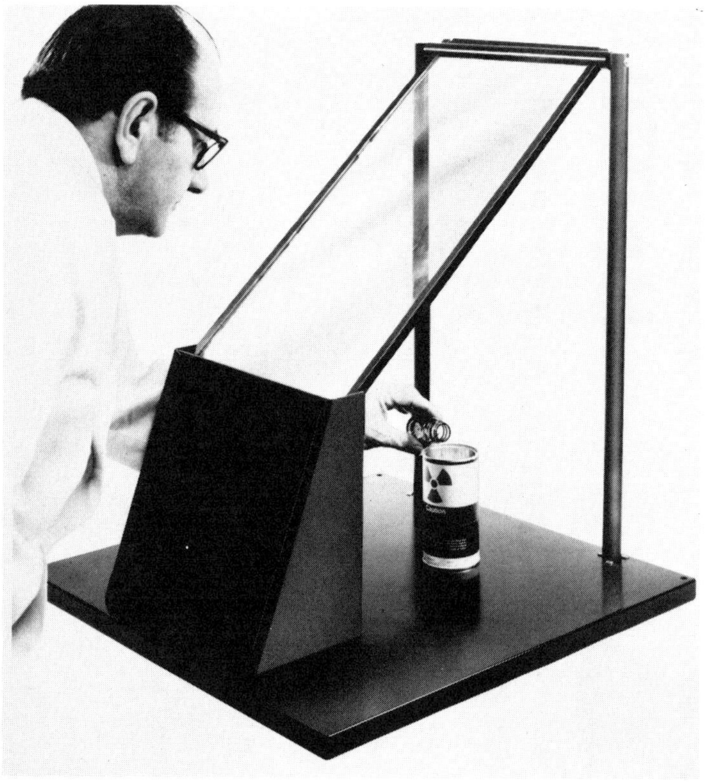

FIGURE 13. Protective lead barrier. (Courtesy of Nuclear Associates, Division of Victoreen, Inc.)

focus is on the radiation safety aspects of the facility. From the health and safety viewpoint, special equipment must be provided for laboratory handling of radioactive materials, administering radiopharmaceuticals to patients, and laboratory and personnel monitoring.

Laboratory Handling Equipment

Equipment that will promote radiation safety includes work trays (for confining

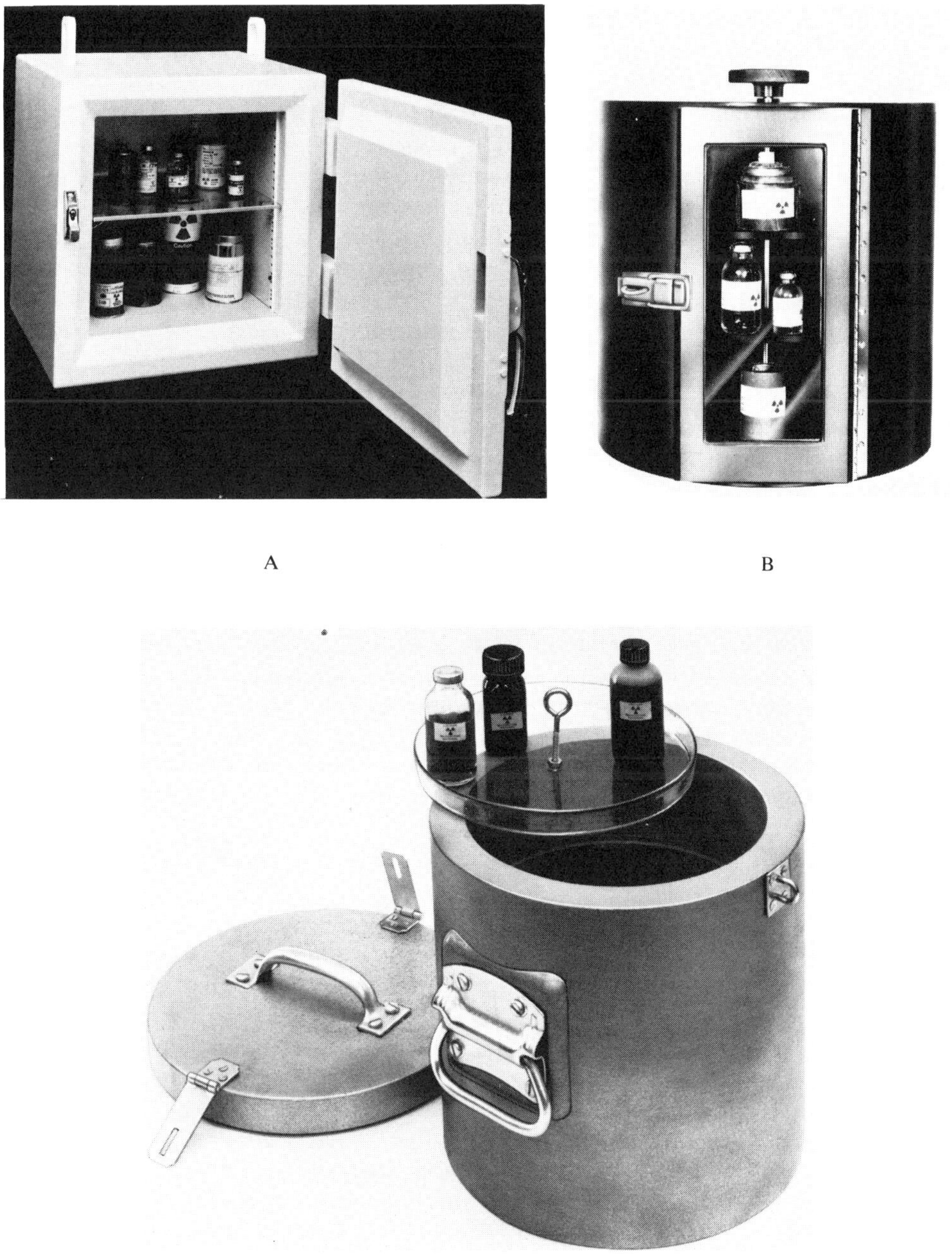

A B

C

FIGURE 14. Typical storage setups. (A) Lead storage safe. (B) Lazy Susan type lead storage cabinet. (C) Lead storage container. (Courtesy of Nuclear Associates, Division of Victoreen, Inc.)

radioactive material and protecting other work surfaces), remote handling tools, shield blocks or portable shields (see previous section on shielding), carts or dollies for transporting materials from dispensing areas to the location(s) of administration, shielded syringes, and suitable radioactive waste-collection cans or containers.

Area Monitoring and Survey Equipment

The purpose of area monitoring and surveys is to determine the direct radiation levels (exposure rates) in radioisotope facilities and to locate areas or spots of radioactive contamination. The measurement of radiation levels can be accomplished by the use of fixed radiation area monitors (RAMs) or portable devices. RAMs that are commonly used include the GM counter type, the ionization chamber type, and scintillation counters. In all cases, the detection probes are coupled with a ratemeter or other readout device calibrated to read in exposure-rate units. Portable survey instruments, such as Geiger counters or ionization chamber instruments, can also be used to measure exposure rates and are generally preferred due to greater flexibility. A typical nuclear medicine laboratory should have at least one high level, ionization-type survey meter capable of reading up to 1 R/hr. Such exposure rates may be found in the vicinity of $^{99}Mo/^{99m}Tc$ generators and for therapeutic amounts of other radionuclides.

For the detection of contamination, sensitive portable instruments are suitable. The Geiger counter is widely used for this purpose, but care must be exercised to recognize the limitations of Geiger counter instruments. For example, ^{125}I widely used in nuclear medicine, is not easily detected with most Geiger counters. A portable thin crystal scintillation counter is recommended for this application. Surveys for contamination are generally directed toward determining the location and extent of contamination on surfaces and equipment, and the degree to which contamination is fixed or removable. Thus, contamination surveys are, at best, only semiquantitative. After locating contaminated areas with a portable survey instrument, the individual conducting the survey may make a wipe or smear of the suspect area to determine if the contamination is readily removable or would easily spread to other areas.

Figures 15 and 16 show typical portable survey instruments with a Geiger-Müller probe and a scintillation probe. A portable ionization chamber is shown in Figure 17. For detailed information on radiation monitoring instruments (including response characteristics and calibration), see NCRP Report No. 57.[31]

Personnel Monitoring

Bioassay

Bioassay refers to the determination of the type, location, and concentration of radioactive material in the human body by direct measurement (in vivo) or by analysis of materials excreted or removed from the body. In vivo measurements are applicable to gamma- or X-ray emitters located in the body whose presence may be determined by external measurements. In vitro measurements are necessary for most beta and alpha emitters and are made on samples of urine, feces, breath, or other suitable materials.

Bioassay measurements become necessary when an individual handles or uses unsealed, open forms of radionuclides in amounts and/or under conditions where there is a definite potential for inhalation, ingestion, or absorption of the material. In a nuclear medicine facility, such conditions are most likely to occur in the use of radioiodine (^{125}I and ^{131}I), but may also involve other radionuclides. Bioassay serves two purposes: (1) it provides a means of ascertaining the effectiveness of contamination-control procedures and the need to modify and improve such procedures and (2) it enables the health physicist to determine the worker's dose commitment (whole body or specific organ) for purposes of dose control and monitoring.

Nuclear medicine programs operating under NRC licenses will find it useful to refer to NRC Regulatory Guide 8.20 for guidance on ^{125}I and ^{131}I bioassay.[60] This guide specifies the conditions under which iodine bioassay is considered necessary, the types of bioassays that should be performed, the frequency of bioassay, and the action to be taken if certain levels of radioiodine are measured in personnel. Table 16 gives NRC guidance for determining when iodine bioassay is necessary. The NRC recommends

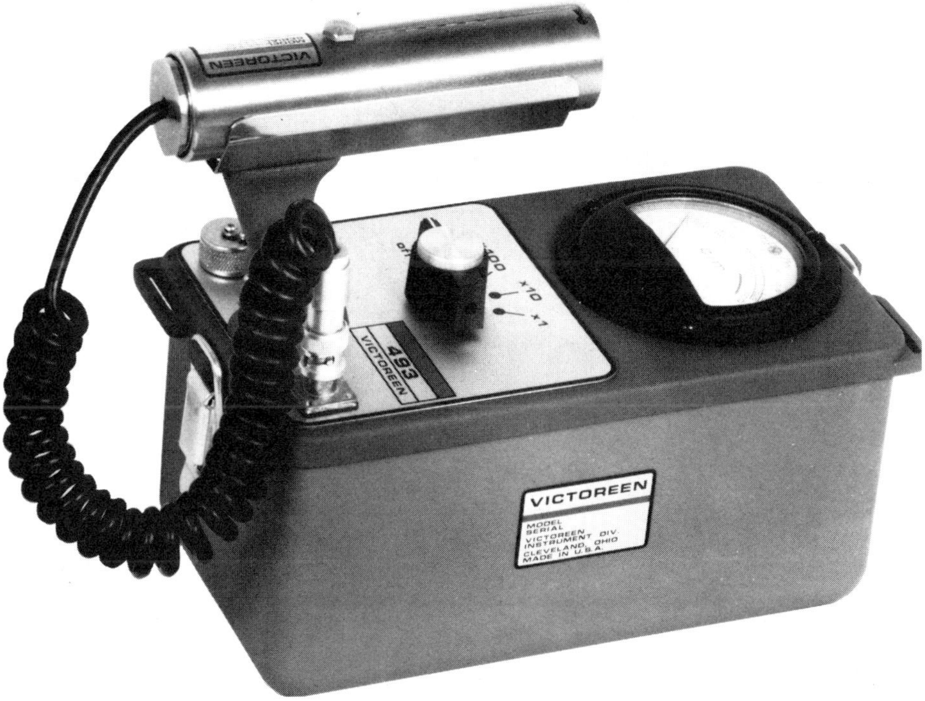

FIGURE 15. Portable survey meter with Geiger-Müller probe. (Courtesy of Victoreen Instrument Co.)

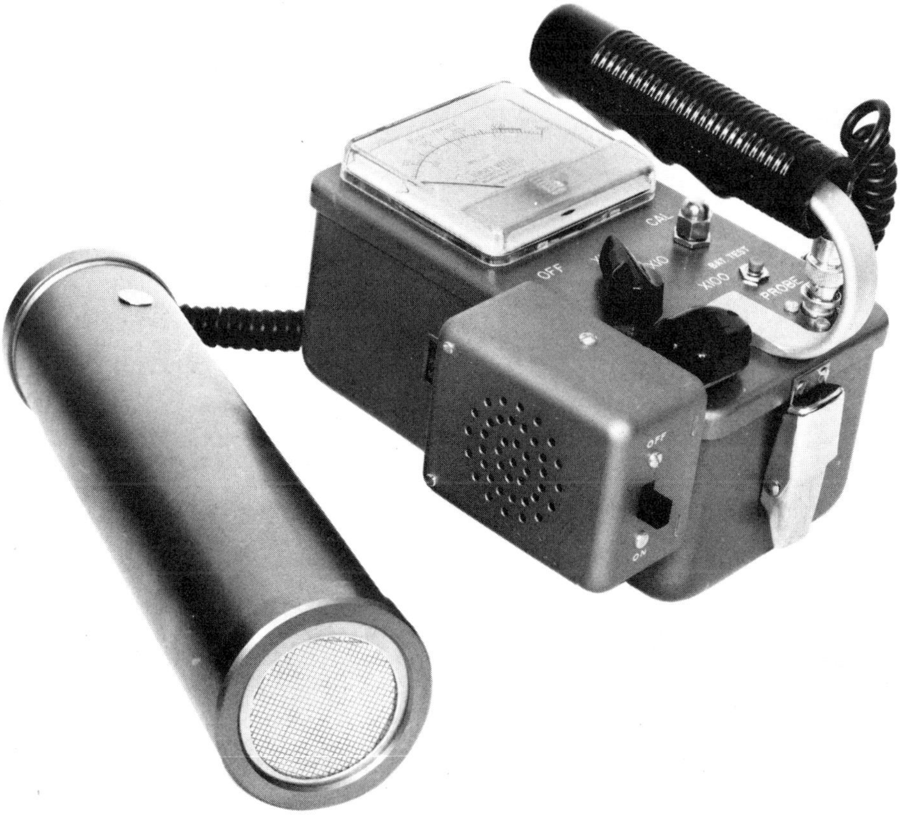

FIGURE 16. Portable survey meter with scintillation probe. (Courtesy of Wm. B. Johnson Associates.)

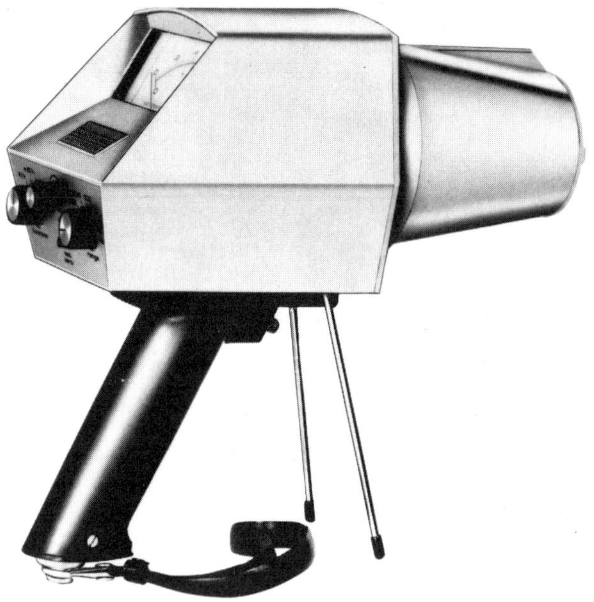

FIGURE 17. Portable ionization chamber-type survey meter. (Courtesy of Victoreen Instrument Co.).

that if thyroid burdens of 0.12 μCi of ^{125}I or 0.04 μCi of ^{131}I are measured in a routine bioassay, an investigation should be made by the user to determine the causes of exposure and the potential for further exposure. Corrective actions to lower the potential for further exposure should be implemented. If the thyroid burden at any time exceeds 0.5 μCi of ^{125}I or 0.14 μCi of ^{131}I, it is recommended that in addition to investigating the procedures and taking corrective action, medical consultation should be obtained regarding therapeutic procedures for accelerating removal of the radioactive iodine from the body.

According to the NRC, continuous intake of iodine at the MPC value will result in a quarterly intake of about 3.2 μCi for ^{125}I and 5.7 μCi for ^{131}I.[60] These activities will result in thyroid dose commitments of 7.5 rems. On the other hand, for single ingestions the ICRP indicates that 0.34 μCi for ^{125}I and 0.26 μCi for ^{131}I will result in a total thyroid dose of 1.5 rem.[61] Clearly, the pattern of uptake is important in relating thyroid burden to dose. Orvis has discussed the ambiguities in relating measured thyroid burdens to maximum permissible doses.[62]

Guidelines on conducting routine bioassay for other radionuclides have been given by Brodski.[63] Table 17 is adapted from Brodsky's work for several nuclides commonly used in nuclear medicine. A number of nuclides used in nuclear medicine are not included in Brodsky's tables. However, most of those not listed are in a toxicity class lower than radioiodine (less toxic) and would logically be classified in group II.

External Personnel Monitoring

The various types of personnel-monitoring devices were discussed in a previous section. Several additional comments should be added with respect to nuclear medicine. First of all, for personnel dispensing, processing, or otherwise handling relatively large amounts of radioactive material, monitoring of the hands and fingers is frequently necessary. Finger ring dosimeters are available for this purpose, utilizing small film or TLD packets as detectors. Hand dosimeters of this type are to be used in addition to

Table 16
ACTIVITY LEVELS ABOVE WHICH BIOASSAY FOR ^{125}I or ^{131}I IS NECESSARY[60]

Types of operation	Activity handled in unsealed form making bioassay necessary[a] — Volatile or dispersible (mCi)	Bound to nonvolatile agent (mCi)
Processes in open room or bench, with possible escape of iodine from process vessels	1	10
Processes with possible escape of iodine carried out within a fume hood of adequate design, face velocity, and performance reliability	10	100
Processes carried out within gloveboxes, ordinarily closed, but with possible release of iodine from process and occasional exposure to contaminated box and box leakage	100	1000

[a] Quantities may be considered the cumulative amount in process handled by a worker during a 3-month period; e.g., the total quantity introduced into a chemical or physical process over a 3-month period, or on one or more occasions in that period, by opening stock reagent containers from which radioactive iodine may escape. Quantities in the right-hand column may be used when it can be shown that activity in process is always chemically bound and processed in such a manner that ^{125}I or ^{131}I will remain in nonvolatile form and be diluted to concentrations less than 0.1 mCi/mg of nonvolatile agent. Capsules (such as gelatin capsules given to patients for diagnostic tests) may be considered to contain the radioiodine in nonfree form, and bioassay would not be necessary unless a capsule were inadvertently opened (e.g., dropped and crushed). However, certain compounds where radioiodine is normally bound are known to release radioiodine when the material is in process, and the left-hand column may then be applicable in those laboratories working only with ^{125}I in radioimmunoassay (RIA) kits, the quantities of ^{125}I are very small and in less volatile forms; thus, bioassay requirements may be judged from the right-hand column. In field operations, where reagent containers are opened outdoors for simple operations such as pouring liquid solutions, the above table does not apply; bioassay should be performed whenever an individual employee handles in open form (e.g., an open bottle or container) more than 50 mCi at any one time. Operations involving the routine use of ^{125}I or ^{131}I in an open room or bench should be discouraged. Whenever practicable, sealed bottles or containers holding more than 0.1 mCi of ^{125}I or ^{131}I should be opened, at least initially, within hoods having adequate face velocities of 0.5 m/sec or more.

Table 17
RECOMMENDED ACTIVITY LEVELS FOR CONDUCTING BIOASSAY PROGRAMS[63]

Nuclide	Relative toxicity[a]	Activity level for which bioassay is recommended (Ci)	Activity level for which spot checks are recommended (Ci)
^{51}Cr	II	10	1
^{198}Au	III	1	0.1
^{32}P	III	0.1	10^{-2}
^{85}K	III	0.1	10^{-2}
^{131}I	III	0.1	10^{-2}

[a] In this classification scheme, the least toxic materials are designated by I, and the most toxic in category VIII. Thus, groups II and III are relatively low in radiotoxicity.

regular whole-body dosimeters, and the results are reported separately as hand or extremity doses.

Next, special attention should be given to the criteria for determining who will be required to wear personnel dosimetry devices. Nuclear medicine activities will generally be subject to NRC regulations which require that personnel dosimetry be provided for individuals who are likely to receive 25% or more of the MPD in any calendar quarter, or individuals who enter high radiation areas. As defined by the NRC, a high radiation area is any area, accessible to personnel, where there exists radiation originating in whole or part from licensed radioactive materials at levels such that a major portion of the body could receive a dose in excess of 100 mrem in any 1 hr. For additional details on personnel-monitoring requirements for licensees, consult Title 10, Part 20, of the Code of Federal Regulations.[31]

In conformance with the ALARA principle, many institutions provide personnel-monitoring devices for individuals whose exposures are well below the levels for which such monitoring is required. Information concerning the absence of exposure may also be useful from a medical-legal point of view in order for a facility to confirm that personnel exposures were low.

Records of personnel exposure should be retained indefinitely. Current NRC requirements are that such records (including both bioassay and external monitoring records) be preserved until disposition is authorized by the NRC. Monitoring records should clearly identify the monitored individuals by name and social security number. Since state and federal regulations specify that an individual (upon request) must be provided with his/her radiation-exposure history, it is important that personnel-monitoring records be maintained in readily retrievable form.

Radioactive Waste Disposal

There are several categories of radioactive wastes that may be generated in a hospital. These include

1. Patients' excreta
2. Laboratory wastes
3. Animal carcasses and wastes
4. Contaminated supplies
5. Spent radionuclide generators

As a general principle, it is desirable to collect radioactive wastes and then either hold them for decay (in the case of short-lived materials), or process them for disposal in an approved manner. Land burial of wastes is still the method of choice, although the availability of commercial, low level waste-burial sites has become a serious problem in the U.S. in recent years. Alternate methods of disposal include incineration, and, for liquids, dilution and dispersion into the sanitary sewage system. As a practical matter, excreta from patients who have received diagnostic or therapeutic doses of radionuclides are permitted to be disposed of in the sanitary sewage system and are exempt from the restrictions otherwise imposed on radioactive wastes.

Laboratory wastes include contaminated glassware, gloves, syringes, absorbent paper, and other paraphernalia. Such solid wastes should be placed in specially designated containers in the laboratory for eventual collection and processing by radiation safety personnel. A convenient method for handling solid wastes is to use a metal or plastic container with a polyethylene bag liner. When it is filled, the bag should be tightly closed (with a wire-twist closure or the equivalent), marked as to content, and removed from the laboratory. Bags of long-lived solid waste are packed in larger containers, such as 55 gal steel drums, for eventual shipment to a burial site. Because

Table 18
CRITERIA FOR RELEASE OF RADIOACTIVE MATERIALS INTO THE SANITARY SEWAGE SYSTEM

Nuclide	Daily release limit (μCi)	Concentration limit (μCi/mℓ)
^{18}F	10,000	2×10^{-2}
^{32}P	100	5×10^{-4}
^{75}Se	100	9×10^{-3}
^{113}Sn	100	2×10^{-3}
^{113m}In	1,000	4×10^{-2}
^{125}I	10	4×10^{-4}
^{131}I	10	6×10^{-5}
^{198}Au	1,000	2×10^{-3}
^{201}Tl	1,000	9×10^{-3}

From Standards for Protection Against Radiation, Title 10, Code of Federal Regulations, Part 20, December 1, 1978.

waste-burial costs are based largely on volumes, many institutions find it advantageous to use trash compactors for volume reduction of solid wastes.

Liquid radioactive wastes are generated from washes of contaminated glassware, unused radioactive solutions, or various chemical procedures used in processing or preparing radiopharmaceuticals. Such liquids may be collected in jugs for eventual pickup and processing by radiation safety personnel. Generally, liquids are not accepted for burial at commercial waste-burial sites and must be processed and solidified prior to disposal. A variety of methods are used to solidify liquid wastes, including mixing with absorbing materials (diatomaceous earth, Pel-E-Cel®, or Microcel-E®), or solidifying with concrete.

Federal regulations permit disposal of radioactive wastes into the sanitary sewage system provided: (1) the waste is readily soluble or dispersible in water, (2) the quantity of radioactive material released into the system in any one day does not exceed specified amounts, and (3) the quantity of radioactive material released in one month, if diluted by the average monthly quantity of water released, does not exceed the maximum permissible concentrations for the nuclides in question, and (4) the gross quantity of radioactive material does not exceed 1 Ci/year. With respect to items (2) and (3), Table 18 gives the appropriate values for many of the radionuclides commonly used in nuclear medicine. The daily release limit may not exceed the larger of column 2 or the quantity which, if diluted with the average daily quantity of sewage released, would not exceed the concentrations specified in column 3. On a monthly basis, the quantities released may not exceed the quantity which, if diluted by the average monthly quantity of sewage released, would not result in concentrations exceeding the values specified in column 3. In some cases, state environmental regulations may be more restrictive.

Liquid wastes in the form of organic solvents pose particular problems in handling and disposal. Organic solvents containing radioactive contaminants arise mainly in those institutions conducting research involving liquid scintillation counting in which toluene and similar compounds are used as scintillation solutions. Since toluene is not miscible with water, used scintillation solutions cannot be disposed of into the sanitary sewage system. Furthermore, these solutions are difficult to solidify in a manner that will meet the requirements of commercial burial grounds. Facilities that generate these types of wastes will need to check carefully on the regulations of the particular waste disposal facility where they intend to ship waste, to determine the particular requirements for treatment and disposal. According to Beck et al., in a 1977 survey of institutional radioactive wastes from hospitals, schools of medicine, and universities, over 43% of the wastes shipped for commercial burial were liquid scintillation wastes.[64] Some of the disposal methods currently being used for organic solvent disposal follow.

Incineration — The organic solvent is burned, and the radioactive materials are generally released to the environment. In most cases, this method requires either a federal (NRC) or state permit for incineration of radioactive materials, or both.

Solidification — Attempts have been made with varying degrees of success, to solidify toluene and similar organic solutions. Granlund and Hayes have reported on a cement-silicate process that is described as being able to solidify wastes, including those that contain organic materials.[65] Absorbing organic solutions on diatomaceous earth or similar material has been used as a solidification method but is not generally satisfactory since it does not seem to really fix the material very well.

Evaporation — Reduction of waste volume by evaporation may be feasible for some facilities. Attention must be given to potential fire problems for evaporation of toluene or similar organic solvents. Also, the chemical toxicity must be considered both with respect to concentrations in working areas and environmental releases.

Distillation — Wright et al. have described a system whereby the radioactive liquid scintillation waste is distilled, leaving a substantially reduced concentrate that contains most of the radioactivity.[66] The distillate may be processed further to obtain reagent-grade toluene. Thus far, it is not clear whether or not this method is economical or whether, in fact, the recovered toluene can be readily used.

Burial in Vials — One method of disposal of liquid scintillation solutions that is attractive from the user's point of view is to package the scintillation vials or containers directly in drums for shipment and subsequent burial. In this method, layers of vials are alternated in a drum with layers of absorbent material. Vermiculite has often been used for this purpose, although diatomaceous earth or similar materials are preferable. The principle advantages of this method are (1) handling of bulk solutions is eliminated; instead one may simply process sealed glass, plastic, or filmware vials which contain on the order of 5 to 15 mℓ of solution each, (2) the fire hazards are reduced since large volumes of scintillation fluids are not opened for processing, (3) the problem of solidifying the waste is eliminated; the solidification method usually involves absorbing the scintillation solution by a suitable material, a procedure that is not generally satisfactory as evidenced by the fact that even when solidified the scintillation solution is not fixed, and readily escapes by evaporation or leaching after burial, and (4) burial directly in vials or scintillation containers has the advantage of keeping the solution immobile for relatively longer periods of time. For all of the methods named, consideration must be given to the potential fire hazards involved in the storage of toluene and other flammable scintillation solutions. A fire or safety engineer should be consulted for advice concerning the storage and processing of such waste.

Patient Dose Considerations

In diagnostic nuclear medicine, every effort should be made to minimize patient dose when this can be done without unduly sacrificing diagnostic information. This can frequently be accomplished by the careful and proper selection of nuclide and radiopharmaceutical form. Risks to individual patients in nuclear medicine are relatively low. However, because of the increasingly large numbers of persons so exposed, population doses become an important issue in risk-benefit analysis. Accordingly, it is important to know the patient doses from various nuclear medicine procedures and to minimize doses through optimum use of nuclides and instrumentation. Wagner has discussed the properties of ideal radiopharmaceuticals that are intended to give maximum diagnostic information while minimizing patient dose.[67,68] The methods of dose calculation from radiopharmaceuticals have been described in detail by Cloutier and Watson.[69] Information on the dose to standard man and how the dose may vary with age and route of administration is given in ICRP Publication 17.[70]

The method usually used for calcuating radiation dose to the patient for radiopharmaceuticals is that recommended by the Medical Internal Radiation Dose (MIRD) Committee of the Society of Nuclear Medicine. The method of the MIRD committee is given by Loevinger and Berman, and the nuclear parameters used in the calculations are given by Dillman and Von der Lage.[71,72] The method of calculation involves use of the equation

$$\bar{D}_{(t \leftarrow s)} = \frac{\tilde{A}_s}{m_t} \Sigma \Delta_i \phi_i(t \leftarrow s) \qquad (6)$$

where $\bar{D}$ is the average dose to the target organ t for activity located in a source organ s, $\tilde{A}_s$ is the cumulated activity in the source organ expressed in microcurie hours, and m_t is the mass of the target organ in grams. The value of $\tilde{A}_s$ is equivalent to the total number of decays that take place in the source organ. $\tilde{A}_s$ is obtained by integrating activity in the source organ over time. The value of $\tilde{A}_s$ is dependent on both the physical half-life and biological half-time of the material in the body. The symbol Δ represents the equilibrium dose constant and has units of g-rad/μCi-hr. It is a measure of the amount of energy released per decay. The other factor in the equation, $\phi_{(t \leftarrow s)}$, is called the "absorbed fraction" and expresses the ratio of the energy absorbed in the target organ to the energy released in the source organ. The MIRD committee has published detailed tables of values for Δ and ϕ.

RADIATION SAFETY IN RADIOTHERAPY OR RADIATION ONCOLOGY

Facility Design for High Energy Therapy Devices

High energy devices frequently require custom-made protective barriers or unique facility designs. Consideration must be given to a number of economic, architectural, and radiological factors in developing an adequate and acceptable design. Details on determining barrier-thickness requirements will not be discussed here inasmuch as complete information for design of shields for medical facilities is given elsewhere.[32] An appreciation for the complexity of factors that must be considered in the design of protective barriers is provided by the American Hospital Association.[54]

Calibration and Maintenance of Therapy Equipment

An important concern with respect to radioactive sources (such as ^{60}Co or machine-produced radiation) used in therapy is source or beam calibration. Controlling patient dose in therapy is important both from a medical and health physics point of view. An incorrect or faulty knowledge of radiation doses from the source will lead to underdosing or overdosing of the treatment area, either of which could be extremely detrimental to the patient. An example of such an occurrence involved a ^{60}Co therapy unit located in a large midwestern hospital.[73] Instead of making periodic measurements of the radiation output of the source, the hospital physicist is reported to have plotted the decay of the source and provided the resulting information for technicians to adjust the exposure times for patients in order to provide the doses prescribed by the physicians. Unfortunately, the source decay was plotted incorrectly, and over a period of some 27 months, the error between the true dose and the calculated dose gradually increased until patients were receiving doses as high as 40% over the desired values. Nearly 400 patients were reported to have been subjected to exposure 10% or more higher than called for, with those toward the end of the 27-month period being subjected to what has been described as substantial overdoses. A large number of lawsuits resulted from this situation.

The solution to preventing the type of situation described is for hospitals to require a periodic check and calibration of their radiation-therapy units. Most hospital physicists use a precision ionization chamber probe connected to an electrometer to measure beam output. A cross-check with a second probe and an electrometer is highly recommended. The measured values should in turn, be rechecked against calculated values in the case of a ^{60}Co source whose output should decrease at a known rate based on its physical half-life. Not all experts agree on the needed frequency of calibration for ^{60}Co sources. Some use a monthly calibration frequency while others feel that every 3 to 6 months is adequate. For machine-produced radiation (accelerator), the beam output should be checked on a daily basis, with a detailed calibration conducted every month.

Routine maintenance of therapy equipment may also have a bearing on radiation safety. Lane and co-workers have reported on a series of radiation incidents associated with source drive failures on a ^{60}Co teletherapy unit.[74] The first incident resulted from the source drive mechanism remaining in the "beam on" position at the end of the treatment. A second incident occurred less than a year later when the source failed to return to the off position at the end of the treatment. In yet a third incident shortly thereafter, the source again stuck in the on position. In the first situation, the failure was found to be due to wear of the source drive mechanism, and replacement of drive gears was required. In the second instance, the failure was due to a crack in the source-positioning stop arm attached to the drive shaft of the source wheel. The third incident was found to have been caused by the misalignment of source drive gears, a condition that resulted from the mounting plate of the source drive mechanism not being securely fastened to the treatment head. In all of the cases cited, the patients received somewhat higher doses than intended (an 8 to 20 rad additional tumor dose), while operating personnel received only slight doses (1- to 10-mrad range) in removing patients from the treatment area. As a result of these incidents and subsequent problems with the same unit, Lane and his colleagues recommended that facilities using such equipment "establish a routine preventive maintenance schedule which includes checking the alignment of the source drive gears, the adjustment of the source with the collimator system, and the time required for source movement from the off position to the on position and return." They further recommended that the entire source drive mechanism be replaced every 5 years since a visual inspection may not detect metal fatigue that may have occurred.

Safe Use of Brachytherapy Sources

Brachytherapy refers to radiation therapy using an encapsulated source to deliver gamma or beta radiation at or near body surfaces or by intracavitary or interstitial application. Historically, brachytherapy was carried out with either radium or radon sources. More recently, other radionuclides have come into widespread use in brachytherapy, including ^{137}Cs, ^{51}Cr, ^{60}Co, ^{198}Au, ^{125}I, ^{192}Ir, ^{182}Ta, and ^{90}Sr. Typically, sources used in brachytherapy are in the millicurie to curie range. Exposure rates per curie at unit distance and at the surface of the source for these sources are given in Table 19.

The NCRP has identified five operational stages in the clinical use of brachytherapy sources during which personnel radiation exposures may occur:[75]

Table 19
APPROXIMATE GAMMA-RAY DOSE RATES TO THE HAND FOR 1 Ci IN A SEALED SOURCE

Nuclide	β max (principal), MeV	γ (principal), MeV	Γ, R/mCi-hr at 1 cm	Surface dose rate,[a] R/min	Dose rate at 1-cm tissue depth, R/min	Dose rate at 3-cm tissue depth, R/min
^{137}Cs	0.51, 1.2	0.662	3.26	513	28	3.7
^{60}Co	0.31	1.17, 1.33	13.00	2075	114	16.0
^{192}Ir	0.67	0.468	4.80	813	43	5.5
^{226}Ra	0.4—3.2	0.04—2.4	8.25	1310	72	9.7

Note: Industrial source housings are usually of stainless steel, and for the purpose of the calculations, the activity is considered to be a point source. In considering these dose estimates, there is assumed a capsule of outside diameter ¼ in., with a wall of stainless steel (type 304) that is 1/32 in. thick.

[a] The total surface dose rate for the ^{226}Ra source is 1900 R/min based on a 45% increase due to electron production in the stainless steel wall.[1] For the other nuclides given in the table, the increase in surface dose rate due to electron production in the stainless steel wall is estimated to be between 25—45%.

From Protection Against Radiation from Brachytherapy Sources, NCRP Rep. No. 40, U.S. National Council on Radiation Protection and Measurements, Washington, D.C., March 1, 1972. With permission.

1. Transfer of sources from storage and preparation for use on patients
2. Transfer from preparation area and application to patient
3. Irradiation of patient
4. Removal of sources from patient and transfer back to preparation area
5. Removal of sources from applicators, and the subsequent cleaning and transfer back to storage

NCRP Report No. 40 provides a list of safety precautions that should be observed for each of these stages.[75] Basically, the precautions involve: (1) care in keeping track or accounting for all sources at all times, (2) proper use of distance and shielding in source manipulations and transfers, (3) careful planning of all stages of source usage, (4) conducting radiation surveys, (5) exercising control over radiation areas (including the patient) during treatment, and (6) maintaining careful records of source use and radiation surveys.

Source, Handling, and Loading

Care must be exercised in identifying and maintaining an inventory on sealed sources. The NCRP recommends that identification be based on physical size, shape, and general appearance, although additional identifying marks or engraving have also been used with varying degrees of success.[75]

Shielded, locked storage vaults are recommended for storage of brachytherapy sources. Shielding thicknesses may be determined from tables provided in NCRP Report No. 40.[75] A condensed version of the NCRP tables is given in Table 20. The source storage vault should provide separate compartments for sources of different activities, and each compartment should be labeled to identify its contents. The shielding should be adequate to insure that the dose to an individual working in front of the vault in performing required duties will be as low as reasonably achievable. Figure

Table 20
PROTECTION REQUIREMENTS FOR VARIOUS GAMMA-RAY SOURCES

Thicknesses of Lead or Concrete Required to Reduce Radiation Exposure to 100 mR at Distances Specified

Millicurie hours	Distance from source 30 cm	1 m	2 m
^{137}Cs[a]—Thicknesses of Lead Required (cm)			
100	1.1	—	—
1,000	3.2	1.1	—
10,000	5.3	3.2	1.9
^{60}Co[b]—Thicknesses of Lead Required (cm)			
100	4.5	0.4	—
1,000	8.6	4.4	2.4
10,000	12.6	8.4	6.0
^{60}Co—Thicknesses of Concrete Required (in.)			
100	9.3	0.9	—
1,000	17.4	9.2	4.3
10,000	25.5	17.0	12.2
^{198}Au[c]—Thicknesses of Lead Required (cm)			
100	0.5	—	—
1,000	1.5	0.4	—
10,000	2.7	1.5	0.8
^{198}Au—Thicknesses of Concrete Required (in.)			
100	2.3	—	—
1,000	7.4	2.0	—
10,000	12.7	7.2	4.2
^{192}Ir[d]—Thicknesses of Lead Required (cm)			
100	1.5	—	—
1,000	3.4	1.4	0.2
10,000	5.5	3.4	2.2
^{137}Cs—Thicknesses of Concrete Required (in.)			
100	3.4	—	—
1,000	9.6	3.2	—
10,000	15.7	9.3	5.7
^{192}Ir—Thicknesses of Concrete Required (in.)			
100	4.3	—	—
1,000	10.0	4.1	0.6
10,000	16.0	9.8	6.4
Ra[e]—Thicknesses of Lead Required (cm)			
100	4.6	—	—
1,000	9.0	4.2	1.4
10,000	13.5	8.8	6.0
Ra—Thicknesses of Concrete Required (in.)			
100	8.7	—	—
1,000	18.0	8.4	2.9
10,000	27.0	17.6	12.0
^{182}Ta[f]—Thicknesses of Lead Required (cm)			
100	3.5	—	—
1,000	7.4	3.3	1.0
10,000	11.4	7.3	4.9
^{182}Ta—Thicknesses of Concrete Required (in.)			
100	7.4	—	—
1,000	16.0	7.2	2.0
10,000	24.6	15.7	10.6

[a] TVL = 2.1 cm lead, or 6.2 in. concrete.
[b] TVL = 4.0 cm lead, or 8.1 in. concrete.
[c] TVL = 1.1 cm lead, or 5.3 in concrete.
[d] TVL = 2.0 cm lead, or 5.8 in. concrete.
[e] TVL = 4.6 cm lead, or 9.2 in. concrete.
[f] TVL = 4.0 cm lead, or 8.6 in. concrete.

Modified from Protection Against Radiation from Selected Gamma Sources, NCRP Rep. No. 24, National Bureau of Standards Handbook 73, U.S. Government Printing Office, Washington, D.C., 1960, in Protection Against Radiation from Brachytherapy Sources, NCRP Rep. No. 40, National Council on Radiation Protection and Measurements, Washington, D.C., March 1, 1972. With permission.

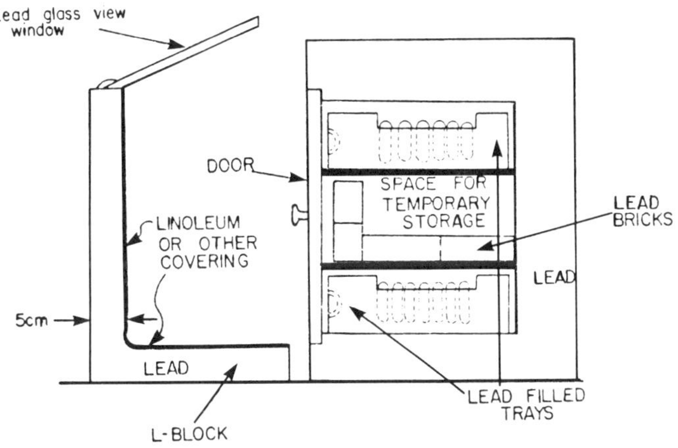

FIGURE 18. Suggested arrangement of preparation bench with L-block and source storage. (From Protection Against Radiation from Brachytherapy Sources, NCRP Rep. No. 40, U.S. National Council on Radiation Protection and Measurements Publications, Washington, D.C., 1972. With permission.)

18 shows the arrangement for source storage recommended by the NCRP. The storage enclosure is positioned behind a protective "L-block" which is a lead shield with a viewing window. The L-block shields the body of the operator during source manipulation or the preparation or dismantling of source applicators. In using the L-block, the operator's hands and forearms will not be shielded, and dose to the hands is often the limiting factor in establishing working times. Brachytherapy sources should not be touched or handled directly with the hands. Rather, they should be handled or manipulated with forceps, tongs, or other handling tools so as to provide as much distance between the source and the hands as practical. The dose limit to hands of 75 rem/year corresponds to a practical weekly working limit of 1.5 rem. Since for gamma emitters an exposure of 1 R results in a dose equivalent to about 1 rem, the working time if the hands are a minimum of 30 cm from a 100-mCi source would be ^{226}Ra, 1.6 hr; ^{60}Co, 1 hr; and ^{137}Cs, 4 hr.

Another way of expressing this is that the number of millicurie-hours to give the hands a 1.5-rem dose (for a source-to-hand distance of 30 cm) is ^{226}Ra, 160 mCi/hr; ^{60}Co, 100 mCi/hr; and ^{137}Cs, 400 mCi/hr.

A variety of devices are available for source handling, including forceps, magnetic handling devices, pneumatic devices, and electromechanical devices. The choice of device is dependent on the physical size and composition of the sources, as well as the amount of radioactivity involved.

The storage safe or enclosure for brachytherapy sources should be located in a secure, restricted area. In addition to the shielding requirements, if radium sources are being stored or used, the source storage room should be provided with a ventilation system similar to that of a nuclear medicine laboratory. Provision of such ventilation serves as a safeguard in case of radon leaks from radium sources. Ventilation, including a filtered exhaust, is also recommended if the sources in use are encapsulated powders or microspheres. If sources for intracavity or interstitial applicators are included, a sink in the storage area may be required for cleanup. Such a sink should have a readily accessible filter or trap for easy retrieval of sources accidentally lost into the drain.

Frequently, brachytherapy sources have to be transported away from the storage area to another location in the hospital. For this purpose, the facility should have on

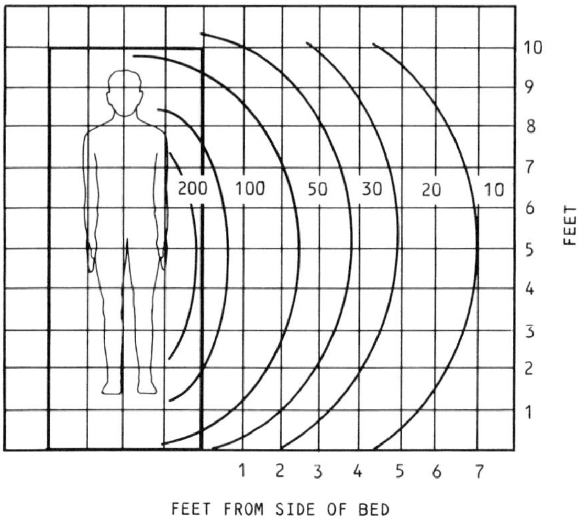

FIGURE 19. Approximate exposure rates (mR/h) in region around bed of patient containing 100 mg of radium, 300 mCi of gold (^{198}Au), or 300 mCi of iodine (^{131}I). (From Radiation Protection for Medical and Allied Health Personnel, NCRP Rep. No. 48, U.S. National Council on Radiation Protection and Measurements Publications, Washington, D.C., 1976. With permission.)

hand suitable shields that can be readily carried by hand or transported by cart to the desired location. The shields used in transport should be secured to prevent the source(s) from dropping or spilling out during transfer from one location to another.

Precautions During Treatment

Immediately after brachytherapy sources have been inserted, the exposure rate at standard distance (usually 1 m) should be determined with an appropriate survey meter. The exposure-rate value is entered on the patient's chart and should be compared to the expected exposure rate for the source in question. Table 7 gives the specific gamma ray constants (exposure rate at 1 cm for 1 mCi of activity) for typical gamma emitters. The observed reading would be expected to be somewhat lower than the value calculated from the exposure-rate constant due to attenuation of the gamma rays by the patient's body. A higher reading, or one considerably different from the expected value, is cause for concern and suggests the need for rechecking the source (for correct nuclide and activity) and the measured exposure rate. Figure 19 illustrates exposure-rate patterns around a patient treated with radium.

The bed or room of the patient must be posted with appropriate radiation caution signs. If it is not practical to provide physical shielding for adjacent areas, it may be necessary to segregate the patient or restrict time and access distances for other patients or visitors. NCRP Report No. 39 provides guidance on the exposure of hospital patients to radiation from adjacent patients. While recommending that such exposures be kept at a practical minimum, the council suggests that as a numerical guide such exposure "should not exceed 0.5 rem during a single hospital admission." In the case of sources covered by a NRC license, radiation levels in unrestricted areas must comply with the limits specified in paragraph 20, 105 (b) of 10CFR20. In practice, with careful planning of patient locations, it should be possible to maintain exposures to adjacent patients well below these levels.

NURSING INSTRUCTIONS FOR PATIENTS TREATED WITH BRACHYTHERAPY SOURCES

Patient's Name: ______________________________

Room Number: ____________ Physician's Name:

Isotope Activity: ______________________________

Date and Time of Administration: ______________________________

Date and Time Sources Are To Be Removed: ______________ Isotope:

Exposure Rates in mR/hr

Bedside	3 feet from bed	10 feet from bed

(Comply with all checked items.)

____1. Wear film badge.

____2. Wear rubber gloves.

____3. Place laundry in linen bag and save.

____4. Housekeeping may not enter the room.

____5. Patient may not have visitors.

____6. Patient may not have pregnant visitors.

____7. Patient may not have visitors under 18 years of age.

____8. A dismissal survey must be performed before patient is discharged.

____9. Patient must have a private room.

____10. Other instructions.

RSO ______________________, ____________/____________

Name ——— On-duty/Off-duty/Telephone Numbers

Date:

FIGURE 20. Nursing instructions for patients treated with brachytherapy sources. (From Regulatory Guide 10.8, U.S. Nuclear Regulatory Commission, Washington, D.C., 1979.)

Hospital personnel involved in the care of patients during the time when sources are implanted must be limited in the length of time they are in attendance with brachytherapy patients. NRC Regulatory Guide 10.8 includes a suggested form that may be convenient to use in providing nursing instructions for patients treated with brachytherapy sources. A copy of this form is reproduced in Figure 20. The guide also includes a list of useful instructions to nurses that should be consulted when brachytherapy is planned.

Leak Testing

The potential always exists for a sealed source to rupture or develop a leak. A leaking source presents a contamination hazard not only for the hospital facility, but also for the patient. The record for leakage has been particularly poor for radium sources. It has been postulated that a factor contributing to leakage of radium sources is the buildup of internal pressure from helium gas resulting from alpha decay of the radium-226. In a survey made of some 70 medical radium installations in Wisconsin, half had leaking or unwanted radium sources.[76] Alpha contamination in these facilities was found on the floors and on handling equipment.

Periodic leak tests of all sealed sources is mandatory for confirming the integrity of sources and spotting leaking sources in a timely fashion. Removable contamination in excess of 0.005 μCi is considered evidence that a source is leaking. In the case of radium, the escape of radon at the rate of 0.001 μCi or more per 24 hr is considered evidence of leaking. In most cases, leak tests are required by federal or state authorities at intervals not exceeding 6 months. A variety of leak-test methods are considered acceptable.

Wipe test — The surface of the source is wiped with absorbent material (using forceps or tongs). The absorbent material is subsequently counted for radioactivity.

Reverse wipe test — A storage container is lined with absorbent material so that the source fits snugly in place. The source is then placed in the container and removed, being wiped by the absorbent material in the process. The material is then counted for radioactivity.

Wash test — The source is immersed or rinsed with a mild detergent solution. An aliquot of the solution is then counted with a suitable detection device.

For radium sources where radon leakage may occur and not be detected by conventional leak tests, a number of special tests have been devised. A number of radium leak-test methods have been reported in the literature.[77-83] One of the simplest methods is that of Benson and Fetz.[82] The radium source is first cleaned and then sealed in a small jar for 24 hr. The lid of the jar is then removed and its inside surface immediately checked for alpha activity with a suitable survey instrument. Radon leakage is evidenced by alpha-emitting radon daughter products which plate-out on the inside surface of the jar and lid. The method is reported to be sensitive to 10^{-4} μCi of radon. If a source is found to be leaking, it should be immediately removed from use and sealed in a container to prevent further spread of contamination. Leaking sources must either be disposed of in an approved manner or returned to the original supplier for repair, re-encapsulation, or replacement. In most cases, the user (the hospital or its personnel) is not permitted to repair leaking sources under either federal or state regulations.

Source Cleaning or Sterilization

Frequently, brachytherapy sources must be cleaned or sterilized. There are several concerns when this occurs, namely, exposure of personnel, source damage, and source loss.

Personnel exposure is controlled by means of distance and shielding as in other types of handling and use. The sterilization method chosen is dependent on the type of source. If boiling is used, care must be exercised that unacceptably high temperatures do not occur if the sterilizer boils dry. For radium sources, 110°C is the maximum temperature that should be permitted. The limits for other sources should be provided by the source supplier. If chemical sterilization is used, care must be taken to use only those solutions that will not attack the encapsulation material. Hot-air sterilization is acceptable in many cases, but not for radium or encapsulated powder sources where leakage could give rise to airborne radioactivity. Abrasive substances and polishes should never be used in cleaning sources.

Precautions for Patients Who Have Received Therapeutic Amounts of Radionuclides

Patients to whom large amounts of radioactive material have been administered for therapeutic purposes may be a source of significant exposure for nurses and other personnel who have to care for such patients on a regular basis. The National Council on Radiation Protection and Measurements has identified four situations for which specific types of precautions and protective procedures must be followed for such patients.[84] These are

1. The patient is receiving regular nursing care in the hospital
2. The patient is referred for emergency surgery
3. The patient is released from the hospital while still containing an appreciable quantity of the radionuclide
4. The patient dies while still appreciably radioactive

Therapeutic use of radionuclides can be categorized as: (1) treatment with encapsulated sources that are mechanically inserted into the desired locations and (2) treatment with solutions, colloidal suspensions, or microspheres that are administered orally or by injection. The mechanically inserted sealed sources that are removable have already been discussed in the section on brachytherapy sources. Sealed sources that are inserted as permanent implants include radon seeds; ^{198}Au, ^{192}In and ^{182}Ta wires; and ^{90}Y pellets. Radionuclides in the category of solutions, colloidal suspensions, and microspheres include ^{32}P and ^{198}Au suspensions and ^{131}I solutions.

Whenever a patient has received a therapeutic amount of a gamma-emitting nuclide, the exposure rate at a specified distance (usually 1 m) should be measured with an appropriate survey instrument. This measurement is basically identical to that previously described for brachytherapy sources and is used to confirm calculated exposure rates and to establish acceptable working times and distances for staff personnel and visitors. Figure 19 gives an example of the expected exposure rates near a patient undergoing treatment. The NCRP recommends that radioactive patients not be concentrated in one area of the hospital, but instead dispersed so that individual hospital staff members have a minimal number of contact hours with radioactive patients.[84] For patients who have been treated with encapsulated sources, the only risk to working personnel and visitors is from exposure to radiation emitted by the material in the patient. This exposure can be readily controlled by limiting the time duration in the vicinity of the patient, and if necessary, the distance from the patient. Refer to Table 20 in the section on brachytherapy for time-distance relationships for dose control.

For patients treated with solutions, colloidal suspensions, or microspheres, there is concern for direct radiation levels as for the sealed sources. Also, there is concern for possible radioactive contamination of personnel from direct contact with the patient or the patient's excreta. Contamination control involves good housekeeping procedures, such as wearing rubber or plastic gloves when handling the patient or other items that have been in direct contact with the patient, including linen, utensils and dinnerware, etc. Items that may be contaminated must be collected and sealed in plastic bags for appropriate disposal. NRC Regulatory Guide 10.8 gives an example of a convenient form that may be used to provide nursing instructions for patients treated with solutions or suspensions of ^{32}P, ^{198}Au, or ^{131}I (see Figure 21).

Doses to other patients and to visitors must be controlled using the same approach as previously discussed for brachytherapy sources. The NCRP recommends that pregnant women and children not, in general, be allowed to visit patients who contain an appreciable amount of radioactivity. Doses to other patients in the vicinity of those being treated should be kept below 100 mrem through the use of distance and time limitations.

For nonsealed radioactive sources (solutions, suspensions), the NRC generally requires that patients not be permitted to be released from the hospital until they contain

NURSING INSTRUCTIONS FOR PATIENTS TREATED WITH PHOSPHORUS-32, GOLD-198, OR IODINE-131

Patient's Name: ______________________________

Room No.: ____________ Physician's Name: ____________________

Radioisotope Administered: ______________________________

Date and Time of Administration: ______________________________

Dose Received: ____________ Method of Administration: ____________________

Exposure Rates in mRem/hr

Date	3 feet from bed	10 feet from bed

(Comply with all checked items.)

_______ 1. Visiting time permitted: ______________________________

_______ 2. Visitors must remain ______________________________ from patient.

_______ 3. Patient may not leave room.

_______ 4. Visitors under 18 are not permitted.

_______ 5. Pregnant visitors are not permitted.

_______ 6. Film badges must be worn.

_______ 7. Tag the following objects and fill out the tag:

_____ door

_____ bed

_____ chart

_____ wrist

_______ 8. Gloves must be worn while attending patient.

_______ 9. Patient must use disposable utensils.

_______ 10. All items must remain in room until approved by the Radiation Safety Officer or his designee.

_______ 11. Smoking is not permitted.

_______ 12. Room is not to be released to Admitting Office until approved by the Radiation Safety Officer or his designee.

_______ 13. Other instructions.

In case of an emergency contact:

RSO ______________________________ ____________ / ____________

Name   On-duty/Off-duty Telephone Nos.

FIGURE 21. Nursing instructions for patients treated with ^{32}P, ^{198}Au, or ^{131}I. (From Regulatory Guide 10.8, U.S. Nuclear Regulatory Commission, Washington, D.C., 1979.)

Table 21
RADIOACTIVITY LEVELS FOR DISCHARGE OF RADIOACTIVE PATIENTS FROM HOSPITAL

	No restrictions		All persons in household over 45 years of age[a]		Some members of household under 45 years of age[b]	
Radionuclide	Exposure rate at 1 m (mR/hr)	Activity at discharge (mCi)	Exposure rate at 1 m (mR/hr)	Activity at discharge (mCi)	Exposure rate at 1 m (mR/hr)	Activity at discharge (mCi)
^{51}Cr	0.5	35	5	350	1.5	100
^{198}Au	5.3	23	53	230	16	70
^{125}I	0.2	8—80[c]	2	20—800[c]	0.6	25—250[c]
^{131}I	1.8	8	18	80	11	50
^{222}Rn	3.8	4.6	38	46	15	18
^{192}Ir	0.2	0.4	2	4	0.6	1.2
^{182}Ta	0.1	0.2	1	2	0.3	0.6

[a] These levels are, in general, higher than any likely to be encountered.
[b] These values are rather arbitrarily selected on a basis of the probability of the situation. They represent complete integrated doses of between 1.5 and 2.5 R.
[c] These values cover a large range, due to the variable attenuation of the 35 keV X-rays in the patient.

From Precautions in the Management of Patients Who Have Received Therapeutic Amounts of Radionuclides, NCRP Rep. No. 37, U.S. National Council on Radiation Protection and Measurements, Washington, D.C., October 1, 1970. With permission.

less than 30 mCi of radioactivity. The NCRP recommends (based on exposure rates rather than activity levels) that a patient not be dismissed until his body burden is not likely to result in a dose to other persons in excess of 0.5 rem. Exceptions to this are permitted for situations where the "other persons" exposed by the patient are over age 45. Table 21 summarizes the recommendations of the NCRP for permitting discharge of radioactive patients from the hospital. In the case of emergency surgery or death of a radioactive patient, as well as for autopsy, burial, or cremation, NCRP Report No. 37 should be consulted for additional recommendations on precautions.

GENERAL REFERENCES

Brodsky, A., Principles and Practices for Keeping Occupational Radiation Exposures at Medical Institutions as Low as Reasonably Achievable, Draft, U.S. Nuclear Regulatory Commission Rep. NUREG-0267, Office of Standards and Development, Washington, D.C., 1977.

Braestrup, C. E. and Vikteslof, K. J., Manual of Radiation Protection in Hospitals and General Practice, Vol. 1, Basic Protection Requirements, World Health Organization, Geneva, 1974.

Health Physics Society, Health Physics in the Healing Arts, Proc. 7th Midyear Symp. Health Phys. Soc. U.S. Department of Health, Education, and Welfare Publ. No. (FDA) 73-8029, San Juan, Puerto Rico, 1972.

International Commission on Radiological Protection, Report of Committee Five on the Handling and Disposal of Radioactive Materials in Hospitals and Medical Research Establishments, ICRP Rep. No. 5, Pergamon Press, Elmsford, N.Y., 1965.

American National Standards Institute, Guidelines for Maintaining ^{60}Co and ^{137}Teletherapy Equipment, ANSI N449-1974, American National Standards Institute, New York, 1973.

U.S. National Council on Radiation Protection and Measurements, Medical Radiation Exposures of Pregnant and Potentially Pregnant Women, NCRP Rep. No. 54, National Council on Radiation Protection Publications, Washington, D.C., 1977.

Straub, C. P., Ed., *CRC Handbook of Environmental Control, Volume V, Hospital and Health Care Facilities,* Chemical Rubber Co., Cleveland, 1975.

Bushong, S. C., *The Development of Radiation Protection in Diagnostic Radiology,* Chemical Rubber Co., Cleveland, 1973.

Bond, R. G., et al., Eds., *Environmental Health and Safety in Health-Care Facilities,* Macmillan, New York, 1973.

International Commission on Radiological Protection, Protection of the Patient in X-ray Diagnosis, ICRP Publ. No. 16, Pergamon Press, Elmsford, N.Y., 1970.

International Commission on Radiological Protection, Protection of the Patient in Radionuclide Investigations, ICRP Publ. No. 17, Pergamon Press, Elmsford, N.Y., 1971.

REFERENCES

1. **Daniel, J.,** The X-rays, *Science,* 3, 562, 1896.
2. **Scott, N. S.,** X-ray injuries, *Am. X-Ray J.,* 1, 57, 1897.
3. **Heineke, H.,** Ueber die Einwirkung der Röntgenstrahlung auftiere, *Muench. Med. Wochsenchr.,* 50, 2090, 1903.
4. **Hesse, O.,** Das Rötgenkarzinom, *Fortschr. Geb. Röentgenstr.,* 17, 82, 1911.
5. **Rolleston, H.,** The effects of radiation on patients and radiologists, and protection *Univ. Br. J. Radiol.,* 23, 264, 1927.
6. National Academy of Sciences-National Research Council, The Effects on Populations of Exposure to Low Levels of Ionizing Radiation, Report of the Advisory Committee on the Biological Effects of Ionizing Radiation, National Academy of Sciences-National Research Council, Washington, D.C., 1972.
7. **Stewart, A., and Kneale, G. W.,** Changes in cancer risk associated with obstetric radiography, *Lancet,* 1, 104, 1968.
8. **MacMahon, B.,** Prenatal X-ray exposure and childhood cancer, *J. Natl. Cancer Inst.,* 28, 1173, 1962.
9. **Oppenheim, B. E., Griem, M. L., and Meier, P.,** The effects of diagnostic X-ray exposure on the human fetus: an examination of the evidence, *Radiology,* 114, 529, 1975.
10. **Oppenheim, B. E.,** Genetic damage from diagnostic radiation?, *JAMA,* 242, 1390, 1979.
11. **Stewart, A. M., Mancuso, T. F., and Kneale, G.,** Radiation exposures of Hanford workers dying from various causes, *Proc. 10th Midyear Symp. Health Phys. Soc.,* Northeastern New York Chapter, Health Physics Society, Troy, N.Y., 1976, 204.
12. **Mancuso, T. F., Stewart, A., and Kneale, G.,** Radiation exposures of Hanford workers dying from cancer and other causes, *Health Phys.,* 33, 369, 1977.
13. **Anderson, T. W.,** Radiation exposures of Hanford workers: a critique of the Mancuso, Stewart, and Kneale report, *Health Phys.,* 35, 743, 1978.
14. **Najarian, T. and Cotton, T.,** Mortality from leukemia and cancer in shipyard nuclear workers, *Lancet,* 1, 1018, 1978.

15. **Najarian, T.**, The controversy over the health effects of radiation, *Technol. Rev.*, 80, 74, 1978.
16. **Bertell, Rosalie,** The nuclear worker and ionizing radiation, *Am. Ind. Hyg. Assoc. J.*, 40, 395, 1979.
17. **Spear, F. G., Russ, S., Andrew, C., and Carling, E. R.**, *Br. J. Radiol.*, 26, 553, 1953.
18. **Rollins, W.**, Apparatus for X-light diagnosis, *Electr. Rev. (London)*, 40, 795, 1902.
19. **Rollins, W.**, *Notes on X-Light*, privately printed, Boston, 1902.
20. **Mutscheller, A.**, Physical standards of protection against X-ray hazards, *Am. J. Roentgenol.*, 13, 65, 1925.
21. International Committee on X-ray and Radium Protection, X-ray and radium protection: recommendations of the international Congress of radiology, *Br. J. Radiol.*, 1, 359, 1928.
22. International Committee on X-ray and Radium Protection, International recommendations for X-ray and radium protection, 1934, *Radiology*, 23, 682, 1934.
23. **Morgan, K. Z.**, Maximum permissible exposure levels — external and internal, in *Principles of Radiation Protection*, Morgan, K. Z. and Turner, J. E., Eds., John Wiley & Sons, New York, 1967, 497.
24. International Commission on Radiological Protection, Recommendations of the International Commission on Radiological Protection (Adopted 9, 1958), Pergamon Press, Oxford, 1959.
25. U.S. National Council on Radiation Protection and Measurements, Basic Radiation Protection Criteria, NCRP Rep. No. 39, U.S. National Council on Radiation Protection Publications, Washington, D.C., 1971.
26. International Commission on Radiological Protection, Recommendations of the international commission on radiological protection (revised December 1954), *Br. J. Radiol.*, Suppl. 6, 1, 1955.
27. International Commission on Radiological Protection, Recommendations of the ICPP (Adopted September 17, 1965), Publ. No. 9, Pergamon Press, Oxford, 1966.
28. U.S. Nuclear Regulatory Commission, Personnel Selection and Training, Regulatory Guide 1.8, U.S. Nuclear Regulatory Commission, Washington, D.C., 1975.
29. Bureau of Radiological Health, Regulations for the Administration and Enforcement of the Radiation Control for Health and Safety Act of 1968, U.S. Department of Health, Education, and Welfare Publ. (FDA) 79-8035, Public Health Service, Washington, D.C., 1978.
30. International Commission on Radiological Protection, Report of Committe II on Permissible Dose for Internal Radiation, ICRP Publ. No. 2, Pergamon Press, New York, 1959.
31. U.S. Nuclear Regulatory Commission, Standards for Protection Against Radiation, Title 10, Part 20, Code of Federal Regulations U.S. Government Printing Office, Washington, D.C., 1978.
32. U.S. National Council on Radiation Protection and Measurements, Structural Shielding Design and Evaluation for Medical Use of X-Rays and Gamma Rays of Energies up to 10 MeV, NCRP Rep. No. 49, U.S. National Council on Radiation Protection Publications, Washington, D.C., 1976.
33. **Wade, L., Jr.**, Accidental ^{60}Co exposure at the University of Tennessee — atomic energy commission agricultural research laboratory, *Nucl. Saf.*, 13, 304, 1972.
34. U.S. Nuclear Regulatory Commission, Guide for the Preparation of Applications for Medical Programs, Regulatory Guide 10.8, U.S. Nuclear Regulatory Commission, Washington, D.C., 1979.
35. **Quimby, E. H.**, *Safe Handling of Radioactive Isotopes in Medical Practice*, Macmillan, New York, 1960.
36. U.S. National Council on Radiation Protection and Measurements, Instrumentation and Monitoring Methods for Radiation Protection, NCRP Rep. No. 57, U.S. National Council on Radiation Protection Publications, Washington, D.C., 1978.
37. U.S. National Council on Radiation Protection and Measurements, Medical X-Ray and Gamma-Ray Protection for Energies Up to 10 Mev, Equipment Design and Use, NCRP Rep. No. 33, U.S. National Council on Radiation Protection Publications, Washington, D.C., 1968.
38. Bureau of Radiological Health, BRH Routine Compliance Testing for Diagnostic X-ray Systems or Components of Diagnostic X-ray Systems to which 21 CFR Subchapter J is Applicable, U.S. Department of Health, Education, and Welfare Publ. (FDA) 77-8001, 1976.
39. **Hendee, W. R. and Chaney, E. L.**, Diagnostic X-ray survey procedures for fluoroscopic installation — part 1: undertable units, *Health Phys.*, 29, 331, 1975.
40. **Dunlap, J. H.**, Survey form and techniques for fluoroscopic installations with undertable tubes, *Health Phys.*, 33, 3, 1977.
41. **Collier, W. C.**, Routine evaluation of the diagnostic X-ray equipment in a large hospital, in Health Physics in the Healing Arts, Proc. Health Phys. Soc. 7th Midyear Topical Symp., U.S. Department of Health, Education, and Welfare Publ. (FDA) 73-8027, Bureau of Radiological Health, 1973, 163.
42. **Repacholi, M. H. and Jack, G. C.**, Photofluorographic X-ray machine chest exposure and survey techniques, in Health Physics in the Healing Arts, Proc. Health Phys. Soc. 7th Midyear Topical Symp.,U.S. Department of Health, Education, and Welfare Publ. (FDA) 73-8029, Bureau of Radiological Health, 1973, 185.
43. Bureau of Radiological Health, Radiation Protection Survey Report Manual, Public Health Service Publ. No. 1582, U.S. Public Health Service, Washington, D.C., 1965.

44. U.S. National Council on Radiation Protection and Measurements, Radiation Protection for Medical and Allied Health Personnel, NCRP Rep. No. 48, U.S. National Council on Radiation Protection Publications, Washington, D.C., 1976.
45. **Hendee, W. R., Chaney, E. L. and Rossi, R. P.,** *Radiological Physics, Equipment and Quality Control,* Year Book Medical Publishing, Chicago, 1977.
46. Bureau of Radiological Health, Gonad Doses and Genetically Significant Dose from Diagnostic Radiology, U.S., 1964 and 1970, U.S. Department of Health, Education, and Welfare Publ. (FDA) 76-8034, Public Health Service, U.S. Government Printing Office, Washington, D.C., 1976.
47. **Shleien, B., Tucker, T. T., and Johnson, D. W.,** The Mean Active Bone Marrow Dose to the Adult Population of the U.S. from Diagnostic Radiology, U.S. Department of Health, Education, and Welfare Publ. (FDA) 77-843, Bureau of Radiological Health, Public Health Service, U.S. Government Printing Office, Washington, D.C., 1977.
48. Bureau of Radiological Health, Published Letter to X-ray Users Dated October 10, 1978 from John C. Villforth, Director, BRH, U.S. Public Health Service, Food and Drug Administration, Rockville, 1978.
49. **Koenig, G. F.,** Quality control in radiography, a primary responsibility of the technologist, in Reduction of Radiation Dose in Diagnostic X-Ray Procedures, Proc. Symp. U.S. Department of Health, Education, and Welfare Publ. No. (FDA) 73-8009 BRH/DMRE 73-1, U.S. Government Printing Office, Washington, D.C., 1972, 123.
50. **Koenig, G. F.,** Quality control in radiography, a primary responsibility of the technologist, in Quality Control in Medical X-Ray, Proc. Radiological Health Section of the American Public Health Association Meeting, November 1972, U.S. Department of Health, Education, and Welfare Publ. (FDA) 74-8002, U.S. Government Printing Office, Washington, D.C., 1973, 7.
51. **Shaver, J. W., Hardin, C. H., and Lubenau, M. S.,** Nationwide evaluation of X-ray trends, in Quality Control in Medical X-Ray, U.S. Department of Health, Education, and Welfare Publ. (FDA) 74-8002, Bureau of Radiological Health, U.S. Government Printing Office, Washington, D.C., 1973.
52. **Cameron, J. R. and Bassano, D. A.,** An Improved Method for Quality Control in Diagnostic Radiology, unpublished paper, Department of Radiology, University of Wisconsin, Madison, 1972.
53. **Cameron, J. R.,** The role of the medical physicist in quality control in diagnostic X-Ray departments, in Quality Control in Medical X-Ray, Proc. Radiological Health Section of the American Public Health Association Meeting, November 1972, U.S. Department of Health, Education, and Welfare Publ. (FDA) 74-8002, U.S. Government Printing Office, Washington, D.C., 1973, 13.
54. **Vanderwalker, R. D., Ed.,** *Use of Radioisotopes in Hospitals,* American Hospital Association, Chicago, 1967, 66.
55. U.S. Nuclear Regulatory Commission, Information Relevant to Ensuring that Occupational Radiation Exposures at Medical Institutions Will Be as Low as Reasonably Achievable, NRC Regulatory Guide 8.18, U.S. Nuclear Regulatory Commission, Washington, D.C., 1977.
56. National Bureau of Standards, Safe Handling of Radioactive Materials, National Committee on Radiation Protection Rep. No. 30, NBS Handbook No. 92, U.S. Government Printing Office, Washington, D.C., 1964.
57. International Commission on Radiological Protection, Report of Committee V on the Handling and Disposal of Radioactive Material in Hospitals and Medical Research Establishments, ICRP Publ. No. 5, Pergamon Press, New York, 1965.
58. American Institute of Chemical Engineers, American Standard Design Guide for a Radioisotope Laboratory (Type B), Std. No. 5.2-1963, American Standards Association, New York, 1964.
59. International Atomic Energy Agency, Radiation Protection Procedures, IAEA Safety Ser. No. 38, International Atomic Energy Agency, Vienna, 1973.
60. U.S. Nuclear Regulatory Commission, Applications of Bioassay for I-125 and I-131, NRC Regulatory Guide 8.20, U.S. Nuclear Regulatory Commission, Washington, D.C., 1979.
61. International Commission on Radiological Protection, Report of Committee IV on Evaluation of Radiation Dose to Body Tissues from Internal Contamination Due to Occupational Exposure, ICRP Publ. No. 10, Pergamon Press, Elmsford, N.Y., 1968.
62. **Orvis, A. L.,** What is a reportable thyroid burden, in Operational Health Physics, Proc. 9th Midyear Topical Symp. Health Phys. Soc., Denver, 1976, 268.
63. **Brodsky, A.,** Determination of facilities, equipment, and procedures required for various types of operations, in *Handbook of Radioactive Nuclides,* Wang, Y., Ed., Chemical Rubber Co., Cleveland, 1969, 664.
64. **Beck, T. J., McCampbell, M. R., and Cooley, L. R.,** A profile of institutional radioactive wastes generated in 1977, in Low-Level Radioactive Waste Management, Proc. Health Phys. Soc. 12th Midyear Topical Symp., Environmental Protection Agency Rep. 520/3-79-002, Williamsburg, 1979, 27.
65. **Granlund, R. W. and Hayes, J. F.,** Solidification of low-level radioactive liquid waste using a cement-silicate process, in Low Level Radioactive Waste Management, Proc. Health Phys. Soc. 12th Midyear Topical Symp., Environmental Protection Agency Rep. 520/3-79-002, Williamsburg, 1979, 91.

66. **Wright, C. C., Lowi, A., Fisk, D. P., Harwood, G. E., and Nakamura, R. M.,** Absorption distillation, a new method for the concentration of liquid scintillation waste for focile disposal, paper presented at the 5th Biennial Campus Radiation Safety Officers Conference, University of California, Irvine, August 1975.
67. **Wagner, H. N., Jr.,** The design of new radiopharmaceuticals, in Medical Radionuclides: Radiation Dose and Effects, Proc. Symp., USAEC CONF 691212, Oak Ridge Associated Universities, Tennessee, 1970, 453.
68. **Wagner, H. N., Jr. and Emmons, H.,** Characteristics of an ideal radiopharmaceutical, in Radioactive Pharmaceuticals, Proc. Symp., USAEC CONF 651111, Oak Ridge Associate Universities, Tennessee, 1966, 1.
69. **Cloutier, R. J. and Watson, E. E.** Radiation doses from nuclear medicine procedures, in Health Physics in the Health Arts, Proc. 7th Midyear Topical Symp. Health Phys. Soc., U.S. Department of Health, Education, and Welfare Publ. (FDA) 73-8029, U.S. Government Printing Office, Washington, D.C., 1973, 7.
70. International Commission on Radiological Protection, Protection of the Patient in Radionuclide Investigations, ICRP Publ. No. 17, Pergamon Press, New York, 1971.
71. **Loevinger, R. and Berman, M.,** A schema for absorbed dose calculations for biologically disturbed radionuclides, *J. Nucl. Med.,* 9, (Suppl. 1), 10, 1968.
72. **Dillman, L. T. and Von der Lage,** Radionuclide Decay Schemes and Nuclear Parameters for Use in Radiation Dose Estimation, MIRD Pamphlet No. 10, Society of Nuclear Medicine, New York, 1975.
73. NRC asks licensees to verify teletherapy output, in Health Physics Newsletter IV, No. 10, Health Physics Society, Bethesda, Md., October 1976, 10.
74. **Lane, R. G., Tolbert, B. R., Palival, B. R., and Radtke, R. R.,** Radiation incidents with a cobalt-60 teletherapy unit, *Health Phys.,* 31, 163, 1976.
75. U.S. National Council on Radiation Protection and Measurements, Protection Against Radiation from Brachytherapy Sources, NCRP Rep. No. 40, U.S. National Council on Radiation Protection Publications, Washington, D.C., 1972.
76. **Tapert, A. C. and Lea, W. L.,** The Survey of Medical Radium Installations in Wisconsin, U.S. Department of Health, Education, and Welfare Publ. (FDA) 75-8022, Bureau of Radiological Health, Rockville, 1975.
77. **Hale, J.,** A method for testing radium containers for leakage using the well-type scintillation counter, *Radiology,* 72, 105, 1959.
78. **Rose, J. E.,** Simple test for leaking radium sources, *Am. J. Roentgenol. Radium Ther. Nucl. Med.,* 90, 403, 1963.
79. **Gallaghar, R. G., Evans, R. D., and McAllister, R. G.,** Testing radium capsules for radon leakage, *Am. J. Roentgenol. Radium Ther. Nucl. Med.,* 2, 396, 1963.
80. **Bedrosian, P. H.,** Photographic technique for leak testing radium sources, *Am. J. Roentgenol. Radium Ther. Nucl. Med.,* 102, 207, 1968.
81. **Rozenfeld, M. L. and Mason, E. W.,** Daily leak testing of the entire stock in a radium safe, in A Collection of Radium Leak Test Articles, U.S. Public Health Service Publ. MORP 68-1, U.S. Government Printing Office, Washington, D.C., 1968, 87.
82. **Benson, J. S. and Fetz, R. N.,** A technique in testing radium sources for leakage, *Am. J. Roentgenol. Radium Ther. Nucl. Med.,* 99, 479, 1967.
83. **Villforth, J. C. and McClain, P. W.,** An approach to leak testing of sealed radium sources, in A Collection of Radium Leak Test Articles, U.S. Public Health Service Publ. MORP 68-1, U.S. Government Printing Office, Washington, D.C., 1968, 101.
84. U.S. National Council on Radiation Protection and Measurements, Precautions in the Management of Patients Who Have Received Therapeutic Amounts of Radionuclides, NCRP Rep. No. 37, U.S. National Council on Radiation Protection Publications, Washington, D.C., 1972.

PREVENTION, PRINCIPLES, AND TECHNIQUES IN LIFTING, TRANSPORTING, AND BODY MECHANICS

Ruth Joyce Barnes

INTRODUCTION

Most health care personnel have been exposed to the basic principles of good body mechanics as it applies to lifting and transporting. The main focus expressed here will be reemphasizing body mechanic techniques, injury-prevention measures, and utilization of these principles and techniques to avoid strain or trauma to the patient or personnel.

Many variables are inherent in the approach to the proper selection and implementation of lifting and transporting techniques to be utilized for safe patient care or personnel practices. The appropriate technique must provide consistency with the level of activity designated by the apparent condition of the patient, as well as limitations prescribed by the physician. It is essential as health care personnel, that the utilization of a team approach be implemented in order to provide a safe hospital environment and share in the responsibility of safeguarding patients, visitors, and fellow staff members.

Good rules that prevent injury or trauma begin with a basic understanding and acceptance of general principles of body mechanics, and being able to cope with the every day stress of living. Prevention starts with knowing what occurs within our body as we move during the day. A slight review of anatomy reveals that fluid is between every joint of our body. As we move during the day, we squeeze some of this fluid out. If we strain or make incorrect moves, more fluid squeezes out. If these incorrect moves continue to occur, pains or aches may appear. Do not expect to encounter pain or discomfort every time you abuse good body mechanics. Very often your muscles are able to tolerate abuse to a high degree; eventually, poor body mechanics will tell its toll on you. The ligaments protect every joint in the body and when an injury such as strains or sprains occur, the discomfort and damage that occurs usually manifest itself in the ligaments.[1] Pain is a warning that an injury has occurred; it may mean the bones do not have the lubrication they need.

The discs of the back are between every vertebra, which are filled with fluid. The cervical area is very vulnerable to strain. Without our doing anything at all, one tenth of our weight goes into the cervical discs. Just imagine the number of times during the day that you bend, twist, turn, or reach. Very often, this is the cause for pain in the posterior base of the neck. The low back is the next greatest strain area (think of the weight you are carrying on that area, and how often you bend, twist, turn, sit, and stand).

Gravity is most important in any lifting procedure, whether it be a patient or pencil. In a standing position, the shoulder level is the line of balance. The center of gravity is the mid-body section, and the foundation or base of support is your feet. Always watch your balance range. Muscle usage is the key to good lifting and handling techniques. The arms act as mechanical levers. The muscles in the arms (biceps and triceps), the abdominal and gluteal muscles, and those in the thighs and legs are the stronger muscular groups. When strenuous work is necessary, you can become adequately prepared by learning to use your muscles properly.[2]

The most essential step in good body mechanics begins with the practice of correct posture. Good posture denotes correct body alignment during various position changes and activities. How do we know when we are utilizing good posture? It is functioning

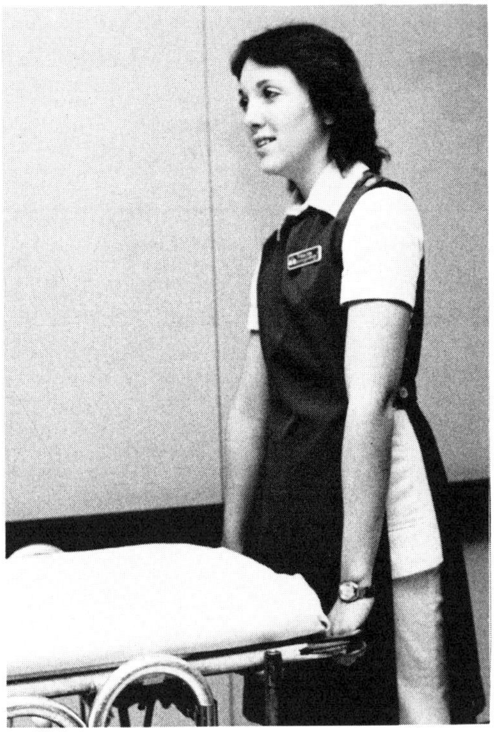

FIGURE 1. Stand close to the subject. (Courtesy of St. Elizabeth's Hospital, Lafayette, Ind.)

when the muscular and skeletal systems are performing efficiently with a minimum of energy use. This efficient performance manifests itself in many ways, i.e., a lessened feeling of fatigue, a more exuberant appearance, and a general overall feeling of well-being.

Lack of good muscle tone has been the leading cause of chronic backache problems. Many well-defined studies show that up to 70 to 80% of the findings of chronic backaches result from the poor muscle tone in the inner girdle area. This area supports all the underlying pelvic structural region.

GOOD ALIGNMENT AND BODY MECHANICS

Good alignment and body mechanics include the following:

- Understand the basis of momentum and gravity, and use both when possible. Pull or slide, but never lift when you do not have to.
- Arms can be like mechanical levers. Utilize a mechanical advantage — brace yourself.
- Keep a good line of balance by keeping all parts of the body as close as possible to the vertical axis of the body.
- Assume a close position to the object or person you must lift. Keep your back straight, do not reach for the load, move in close, and use your leg muscles, not your back. (see Figure 1).
- Return to an erect position as soon as possible when lifting or handling. Do not remain in a bent position when you can accomplish the same thing in an erect stance.

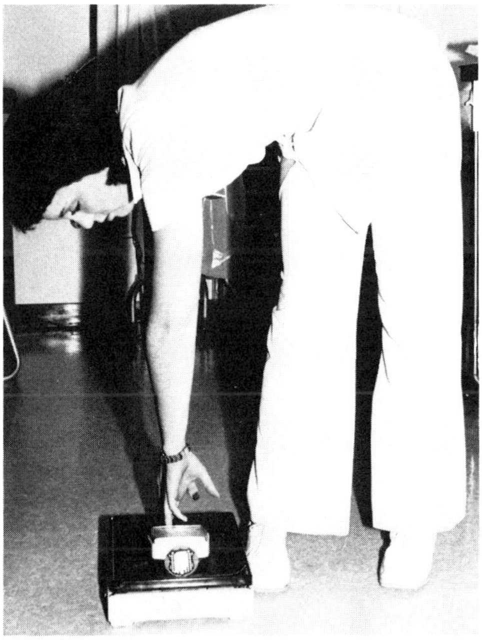

FIGURE 2. Never twist your body. (Courtesy of St. Elizabeth's Hospital, Lafayette, Ind.)

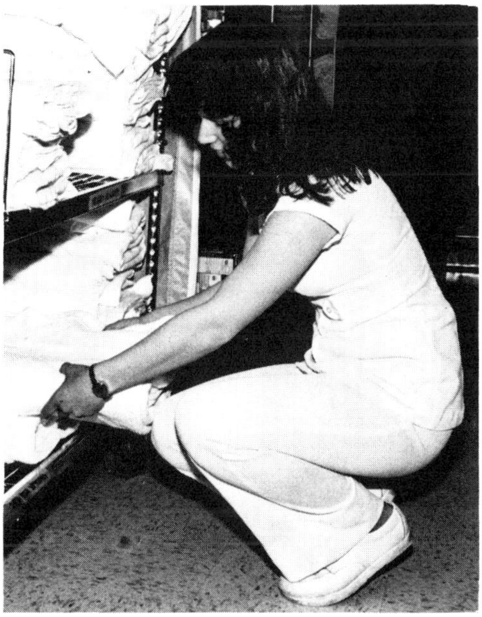

FIGURE 3. Bend your knees. (Courtesy of St. Elizabeth's Hospital, Lafayette, Ind.)

- Never twist when lifting. Keep spine stationary and change the position of your feet. Keep your back straight (see Figure 2).
- Always keep a wide base of support. Spread your feet and advance one leg slightly in front of the other.
- Remember to utilize the strong leg and abdominal muscles when lifting. When possible, pull, do not push, and use your legs, not your arms and back (see Figures 3, 4, 5, and 6).

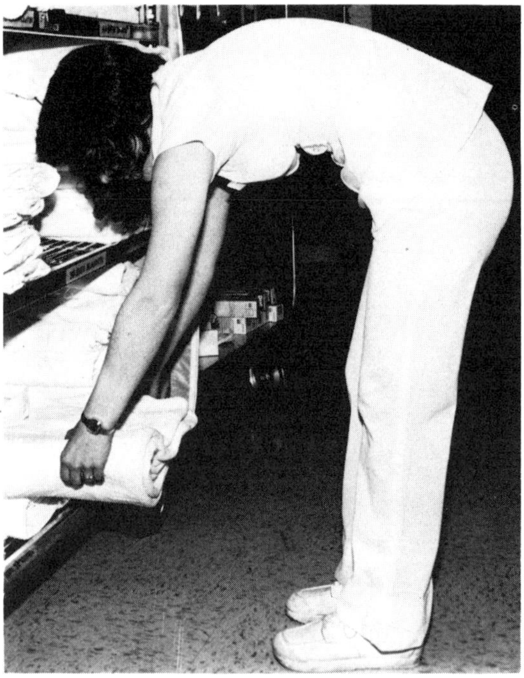

FIGURE 4. Do not bend your back. (Courtesy of St. Elizabeth's Hospital, Lafayette, Ind.)

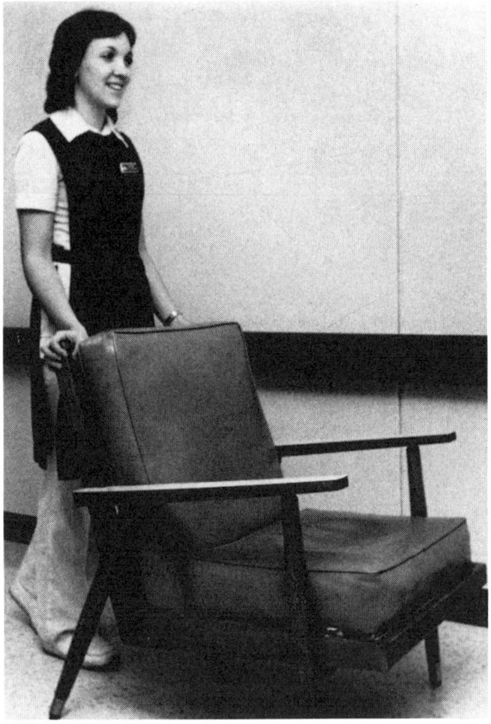

FIGURE 5. Push or pull. (Courtesy of St. Elizabeth's Hospital, Lafayette, Ind.)

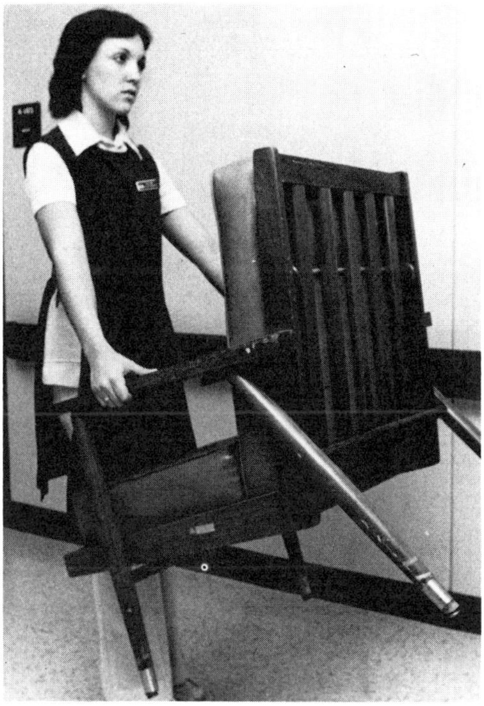

FIGURE 6. Do not lift. (Courtesy of St. Elizabeth's Hospital, Lafayette, Ind.)

- Always squat or kneel when it becomes necessary to work in a lower position.
- Pay close attention to your surrounding area before starting to lift in order to allow unobstructed range and movement.

The key to lifting and handling (whether it be a patient or an object) is planning. Always plan in advance when possible; announce the method to be used. Also, obtain assistance when needed. Always evaluate the load that is to be moved or lifted. Never attempt to lift alone if you have any doubt about your ability to do so alone. If the load requires assistance, lift smoothly and together (it is more effective if you count 1, 2, 3) with the person assisting you (see Figure 7).

TRANSFERRING PATIENTS

In any transferring activity where patients are concerned, the first step is to assess the capabilities of the patient.

1. Are there any restrictions in mobility?
2. What is the basic physiological and psychological condition of the patient?
3. Is the patient capable of understanding your moving instructions?

If possible, when lifting or moving a patient be sure that the patient understands what is going to occur. Explain the details of the lift or move, including the where, when, and how (see Figure 8). For turning or rolling, see Figure 9. Now:

- Face the patient, stand with one leg slightly forward, and get as close as possible to the bed or cart.

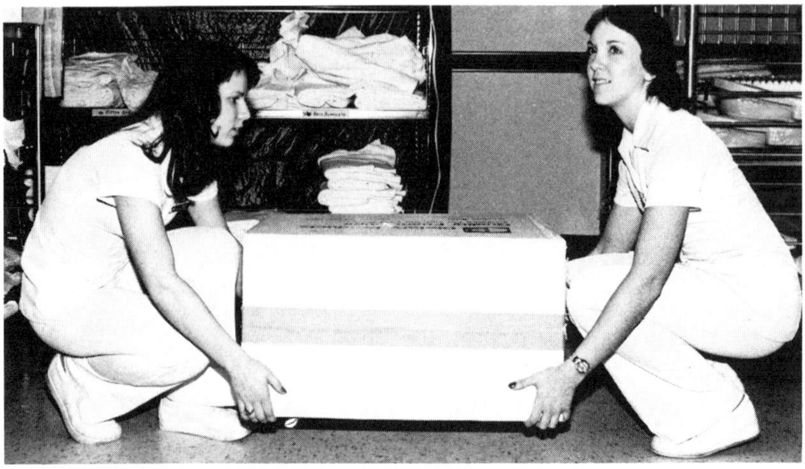

FIGURE 7. Be a team; work together. (Courtesy of St. Elizabeth's Hospital, Lafayette, Ind.)

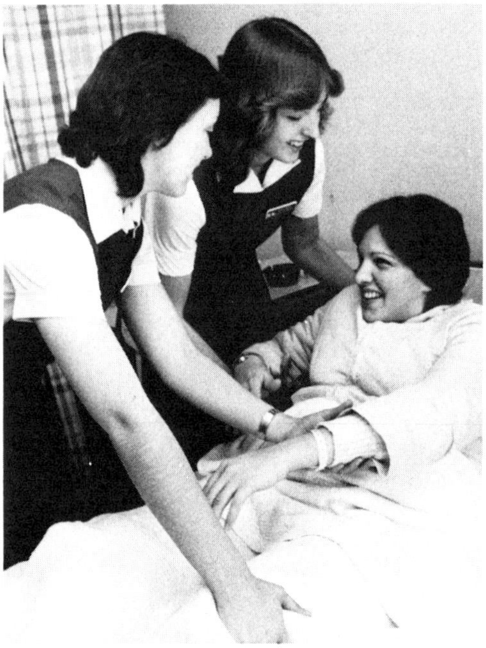

FIGURE 8. Tell your patient what you are doing. (Courtesy of St. Elizabeth's Hospital, Lafayette, Ind.)

- Shift your weight to the advanced leg.
- Working as a team, allow your weight to shift from the forward to the backward leg, at the same time straightening your elbows and turning the patient.
- For transfer to the side, up, or down in bed, turn or transfer sheets are highly recommended.
- Always estimate load. If large, get assistance, using a two- to three-person transfer.
- In a two-person transfer, hand placement is important. Move patient's legs to the side and stabilize arms across abdomen.

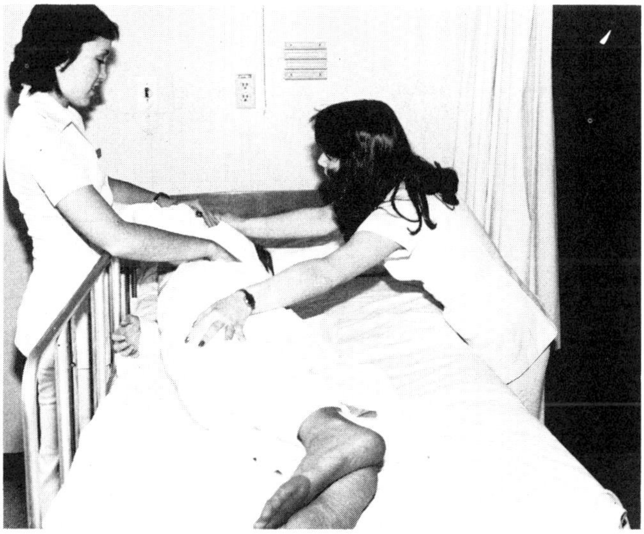

FIGURE 9. Turning or rolling the patient. (Courtesy of St. Elizabeth's Hospital, Lafayette, Ind.)

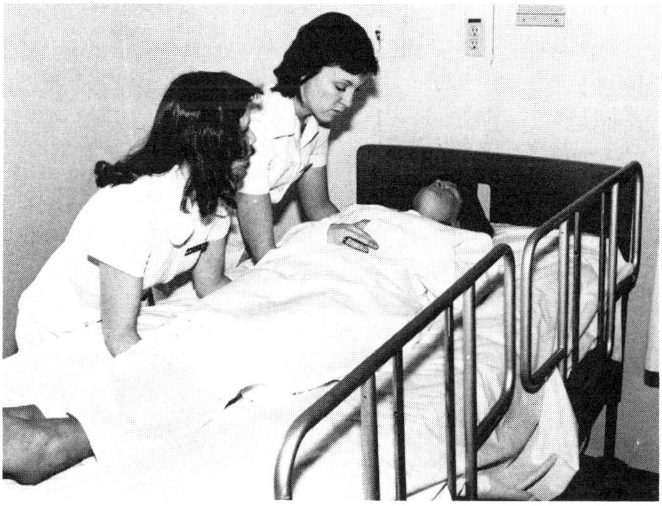

FIGURE 10. Moving the patient to the side. (Courtesy of St. Elizabeth's Hospital, Lafayette, Ind.)

- Number one person, place left arm under neck and grasp opposite shoulder of patient, supporting the head. Place right arm under lower chest, almost waist level, and grasp lower portion of patient's opposite arm.
- Person number two places hands under buttocks as shown in Figure 10 for a side move and Figure 11 for a move up in bed.

There are many other transfer and lifting techniques for you to be knowledgeable about, and they are essential for your personal safety, as well as the safety of the patient. The central theme here is to offer you a preventive mode. Your hospital safety manager can be a valuable resource in gathering material on the proper body mechanic techniques.

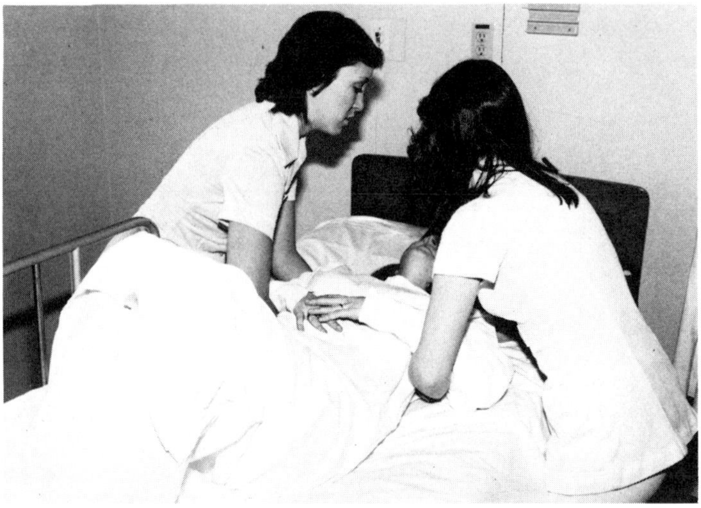

FIGURE 11. Up in bed. (Courtesy of St. Elizabeth's Hospital, Lafayette, Ind.)

SOME CASE HISTORIES

Over a period of years, I have gathered case situations relating to injuries that I would like to share with you. Review them carefully and think about what could have possibly prevented the occurrence. They have been collected from many health care settings, and any direct resemblance is purely coincidental.

Case A

A female employee moved an obese patient up in bed without assistance. The patient became confused as to instructions relating to the move. Severe back pain resulted and was reported by the employee. Extensive treatment and time loss followed. What steps could have been taken to prevent this occurrence?

Case B

A female employee moved a mattress while cleaning a bed. She did not request assistance to move the mattress. She reported severe back pain and extensive treatment was administered, including numerous physician visits and tests. There was prolonged absence from job duties because of recurrent pain. What are the many difficulties you see here?

Case C

A male employee lifted heavy equipment from a shelf higher than his waist level, although he had been instructed to obtain assistance and a ladder. This employee suffered both back and arm injuries. Was this an emergency situation? Could this not have been prevented?

Case D

A female employee lifted a heavy tray in a dish area without requesting assistance. As she turned holding the tray, she twisted her back. Perhaps she could have eliminated the strain had she not lifted and twisted, a common problem in improper body mechanics.

Case E

While observing a patient during labor, a female employee reported that it became urgently necessary to transfer the patient into the delivery room. In pushing the labor bed, the employee sustained low back pain. Many variables entered into this emergency situation, including the need to push, rather than pull the bed in order to observe the patient better. The employee was well aware of the proper techniques to use. This case was prolonged over a 2½-year span. The employee received extensive care and compensation during this time.

The key issue is to constantly make everyone in your organization aware of the need to be ever visual of possible emergency situations, and to train their reactive abilities to be on a constant personal- and patient-safety alert. What could have helped here in Case E? Was there a way to prevent Case E?

There has been much discussion outlined on preventive measures, including examples and reminders of good body mechanics. The whole key to its utilization begins with you as a health care employee. This discussion should be integrated into your total lifestyle.

Fatigue and strain can be prevented, it is largely up to you. The cosmetic effect of excellent posture should be enough in itself to prompt you into the practice of good posture. The efficiency and comfort of good body alignment during your daily activities will reward you through better physiologic functioning. If problems now exist with your current posture status, start corrective action immediately. As a health care worker, your body is your job. The mental and physical demands made on health care workers are great in our society. The usual degree of lifting, walking, standing, and stooping is tremendous in our daily work lives. We are exposed to many opportunities for failure to use our knowledge as it relates to proper body mechanics. Your performance in daily work activities must be more than adequate. When going about your daily tasks as a health care specialist, remember you are needed, and needed in good shape. Prevention is the key.

BODY MECHANICS AND PREVENTIVE CARE FOR EMPLOYEES

Preventive measures are a very important aspect in the field of body mechanics. James I. McKee has written many articles on body mechanics; the following information is but a small part of his extensive knowledge.

One might ask a very solid question after reading the topic denotation: why would body mechanics be any different in the medical field than in other work settings? What is so different about working with patients than moving cartons of soap, lifting groceries, or filing records? These are concrete challenges to the topic which require careful explanation. The medical industry in the U.S. is the third largest manpower work force. It is a profession that is growing: will it not always be a profession that is needed? As technology grows, the health professions expand, research grows, and education advances, yet we still have one common element that will never change — someone has to work with the patient. McKee believes the patient will always need (in some way) physical help at some stage in rehabilitation.

The spine is a most complex engineering creation of 1400 muscles and ligaments, with usually 134 mobile joints (to some degree) surrounding approximately 32 bones. Therefore, the concept of body mechanics is a deceptively simple topic that many great minds have written books on in the area of prevention care.[3]

McKee's list of sharing points that make any work in the medical field complex, constantly challenging, and mandatorily attentive for the worker follow.

1. This is a high-risk work situation because the weight to be moved — the patient

— is a variable. Body weight differs greatly, shifts constantly, and attains thousands of different positions and angles in bed, a wheelchair, commode, etc. Therefore, the object to be moved is not a constant, and the beginning position for motion varies greatly.

2. Working with patients who are medicated can allow for many situations where cooperation is not always prevalent. Mental clarity is usually fuzzy, and a post-operative patient moves differently than he did before, creating apprehension, pain, and stress for both parties.[4]
3. Due to many reasons (some of which are mental), "Why do I have to walk? Is it necessary to sit up? I am sure I will fall, and if I do, then I will sue you."
4. The workers in the medical field are moving a weight from many varying positions to another uncommon piece of equipment. Think of the patients that are moved from beds to chairs, commodes, wheelchairs, canes, other helpers, showers, tubs, whirlpools, parallel bars, etc. Imagine the combination of these heights, angles, fabric covering variations, etc. and we can begin to see the complexities of this section.[5]

The education preparation for personnel lifting and handling patients must be re-emphasized through in-service. Again, we face a barrage of factors here.

1. As hospital efficiency improves, more people have to hustle during work; this creates stress and causes injury rates to go up.
2. As the population grows, all medical settings become crowded, necessitating more equipment, people, and cramped conditions.
3. The training in body mechanics may not have existed to the extent that is necessary for todays sophisticated medical practice.
4. The worker who does the lifting must fully understand what type of injury the patient has, and gain full patient cooperation due to the patient's apprehension and insecurity.

We now approach the concept McKee initially denoted. We must think preventive. Why?

1. We must teach specific workers how to handle the patients physically.
2. We must teach them body mechanics and a knowledge of how to move patients (understanding why) with certain injuries.
3. We must help these workers with good body posture awareness.[6]
4. We must teach them how to use assistive equipment.
5. We must, as managers, keep open communication so they will ask for help when needed.
6. These workers deserve decent working hours and controlled shifts.
7. We must teach them how to get cooperation from the patient, and how to know when they will not get cooperation.
8. We must help them with proper foot dress and shoe structures.
9. We must help them care for their back; their back will be involved in their job.

McKee's basic rules of preventive care for the back follow.

1. Never bend from the waist only; bend with the hips and knees when lifting an object from the bed or floor.
2. Never attempt to lift a heavy object higher than your waist — especially not over your head — unless you have help.

3. Turn and directly face the object you wish to move; avoid lifting with the back twisted.
4. Carry heavy objects as close to your body as you can; do not move an object that can suddenly shift in position and surprise you.
5. Never attempt to move or lift an object that is heavier than you think you can handle.
6. Never lift a patient alone; get help or professional assistance.
7. Avoid sudden movements (which cause overloading of muscle groups) when handling patients.
8. Learn to keep the head in line with the spine when standing, sitting, or lying in bed.
9. Wear shoes with moderate heels, and do not cut costs in good footwear. You will be on your feet many hours, so get solid arch support and sole contact with the floor by wearing high quality shoes.
10. Train yourself vigorously to use the abdominal muscles to flatten your stomach. In due time, this muscular contraction will become habitual and people will be envious of your posture.
11. When sleeping at night, lying on the back definitely makes swayback worse. A firm bed does not give in to curves, and we do not need swayback.
12. Try the side-lying position with bent knees and hips for correct sleeping.
13. Do not let the low back arch or attain that hollow; keep it with a minimal curve.
14. To prevent strain and stress in everyday work with the patient, it is restful to change from one position to another to avoid fatigue.
15. Learn how to use assistive equipment in moving difficult patients. Ask for training sessions.
16. Slow down in your work. Do not create problems with the patient.

Finally, inform the patient of what you desire to do. Keep communication open. Ask the patient to help you all he can. You can both work together. If you have a patient's respect for kindness and love in trying to help him, the difficult transfer or move can be made a lot easier. Explain why you would like to move the patient, including where, how, and for how long. Provide a call button or nurse call bell in case the patient needs you; prevent apprehension. If the task is too large in your opinion, get help. Equipment is made to assist you — use it. Try to move the patient smoothly, efficiently, and with concrete direction and clarity.

If you injure an arm or leg, it can be put into a sling or you can ambulate on crutches. However, injure your back and the recuperation period triples; you will have to heal the back and walk, bend, sleep, twist, etc. all at the same time.[8] The healing period is many weeks and unless you are wealthy, not many of us can take 6 weeks off; do not get hurt. Protect that great piece of equipment that is so strong, so mobile, and so supportive — your spine.

This brief discussion has only touched the surface regarding good body mechanics; it is an ongoing never-ending learning process.

Prevention is the key word towards better health care of our industry workers. In turn, this will result in a better cared for patient. Key areas which must be continually emphasized (regarding lifting, transporting, and body mechanics) to health care employees are (1) the importance of a safe environment for the patient, (2) causes of back strain and pain areas, (3) ambulation and nonambulation in relation to patients, (4) strain areas, (5) work areas, and (6) basic rules.

Health care institutions should have an ongoing preventive program in education for body mechanics and transfer techniques. This program should include basic rules or principles of body alignment, including transporting and transfer techniques with

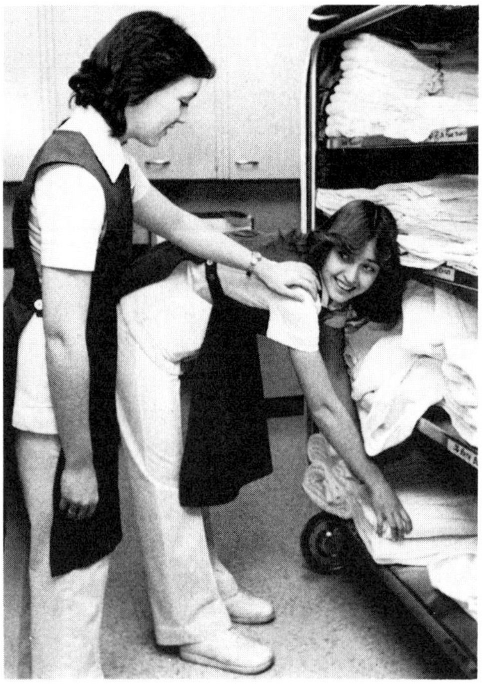

FIGURE 12. Go forth and spread the word to others. (Courtesy of St. Elizabeth's Hospital, Lafayette, Ind.)

demonstration of the correct methodology to use with each technique (e.g., the proper way to move, lift, or turn a patient or an object). Practice sessions should be set up which will enable the learner to give a return demonstration which ensures that learning and understanding has taken place (see Figure 12).

It is essential to reemphasize assessment of load and environment at each session. Often, this assessment can be the initial step in the prevention of injury to staff and patient. Remember the three "Ps" for prevention — planning, posture, and patience — for our health care personnel.

REFERENCES

1. **Larson, C. B. and Gould, M.,** *Orthopedic Nursing,* C. V. Mosby, St. Louis, 1970.
2. **Grollman, S.,** *The Human Body, Its Structure and Physiology,* 2nd ed., Collier MacMillan, Toronto, 1969.
3. **Hoppenfield, S.,** *Physical Examination of the Spine and Extremities,* Appleton-Century-Crofts, New York, 1976, 237.
4. **Tarsy, J. M.,** *Pain Syndromes and Their Treatment,* Charles C Thomas, Springfield, Ill., 1968, 171.
5. **Williams, M. and Worthington, C.,** *Therapeutic Exercises for Body Alignment and Function,* W.B. Saunders, Philadelphia, 1961, 6.
6. **Shands, A., Raney, R., and Brashear, R.** *Handbook of Orthopedic Surgery,* C. V. Mosby, St. Louis, 1963, 81.
7. **Hall, M. C.,** *The Locomotor System — Functional Anatomy,* Charles C Thomas, Springfield, Ill., 1965, 163.
8. **Cailliet, R.,** *Low Back Pain Syndrome,* F. A. Davis, Philadelphia, 1965, 49.

HOSPITAL FACILITY SAFETY AND SECURITY

Robert H. Bartels and Steven O. Beaudoin

HOUSEKEEPING SAFETY

A great portion of the responsibility for maintaining a safe and healthful environment within the hospital rests with the housekeeping department. Some of the things the housekeeping department must deal with on a daily basis include safe storage practices for the prevention of accidental injury and fire, disposal of hazardous wastes, and pest management. All of these things have a great effect on the safety and health of all who enter the hospital. Without a good, well-trained housekeeping department, the opportunity for fire, accidental injury, or infection is greatly increased.

Protection of Employees

It may well be that the housekeeping employee is exposed to more hazardous conditions and is provided with less safety education and personal protective equipment than any other employee in the hospital. All too often, one can walk through the hospital and see a housekeeping employee moving heavy boxes while wearing canvas shoes or sandals. Frequently, a housekeeper can be seen using harsh cleaning solvents with no kind of hand protection. How often does a housekeeper enter a patient's room that has been previously used for isolation, yet is not properly dressed nor wearing any kind of mask or respiratory protection?

To insure that proper equipment is provided and worn is the responsibility of the supervisor. Unfortunately, it is not enough for the supervisor to tell an employee that gloves are required when using cleaning solvents. The supervisor must take the time to explain to the employee why this equipment is required and where it may be obtained. Once this has been done, policies regarding the use of personal protective equipment must be strictly enforced. The most common types of personal protective equipment used by housekeeping employees include proper footwear, gloves, respiratory protection, eye protection, and hearing protection if the employee is required to work in noisy areas such as a trash-compactor room. When considering the protection of an employee, it is equally important to consider what things should not be worn. This could include loose-fitting clothes, jewelry, and improper footwear like clogs and high heels.

Waste Disposal

It is a known fact that refuse collectors have one of the highest accident frequency and severity rates of any type of employee. It stands to reason, therefore, that the collection of refuse in the hospital may be a very dangerous job. In order to properly protect the employee, the size of containers should be limited to help prevent back injury and other muscle strain-type injuries. Trash receptacles containing sharps (needles, etc.) should be properly identified to prevent puncture wounds and lacerations to the employee picking up the trash. It is of greatest importance that radioactive waste and biologically hazardous waste be properly labeled, and that reputable service companies be contracted for the removal of such waste from the hospital premises. In addition to this, a program for the disposition of unwanted chemical waste should be established. Such a program will reduce the chance of toxic or highly flammable chemicals from being dumped down the drain or allowed to sit on shelves waiting for an accident to happen. Such a program should be conducted under the supervision of the safety director and should include the use of a reputable chemical disposal firm and a qualified chemist, if possible. In any case, the disposal program for all wastes generated within the hospital should be in complete compliance with guidelines and regulations established by the U.S. Environmental Protection Agency.

Storage

Proper storage plays a very important role in the prevention of accidental injuries and fires. The following is a list of things to consider when deciding how and where to store materials, equipment, and supplies:

1. Storage areas should be kept in an orderly condition at all times.
2. Aisles and doorways, especially fire doors, must be unobstructed.
3. Pallets and skids should be kept in neat piles not over 4 ft high.
4. Trash should not be allowed to accumulate and create a sanitation or fire hazard.
5. Stored materials should be secure so as to not create a falling hazard.
6. Shelves and racks should be kept in good repair and not overloaded.
7. Special materials such as flammable liquids, toxic materials, and chemicals should be handled and stored according to applicable standards and regulations.
8. Storage in corridors or in exits should be forbidden.
9. All permanent storage areas should contain automatic fire-detection and/or fire-extinguishing systems.

PEST MANAGEMENT

The problems insects and rodents have caused mankind throughout time will not be itemized here; enough can be said by merely mentioning the plagues and epidemics that have dotted history. Not all of these sicknesses were carried exclusively by pests, but the conditions that created an inviting environment for them then still exist today.

The institutions that exist to care for the sick and injured are often confronted with insect and rodent problems. From health, sanitation, and psychological viewpoints, the pest in a health care facility is undesirable and unallowable. Possibilities of prevention, control, and elimination of insects and rodents in a facility must be considered to achieve the desired end result — a pest-free health care facility.

General Conditions

Insects and rodents have the same reason for setting up housekeeping in health care facilities as they do anywhere else; the conditions for their existence are favorable. Unless provided with a place to hide, food to eat, and water to drink, pests have a most difficult time establishing residencey.

Often, the pest problem in a clean, well managed and operated facility is caused by incoming items. Pests should be stopped before they enter the building. A few ways to accomplish this are

1. Mechanical barriers (screens, weather stripping, and air curtains)
2. Traps (for rodents and insects)
3. Chemicals (application of insecticides and rodenticides around building perimeter and at entrances, particularly at grade level)

An incubation area where proper treatment can be applied should be utilized whenever goods coming into the health care facility are discovered to be infested. The receiving and trash disposal areas of a facility are usually high entry ports for pests.

Once the pests arrive, they may be transported throughout the facility in goods or carts, or they might even migrate under their own power. Within the facility, the pests will look for a place to live that is convenient to food and water.

If an area is found to contain pests, a systematic approach to their elimination should include

1. An established and thorough cleaning program that includes all areas
2. Repairing of all leaking piping and the insulation of piping prone to "sweating"
3. The cleaning of mechanical areas including the space above drop ceilings
4. The patching of all cracks and openings in wallsand floors (especially around openings where pipes or ducts pass between walls or floors)

The above items can provide good protection against inviting unwanted pests, too. When pest-proofing to make the facility undesirable to insects and rodents, it is wise to pay special attention to areas prone to dampness, moistness, or dirtiness, such as refrigerators, ice machines, sinks, and water closets. Linen and trash chutes and their collection rooms are excellent targets for preventive treatment.

Specific Areas

Should pests persist after thorough cleaning and sealing of an area, the need for insecticides or pesticides is indicated. At this point, one should include medical personnel in order to assure that any treatment is compatible with employee and patient health.

General areas should be treated with the following precautions:

1. Never place or use chemicals where they can be carried by feet or wheeled vehicles to areas where they should not be.
2. Shut down or block off air-handling systems that can spread or dilute the application.
3. Special precautions should be taken in any area where food, linen, sterile goods, or medication is stored.

Food-handling areas should be treated with the following precautions:

1. All food preparation must be stopped before treatment and the type of treatment considered must be compatible with the restoration of food processing.
2. All food-preparation surfaces must be washed after treatment.
3. Removal of utensils from the area is required. Cabinets, drawers, or cupboards do not provide adequate protection from contamination.

Patient areas should be treated with the following precautions:

1. Any movable equipment should be treated away from the patient area.
2. If the area must be treated, the patients must be removed. A nonresidual chemical must be used, followed by adequate ventilation of the room; some patients or employees can have allergic reactions to chemical pesticides.
3. The use of a more powerful chemical treatment should be followed by a cleaning and painting of the area.
4. Never treat linen, sterile materials, or mattresses without knowing the proper use of a particular pesticide.

Whenever using any chemical pesticide:

1. Never use a pesticide without contacting the users of the area and notifying the proper authorities of the facility.
2. Never use a chemical pesticide stronger than that actually needed to do the job.
3. Never use a chemical pesticide without knowing exactly what type of pest is to be dealt with.
4. Never use a chemical pesticide that is not approved for the intended application.

The use of commercial pest control vendors is often appealing to the health care facility because of the various considerations involved. For the most part, these people are honest and knowledgeable professionals. However, it is prudent to monitor exactly their procedures and materials to assure proper application of and protection from chemical pesticides.

PHYSICAL FACILITY SAFETY

While the relationship between employees, staff, and visitors greatly affects the level of safety achieved in the hospital, of at least equal importance is their relationship with the physical plant, their working and living environment. All too often, the significance of a properly designed and maintained hospital is overlooked and all safety efforts are concentrated on training and committees. Often, the need for more space causes the conversion of a floor or unit in order to house a department that it was never designed to handle. A good example of this situation is when an area currently designed for offices is remodeled to house patients on an overnight basis. In this case, due consideration may not have been given to the number of air changes now required in the rooms, the width of door openings and aisles, or the appropriate lighting that is needed for the tasks that must be performed. All of these things and many more are potentially hazardous to patients and staff.

Proper maintenance of a unit or building is of paramount importance. Even the most perfectly designed and constructed facility can become a highly dangerous area in a relatively short period of time if a good maintenance program is not implemented. Without an effective maintenance program, it is only a matter of time before equipment begins to fail, repair costs escalate, and the number and severity of patient incidents directly related to equipment failure or faulty equipment greatly increases. A good example of this is the hospital that never tests or maintains its power distribution equipment and emergency generator. Eventually, the hospital may have a power failure in some portion of the building, possibly due to the lack of adequate preventive maintenance of some part of the distribution system. When the power does fail, the emergency generator is not capable of picking up the load. As a result of the emergency-generator failure, the hospital will be without power for an indeterminate period of time. Patient safety is greatly compromised because electrical power can no longer be delivered to patient electrical equipment, task illumination, and alarm signaling systems, etc.

Designing for Safety

Before the first shovelfull of earth is ever taken out of the ground, architects, engineers, and building planners can do a great deal to provide a safe and healthful environment for those who will eventually inhabit the building.

The architect has the initial responsibility to design a facility that complies with federal, state, and local regulations. Standards for safety that must be met may include those of HEW, OSHA, NFPA, municipal building codes, and municipal fire codes. A hospital should be careful to select an architect who is totally familiar with all pertinent safety standards. Once the architect is selected, he should maintain regular contact with the chief engineer and safety director of the hospital. The engineer and safety director should be given ample opportunity to review and comment on all drawings to make sure hazardous conditions are not being designed into a new facility. If the engineer or safety director discovers a hazardous situation or code violation, this should be properly documented and forwarded to the architect's office.

Once construction has begun, the architect or project manager should make regular inspections with the engineer and safety director to insure construction and installation is being done according to specification. At the same time, the safety director should be inspecting the job site for hazardous conditions that might cause injury to workers. The frequency of these inspections should increase with the degree of completion of the project.

When reviewing plans for code compliance and safety, many things must be taken into consideration. Some of the areas to be considered and a partial list of items to look for are shown below.

Fire Protection

- Are adequate numbers and types of exits provided?
- Are exit travel distances appropriate?
- Does the fire alarm system transmit a signal directly to the fire department?
- Do corridor walls and smoke partitions extend from the floor slab below to the floor or roof slab above?
- Are interior finishes in exit corridors proper?
- Are penetrations between floors protected by "B"-labeled 1½-hr doors?
- Are vision panels in corridor doors and walls of proper size and made of wired glass set in approved steel frames?

Electrical

- Are sufficient receptacles provided in patient rooms?
- Are wet locations provided with either ground fault circuit protection or isolated power systems?
- Does the emergency generator serve all required areas?
- Are flammable anesthesizing locations provided with isolated power systems and line-isolation monitors?

Plumbing

- Are vacuum breakers provided where required?
- Are drain pipes that will carry corrosive materials made of glass?
- Are sprinkler systems designed for proper pressures?
- Can the hot water system be controlled to insure that temperatures in patient rooms/areas won't exceed 110°F?

Miscellaneous

- Are emergency call systems provided in patient rooms, showers, and toilets?
- Are grab bars provided in all patient shower rooms and toilets?
- Have adequate provisions for the handicapped been made?
- Do floor coverings present a slipping or tripping hazard to the elderly and handicapped?
- Are linen and rubbish chute doors designed to prevent accidental entrance?

These are but a few of the items that need to be considered when designing a hospital and reviewing plans. The hospital engineer and safety director should develop a complete list of items that need to be reviewed during construction.

Once construction of the facility is completed, acceptance tests should be conducted on all major building service equipment, including, but not limited to, fire warning systems, fire alarm systems, emergency generator, elevators, medical gas systems, power distribution systems, etc. If possible, these tests should be performed in the presence of municipal authorities and insurance company representatives. Records of the results of such tests should be maintained by the hospital.

SAFETY AND PREVENTIVE MAINTENANCE

Once construction of a facility is completed, responsibility for the upkeep of that facility is transferred to the hospital engineer. In order to achieve an acceptable level of safety for patients, staff, and visitors, an effective plan for preventive maintenance is necessary. An effective preventive maintenance program is one that insures through testing, inspection, and scheduled maintenances increased equipment service life and decreased likelihood that a given piece of equipment will injure or cause injury to any patient, visitor, or staff member due to the faulty manufacture or physical damage of the equipment.

To suggest that a hospital that has a good preventive maintenance program will never experience an injury to a patient, visitor, or employee is, of course, absurd. The presence of such a program will, however, greatly reduce the frequency with which such incidents happen.

Organizing a Preventive Maintenance Program

The first step in organizing a preventive maintenance program is equipment identification. The engineering department should develop a list of all equipment within the facility that requires preventive maintenance. This list should show the type of equipment, name of the manufacturer, model or serial number of the equipment, any hospital identification numbers, and any other pertinent information such as RPMs, normal operating pressures, etc. Once this is done, policies and procedures for each type of equipment need to be developed. These policies and procedures will help insure that the person responsible for doing maintenance on a particular piece of equipment knows exactly what to do. They may also be used as supportive documentation should a claim regarding faulty equipment ever be filed.

The policy and procedure manual should define exactly what is to be done, at what frequency, and how it is to be accomplished. In addition, it should show that the policy has been formally approved by the department head, including how often it is reviewed. A checklist appropriate to each piece of equipment should be provided, and a record form prepared each time a service is carried out. Such a form will serve as a record of the testing and inspection. It should be kept in a central filing system with all other preventive maintenance records when completed. See appendix for an example.

Scheduling Preventive Maintenance

The next task when developing a preventive maintenance program is scheduling of work. In order to do an effective job of scheduling maintenance, one must look at all of the tasks to be performed during the year and determine the estimated man hours required for the completion of each task. Such estimates may be obtained by calling other hospital engineers, contacting manufacturers, or contacting service organizations or consultants for estimated man-hour requirements. It is wise to try to divide the number of man hours used for preventive maintenance as evenly as possible over the course of the year. For example, if the total man-hour requirement for 1 year was 1800 hr, it would be far better to try to do 150 hr preventive maintenance per month than 50 hr 1 month and 250 hr the next. One must recognize, however, that it is unlikely that exactly the same number of hours will be used each month because some work is seasonal.

Probably the most difficult problem facing the hospital engineer is convincing hospital management that preventive maintenance is necessary and can be a cost-saving program in the long run. The burden of proving the value of the preventive maintenance program rests, of course, with the engineer. To achieve this end, the engineer must work to develop data that show that preventive maintenance can increase equipment life, reduce equipment failure, and thereby reduce operational cost and risk exposure. If these factors can be brought to light, then there are few hospital administrators who would not fully support a preventive maintenance program.

Program Evaluation

The final phase of developing a preventive maintenance program is the constant reevaluation and upgrading of that program. Without regular reevaluation, the program can quickly deteriorate and become obsolete.

DEVELOPING A SECURITY DEPARTMENT

Many security departments are organized haphazardly. Therefore, the functions of this department are usually disjointed, and operational dependability cannot be maintained. When organizing a security force, one must always remember that it is a professional organization and should be developed accordingly.

Private or Contract Force

Before developing a department, one should begin by discussing the pros and cons of private vs. contract security forces. When deciding on a private force or a contract service, needs must be surveyed. If circumstance dictates the need for manpower to control traffic (vehicle or pedestrian), and patrol only limited areas, then it may be advantageous to use a contract service. If the needs of the hospital are on a larger scale, then the hospital should consider a private force. With a private force, the hospital will not have to be concerned with orientating personnel to the facility every other month, and control can be maintained over hiring, policy and procedures, and many other areas.

The ultimate decision to use contract or private service rests with the hospital. This decision should be based on the size and complexity of the institution and the services that need to be provided. To assist in making this decision, one might consider using a survey sent to other hospitals in the area. This will aid the hospital in sorting out the services and manpower that need to be provided to allow the department to do a thorough job.

Statement of Purpose

Service departments are normally required to state their purpose. The statement of purpose should be clear and direct. For a security department, this statement could be easily summed up as follows: "The purpose of this department is to safeguard all patients, visitors, and employees from unwarranted harm, or theft of personal property." A statement should also be made concerning the protection of hospital property, but it should carry considerable less importance than the protection of patients, visitors, and staff.

Objectives

Departmental goals and objectives should be established with both short- and long-range goals in mind. When writing long-range goals and objectives, consideration should be given to the possible expansion of the facility and, therefore, increased demand on the department. Consideration should also be given to the possibility of additional responsibilities being assigned to the department. If the hospital expands as planned, accurate long-range planning will allow for an easy transition from a small department to a large force. This will help insure that the level of security provided does not decrease with the growth of the facility.

Statement of Authority

A statement of authority gives a department the authority to carry out the purpose, goals, policy, and procedures authorized by hospital management. As the management's agent, the security department is required to enforce rules and regulations. The statement of authority should be written by administration and approved and signed by the board of directors and the director of the medical staff.

Chain of Command

Reporting relationships may vary depending upon whether or not a contract force is used. If a contract service is used, they will usually supply the field officers and supervisors. The service will usually supply the department head. The contract service should also supply any protective equipment upon approval of the particular hospital they are serving. If a private force is chosen, the chain of command could be administrator, director of security, assistant director, supervisor (for each shift), officers (for each shift), and any ancillary staff necessary.

Job Descriptions

The job description should be a detailed outline of all responsibilities of the position, the reporting relationships, and all other information pertinent to the performance of that job. It is essential that the job description clearly state the responsibilities of each employee. An example follows.

The supervisor is required to:

1. Report all activities of the shift to the director or assistant director
2. Supervise the activities of staff assigned to his/her shift
3. Review and approve all reports turned in by his/her shift

This type of description should be developed for all positions in the department. If a new position is added, there must be a job description written and added to the departmental manual.

SECURITY EMPLOYMENT-SCREENING PRACTICES

Application

Before an officer is hired, the individual should be required to fill out an application, or submit a resume where applicable. The application should be the standard form used by the personnel department. It is essential for this position that past work histories be verified and all time previous to this employment be accounted for.

Age requirement — These requirements will vary depending on what type of security services are being provided. If members of the staff carry any type of weapon, they must be insurable and bondable. If a person is hired for a cadet position (usually for training), then the person may be younger than the minimum age. In the case where the job requires officers to be armed, the officer in question must meet applicable age requirements.

Polygraph test — Polygraph tests can be given before or after employment with the prospective employee's consent. An applicant, however, cannot be denied employment on the grounds of his/her refusal to sign the polygraph consent form. If the individual does sign the consent form, then he/she is obligated to take the test when required. Information attained from the polygraph test is inconclusive. Failure of a polygraph test does not necessarily prohibit employment.

Psychological exams — This type of test was used extensively in the past, but due to discrepancies between test results and actual behavior, its use has become limited. The test usually consists of 500 standard questions and an oral interview. The candidate may be required to answer part or all of the questions. One purpose of this test is to expose any hidden complexes, such as a persecution complex or irrational behavior. As stated earlier, this exam is now in limited use due to the fact that many people pass the test, but at a later time are found to have psychological problems that interfere with job performance. This does not mean that the psychological exam is useless to the employer. Certain cases may warrant such an exam.

Physical examinations — The physical examination can be of two forms: a medical exam or a physical agility test. The employee's medical history as well as a physical examination, are usually required by most hospitals and industry. A medical examination is usually conducted on an annual basis, depending on the policies of the particular institution.

SECURITY STAFF ORIENTATION

Prior to beginning work, all security employees should be required to attend a period of orientation to familiarize them with their job. The period of time spent will depend mainly on the individual's ability to grasp what is being taught. The employee should be made familiar with all shifts and should work for a specified period of time on each shift under the direct supervision of a supervisor or other capable person. Included in the program should be the following topics.

Policies and Procedures

During the orientation, all policies and procedures pertaining directly to employment are discussed. In most cases, there are a set of general hospital policies and procedures. It should be understood, however, that each department has the responsibility to develop its own. These departmental policies and procedures should be developed in conjunction with the minimal general requirements and may be more restrictive, but never less. For example, when calling in sick, the hospital requires that a minimum 1-hr notice be given before the start of an employee's shift. However, the department requires at least a 2-hr notice before the start of an employee's shift. During employees' departmental training, they should be made aware of any differences between the general requirements and departmental requirements.

Attendance

In order for the department to operate well and serve the hospital to its fullest, all officers must be required to report to work on time for their tour of duty. Sick calls should be carefully screened and attendance patterns observed. If an officer is unable to report to work, whether late or sick, departmental procedures must be followed. A list of each shift schedule should be supplied in the policy manual, and each officer should be familiarized with the list. This will assist in assuring proper attendance.

Duties Per Shift

As part of orientation, each officer should be required to work for a period of time on all three shifts. The length of time spent on each shift can be fixed, or may vary according to the employee's ability to grasp what has been taught. During this period, the officer should be made familiar with the officer's duties on the shift, such as post locations, report writing, and special assignments. During this orientation period, the employee should be under the direct supervision of an experienced supervisor or training officer. Upon completion of training, the officer should be capable of working on any assigned shift with minimum supervision.

Dress Code

Security officers, in most cases, are required to wear a uniform. When a uniform is worn, it should meet general requirements set down by the department. All staff will be required to wear identical uniforms. Supervisors' uniforms should distinguish them from regular officers. For example, line officers may wear blue shirts while supervisors wear white. The uniform may vary according to seasons, e.g., long-sleeve shirt and tie during the winter months and short-sleeve shirt and no tie during the summer. A description of the uniform, as well as the proper time to wear it should be in the departmental policies and procedures. Many people respect a person and his/her authority when a uniform is worn. Due to daily contacts with employees, patients, and visitors, the security officer often functions like a public relations officer; his/her appearance should be perfect. The officer should report to work clean-shaven, well rested, and with a clean, pressed uniform.

Weapons/Self-Defense Training

The security department should institute a program to train officers in weapons use and self defense. Part of this training should include an explanation of legal requirements governing the use of weapons and force. After training, personnel should be drilled regularly to insure they understand when and when not to use weapons and or physical force. This portion of the program cannot be overemphasized. Employees taught to use a weapon or self defense must meet various requirements prescribed by municipal, state, and federal legislation. Employees should be required to periodically requalify with weapons. Records of program content and attendance should be kept in departmental and personnel files indefinitely.

Legal Aspects

Many cities in the U.S. have rules and regulations governing the actions of a private security force. Persons employed as security officers are required by law and often by their employer to learn these regulations.

FUNCTIONS OF THE SECURITY DEPARTMENT

New Employee Orientation

All new employees of the hospital staff should attend new-employee orientation. Part of this orientation should include a discussion of the services provided by and purpose of the security department given by a representative of the security department.

Exit/Entry Control

Most industry and some hospitals try to control the movement of employees by requiring them to exit or enter through one doorway. This is usually done to set up some kind of control of who and what enters and leaves the hospital. Another step in aiding exit or entry control is the identification badge. The most widely used type is the photo ID. This badge should be issued by the security or personnel department, and a duplicate picture should be kept in the employee's file. The ID badge should be worn at all times while the employee is at work. To enforce the use of the ID badge, hospital policy should include action to be taken for not having an ID badge.

Patient/Visitor Pass

All hospitals use some type of pass to allow visitors to enter upon the floors. This pass should show any information pertaining to the use of the facility, smoking, and visiting times. Guests should have the pass with them at all times.

Personal Effects of Employees

All employees, regardless of position, like to bring personal items to work. These items will range anywhere from a small radio to a television. Any items other than those needed to perform the job should be left at home.

If an employee receives permission to use his/her personal items at work, then this permission should be documented and a record kept in a file in the security office. A copy should also stay with the department head granting the permit to the employee. If the employee wishes to remove the item, he/she must show proper documentation of ownership.

Personal Property

Regardless of the length of stay, patients often bring articles with them to the hospital. The patient, much like the employee, should be discouraged from bringing radios, televisions, hairdryers, and other such items into the hospital. In some cases, substantial amounts of money, as well as expensive jewelry, are brought into the hospital. The hospital should have some type of safe set up to hold these items. The amount of cash and other items should be documented. A copy should be given to the patient or put with their chart, and a copy kept with the department holding these items. The patient should be allowed to remove part or all of the items at any time.

Management of Prisoners

At some time, the department will have to detain a person or persons, or watch a prisoner while at the institution. Policies and procedures regarding prisoner management should be developed only after checking with the local police agency for appropriate precautions. All staff should be properly trained in the detention of prisoners.

COMMUNICATIONS SYSTEMS

When choosing communications equipment, it is important to have equipment tailored to meet the needs of the hospital. Equipment should be tested in the facility before purchase. Once the equipment or system has been accepted, each person using it should be trained in its proper operation. Employees should also be trained in the proper use of codes and verbal conduct to be observed when using this equipment. All of the above information should be included in the departmental manual.

SURVEILLANCE EQUIPMENT

Surveillance equipment, much like communication equipment, should be tailored to the needs of the institution. This equipment can include anything from mirrors and cameras to a sophisticated computerized system. All personnel in the department should be trained in the proper use of surveillance equipment. Training all staff will help insure proper coverage of the facility when key personnel are absent.

PROCEDURE FOR EMERGENCY GENERATOR TESTING

1. Make all necessary modifications as noted in the Maintenance Department Policy and Procedure Manual.
2. Connect the transfer switch in the basement control panel.
3. Monitor generator for the entire test.
4. After test, disconnect transfer switch
5. Fill out inspection checklist.

EMERGENCY GENERATOR TESTING CHECKLIST

	J	F	M	A	M	J	J	A	S	O	N	D
Anti Freeze Level												
Radiator Level												
Oil Level												
Oil Pressure												
Voltage												
Amperage												
Batteries												
Belts (Fan)												
Belt (Alt.)												
Air Filter												
Running Time												
Time to Date												

FIGURE 1. Policy for emergency generator testing. The emergency generator shall be tested monthly under load conditions for a minimum of 30 min. Upon completion of the test, this inspection report form shall be filled out in total by the person conducting the test.

APPENDIX

Every hospital must have an autonomous emergency power source that is able to provide the essential service when the normal supply is interrupted. Details of such a system are given in the NFPA standard for Essential Electrical Systems for Health Care Facilities and the Accreditation Manual for Hospitals published by the Joint Commission on Accreditation of Hospitals. Figure 1 is a policy statement concerning emergency power as it may be found in a hospital policy and procedure manual.

REFERENCES

1. Accreditation Manual for Hospitals, Joint Commission on Accreditation of Hospitals, Chicago, 1979, 77.
2. Housekeeping Manual for Health Care Facilities, American Hospital Association, Chicago, 1966.
3. Maintenance Scheduling, American Hospital Association, Chicago, 1978.
4. Management Engineering for Hospitals, American Hospital Association, Chicago, 1970.
5. Accreditation Manual for Hospitals, Joint Commission on Accreditation of Hospitals, Chicago, 1979, 11.
6. Security Programs in Health Care Institutions, American Hospital Association, Chicago, 1976.
7. Theft in Hospitals — Cost Effectiveness Enemy No. 1, American Hospital Association, Chicago, 1976.
8. Accreditation Manual for Hospitals, Joint Commission on Accreditation of Hospitals, Chicago, 1979, 45.

OCCUPATIONAL SAFETY AND HEALTH ACT: OCCUPATIONAL SAFETY AND HEALTH ADMINISTRATION REQUIREMENTS

Earle P. Shoub

INTRODUCTION

Prior to December 29, 1970, occupational safety and health was largely controlled by the states. A few laws existed that placed specific industries under federal jurisdiction in connection with work place conditions. The Federal Metal and Nonmetallic Mine Safety Act (enacted in 1966) and the Federal Coal Mine Health and Safety Act of 1969 are two examples of acts that have since been displaced by the Federal Mine Safety and Health Act of 1977. The latter of the two attracted wide attention because it provided for payments and assignments to work in low-dust atmosphere (at the option of the coal miner) for coal miners with respiratory impairment presumably caused by the inhalation of coal mine dust. Despite these and a very few other legislative efforts to provide (on a national level) minimum occupational health and safety standards, prior to passage of the Occupational Safety and Health Act of 1970 (OSH Act), the vast majority of American workers were protected only by the laws of their state and lesser jurisdictions.

During the 1960s, Congress held hearings that resulted in passage of the OSH Act. Testimony at these hearings varied considerably in support of and against national legislation. The need for strong legislation was espoused by some, while the opposite view claimed the states were adequately protecting the worker. Additionally, the issue of states' rights was raised, and there were expressions, pro and con, concerning the desirability of a regulatory agency to perform research leading to the development of regulations.

The resulting OSH Act was a compromise in many respects, reached in the Congress before the final bill was sent to the President for signature. Like all statutes, the OSH Act is interpreted, usually by the courts, in a social environment that is dynamically changing. Two concepts that were not spelled out in the act but this author believes were inherent in it were (1) that the age-old concept of the master-servant relationship—placing all responsibility for controlling occupational safety and health in the employer—was a practical approach to achieving the purposes of the act and (2) that no comparative value for injury, death, or disease was involved in achieving to the utmost the purpose of the act. Both of these concepts are now being challenged in one or more ways. Employees are refusing to work, and are demanding wages when they believe working conditions are unduly hazardous. In some cases, employers are denying that the conditions are hazardous or sufficiently hazardous to warrant this action by the employees. The issue is before the adjudicating bodies and the courts. Presumably, a set of guidelines will emerge as the result of decisions in precedent-setting cases. Economic impact statements or their equivalent are now under consideration to become an ingredient of the rules-making process by being put before the courts as evidence in opposition to regulatory requirements.

These examples, and at least one other that will be discussed later in this chapter, indicate that the interpretation of the OSH Act and the standards and regulations issued under it are not static and do not lend themselves to being listed even during periods when standards and regulations are not overtly being changed. The employer who is subject to the act would be well advised to subscribe to one of the periodicals or services that report, on a current basis, probable impending changes and adopted modifications in interpretations and regulations affecting employers.

COVERAGE OF THIS ACT

Although Section 5(b) of the OSH Act requires employees to comply with the act, there are no penalties (for violations) imposed on employees, whereas penalties are imposed on employers. Thus, the OSH Act places heavier responsibility on employers, with a few exceptions as to its application. These exceptions are largely decreasing, although Congress has provided some temporary relaxation for minor infractions in small businesses. Section 3(5) of the act defines employer as "a person engaged in a business affecting commerce who has employees, but does not include the United States or any State or political subdivision of a State." Standing alone, this would appear to exempt facilities of the federal government, a state, or a political subdivision of a state. Section 19 of the OSH Act, however, makes it the responsibility of the head of each federal agency to establish and maintain an effective and comprehensive occupational safety and health program. This program shall be consistent with the standards promulgated by the secretary of labor under the OSH Act. Furthermore, the secretary of labor is directed to report to the president his evaluations and recommendations concerning the occupational safety and health programs of the agencies.

Section 24 of the act requires the secretary of labor to compile and analyze occupational health and safety statistics. This section specifically requires employers in the private sector to file such reports as may be required with the secretary of labor. The secretary's responsibility in compiling and analyzing occupational health and safety statistics does not stop at this point, but includes (although they are not named) other sources of information of the same nature as is collected from private industry. Any question as to the responsibilities of federal agencies that may arise out of this diverse situation was resolved by Executive Order 11807, dated September 28, 1974. The secretary of labor is required by this executive order to issue record keeping and reporting regulations for the federal establishment such as envisioned by Section 24 of the OSH Act and the heads of agencies are assigned detailed responsibilities to comply. The order also encompasses authority for the secretary of labor to issue regulations and guidelines for the safety and health programs of the agencies.

The intention was emphasized when Assistant Secretary of Labor for Occupational Safety and Health Eula Bingham addressed an AFL-CIO public employee department convention in Washington. The *Occupational Safety and Health Reporter* for September 13, 1979, reported Bingham's remarks as follows:

> "Assistant Labor Secretary Eula Bingham September 11 urged government employees to continue to publicize health and safety hazards present in their workplaces in order to increase public awareness of the problems they face. The injury and illness rate for federal employees has increased from one among every 23 employees in 1974 to one among every 16 workers in 1977, Bingham stated. She added that 'inadequate safety and health conditions in federal workplaces have become an economic burden upon taxpayers', citing direct workers' compensation payments and medical benefits exceeding $626 million for federal workers in fiscal 1978...."

Earlier, Secretary of Labor Ray Marshall had sent a strong recommendation to the Office of Management and Budget urging that the executive order be materially strengthened. Subsequent to the order, 29 Code of Federal Regulations (CFR) 1960, Safety and Health Provisions for Federal Employees, was promulgated. This implements the preceding insofar as occupational safety and health of federal employees is concerned. Job-related accidents, illnesses, and injuries are required to be reported, as well as specific records kept and made available to the secretary of labor (OSHA) and the employees at the establishment involved. This regulation reiterates the provision in Executive Order 11807 that directs the head of each agency to "designate or appoint... an agency official with sufficient authority to represent effectively the interest and support of the agency head,'' and provides for each agency to have an appropriate organization, committees, and dissemination of information. Moreover, 29 CFR 1960 establishes procedures for inspections and abatements by each agency, as well as the issuance of notices of unsafe or unhealthful working conditions that among other things, shall be publicly displayed at the establishment involved. From the foregoing, there seems no doubt that all the authorities involved are united in a desire to provide to federal employees protection in occupational safety and health at least equal to that provided by the OSH Act and regulations under it to employees in private industry.

The OSH Act (Section 4(b)(1)) provides that nothing in it ''shall apply to working conditions of employees with respect to which other Federal agencies,...exercise statutory authority to prescribe and enforce standards or regulations affecting occupational safety or health.'' Section 4(b)(2), however, states:

> ''The safety and health standards promulgated under the Act of June 30, 1936, commonly known as the Walsh-Healey Act (41 U.S.C. 35 et seq.), the Service Contract Act of 1965 (41 U.S.C. 351 et seq.), Public Law 91-54, Act of August 9, 1969 (40 U.S.C. 333), Public Law 85-742, Act of August 23, 1958 (33 U.S.C. 941), and the National Foundation on Arts and Humanities Act (20 U.S.C. 951 et seq.) are superseded on the effective date of corresponding standards promulgated under this Act, which are determined by the Secretary to be more effective. Standards issued under the laws listed in this paragraph and in effect on or after the effective date of this Act shall be deemed to be occupational safety and health standards issued under this Act, as well as under such other Acts.''

The secretary of labor promulgated his ''Rules of Procedure for Promulgating, Modifying, or Revoking Occupational Safety or Health Standards'' in 29 CFR 1911. This regulation makes specific reference to the Walsh-Healey/Walsh-Healey Public Contracts Act, the Service Contract Act of 1965, the Construction Safety Act, the Longshoremen's and Harbor Worker's Compensation Act, and the National Foundation on Arts and Humanities Act. The effect is to bring those persons and organizations coming under the health and safety provisions of the acts to which reference is made under the occupational safety and health standards established in accordance with Section 6 of the OSH Act.

Of the acts mentioned in 29 CFR 1911, the Walsh-Healey Public Contracts Act is probably the best known and of the widest application. In brief and insofar as this presentation is concerned, it is required that most government contracts in excess of $10,000 include occupational safety and health requirements providing for the protection of workers engaged in the work called for or related to the contract. Contracting officers representing the federal agency involved are responsible for including this requirement whenever appropriate and assuring that it is carried out. Thus, some employers who might otherwise not be subject to the OSH Act may be made subject to it by virtue of a contractual relationship with the federal government.

Another route by which facilities owned or operated by a state or a political subdivision thereof may be brought under the OSH Act occurs when a state elects to assume responsibility for the development and enforcement therein of occupational safety and health standards providing at least as effective coverage as the standards of the act. In order for a state to provide for enforcement by its own personnel, it must make an application to the secretary of labor and show that the state and its laws meet all criteria, including occupational safety and health requirements in Section 18 of the OSH Act and regulations. If the secretary concurs, the state ultimately takes over responsibility for conducting its own program subject to audit by and reporting to the OSHA. In addition to the requirements of the OSH Act that are imposed or devolve on the vast majority of employers, one should not complacently and solely rely on compliance with the published standards and regulations. The OSH Act does not deprive states and other jurisdictions from imposing and enforcing additional or more stringent requirements.

The protection of the act applies to employees, not to visitors or others (such as students in schools) who are not employees. However, there can be doubt as to who is an employee and during what time period. Health care facilities, especially those connected with schools, may have volunteers or employ students on a part-time basis. Not all employees receive wages or salaries. Payment may be in kind. A legal review may be necessary to determine the full status of such people. It is clear, however, that when one is concerned with persons in dual or ambiguous capacities, publication of clear rules of conduct and relationship is highly desirable.

REGULATIONS, STANDARDS, AND DUTIES OF EMPLOYERS

The OSH Act provides a standards- or regulation-setting procedure that offers each interested party an opportunity to express himself and have his comments considered before a regulation or standard is promulgated. In simple terms, the first step is for the OSHA to publish its proposed standard in the *Federal Register,* a publication issued every working day by the National Archives and Records Service (General Services Administration, Washington, D.C.). In addition to explanatory material and the proposed standard as an amended standard, the notice must state the period of time allowed for comment and precisely where the comments should be sent. Interested parties may not only file written comments, but may also request a public hearing. Within 60 days after the period for comment and hearings has expired, and after due consideration of all the information presented, the secretary of labor shall: (1) announce that the standard is unnecessary, (2) publish the standard including its effective date in the *Federal Register* or (3) publish a modification of the proposed standard including its effective date in the *Federal Register.* There is nothing to prevent the OSHA from rescinding its proposed standard (course number one above) and publishing a greatly revised version for public comment, etc.

The OSH Act not only created OSHA in the Department of Labor, but also created the National Institute for Occupational Safety and Health (NIOSH) in the Department of Health, Education, and Welfare. NIOSH is authorized to conduct research, experiments, and demonstrations applicable to occupational health and safety. It is intended that NIOSH will, among other things, facilitate the development of health and safety standards to be adopted by OSHA. Thus, it may be that a proposed standard or regulation will arise out of NIOSH information supplied to OSHA, out of information developed solely by OSHA, or from a joint OSHA-NIOSH effort. Additionally, there is provision for other interested parties with sound evidence to present to petition for the establishment of regulations.

The rule-making procedure described above has the advantage of encouraging those who would be affected by the proposed regulation to participate by contributing information from their experience and knowledge, and of obtaining a public answer to the comments, written and oral, as part of the decision-making process. At the same time, it is obvious that the procedure is not rapid nor immediately responsive to urgent situations that may emerge from time to time. To meet urgent situations that become apparent as the result of research, statistical analysis, new technology, etc., OSHA has authority to issue Emergency Temporary Standards (ETS) after it has determined that employees are subject to grave danger due to exposure to the specific hazard(s) to which the ETS applies and that the ETS will provide urgently needed protection. The *Federal Register* also publishes ETS. The notice in the *Federal Register* contains the regulation or standard and its effective date (usually within 30 days from the date of publication). The OSH Act provides the OSHA shall publish a proposed rule applying to adopting the ETS within 6 months of first publication. The proposed regulation undergoes the rule-making procedure, including public participation, described above. The ETS remains in effect until the regular rule-making procedure is completed.

OSHA exercises authority over employers in still another manner that appears to be employed with increasing frequency. This enforcement procedure is based on Section 5(a) (1) of the OSH Act (commonly called the "general duty clause") that says "Each employer shall furnish to each of his employees employment and a place of employment which are free from recognized hazards that are causing or are likely to cause death or serious physical harm to his employees;..."

Most of the OSHA regulations or standards were promulgated shortly after the OSH Act was signed into law. There have been numerous amendments, additions, and deletions. Nevertheless, the regulations are not fully consonant with the most recent information concerning occupational health and safety. In many cases, OSHA compliance safety and health officers (CSHOs) issue citations under the general duty clause when they believe a hazard exists, despite the fact that the employer is not violating any published OSHA standard or regulation.

While any reliable scientific, technologic, or statistical information may be the source of information to guide the CSHO in applying the general duty clause, the Criteria Documents issued by NIOSH are often involved. Over a hundred of these documents, including maximum exposure recommendations and the rationale for each, have already been issued and more are in process. An example of a document issued in March 1977 that could affect health care facilities is "Waste Anesthetic Gases and Vapors". It is recommended that employee exposure on a time-weighted average for the duration of the period during which a mixture of nitrous oxide and halothane is administered not exceed 25 ppm of nitrous oxide and 0.5 ppm of halothane. Neither compound appears in the OSHA regulations, General Industry Standards, Title 29, Code of Federal Regulations, Part 1910.

Any citation may be appealed. Naturally, it is usually more likely that the appeal of a citation based on the general duty clause will be successful. More will be said about this later in this chapter.

Throughout the published OSHA regulations or standards, various concensus standards such as those published by the American National Standards Institute (ANSI), the National Fire Protection Association (NFPA), the American Society for Testing and Materials (ASTM), and the Compressed Gas Association (CGA) are adopted and incorporated into the OSHA requirements. These specifically named standards are integral parts of the regulations just as if they were reprinted in them. However, it is important to recognize that the edition of the consensus standard adopted by reference cannot be more recent than the date of promulgation of the OSHA regulation.

Many of the consensus standards have since been revised. Local jurisdictions often depend on more recent editions than the OSHA regulation. For example, Part 1910.308 of the General Industry Standards indicates that reference (throughout the standards to the National Electrical Codes) is to the 1971 edition. Since the 1971 edition was adopted, there have been at least 3 subsequent editions. Some local jurisdictions have adopted one of the more recent editions of the National Electrical Code with the possible result that a compliance safety and health officer and a local electrical or building inspector might each demand a different configuration. In OSHA Program Directive #200-67, dated December 1, 1977, CSHOs are instructed to cite as a *de minimus* violation any case in which:

> "An employer's workplace is at the 'state of the art' which is technically advanced beyond the requirements of the applicable standard, and provides equivalent or better safety and health protection. An example would be when OSHA standards, derived from such consensus groups as NEC, NFPA, etc.,

have been updated in later consensus publications in accord with new technology or equipment and the updated standard provides equal or greater safety and health protection."

A *de minimus* violation is of minimum significance and applies when a deviation from a standard is of no consequence or does not detract from the protection afforded the workers.

VIOLATIONS, PENALTIES, AND APPEALS

Under the act, there are both serious and nonserious violations. The former include those that are likely to result in serious bodily injury, illness, or death. Serious violations are subject to a mandatory penalty that may be as high as $1000 per violation. The former that are violations not likely to have the serious results enumerated are also subject to the same maximum penalty, but at the discretion of OSHA.

In the event a violation is established during an inspection and the same violation is found in the premises on subsequent inspections, it may be asserted that the violation is willful or repeated. In such a case, additional penalties of up to $10,000 per violation may result. Also, if a period is specified by OSHA for abatement of a violation, a penalty of $1000/day is assessible if abatement is not accomplished in the period allowed. Criminal penalties of up to $10,000 and 6 months in prison are possible in the event a willful violation results in the death of an employee. These penalties become progressively more severe as the offenses are repeated.

Because of the severity of the penalties connected with repeated occurrences (willful violations), it is usually advisable to appeal first offenses if there is any ground for the appeal. Initial offense penalties are often small enough to make it less costly to accept them than to go through the appeals procedures. This may be a penny-wise-and-pound-foolish position in the long run.

Appeals should be handled with expert help in almost all cases. The procedures are available from OSHA; experienced consultants and attorneys can usually be located without difficulty.

RECORD KEEPING AND REPORTING

Each employer is required to maintain for each place of employent a Log and Summary of Occupational Injuries and Illnesses (OSHA Form No. 200). He/she is required to enter all recordable cases in this log within 6 working days of learning of the occurrence. Recordable items are

1. Any occupational death (regardless of the time between the occurrence and death or the duration of illness)
2. Any occupational illness
3. Occupational trauma involving loss of consciousness, restriction of motion or work, assignment to another job, or medical treatment (first aid excluded)

OSHA Form No. 200 may be replaced with any other form that provides the same information. Thus, many Worker's Compensation First Report of Injury forms will suffice. Details of what is required are in 29 CFR 1904.2. It is also mandatory that OSHA Form No. 101, Supplementary Record of Occupational Injuries and Illness, or a surrogate form, be completed for each recordable injury or illness. The requirements for an alternative or surrogate form are contained in 29 CFR 1904.4. An annual summary of log entries appearing on the OSHA Form No. 200 (or equivalent) shall be prepared at the end of each calendar year for each establishment. A copy of the summary for the preceding year shall be displayed in an appropriate location from February 1 (or earlier) until March 1 (or later).

OSHA requires that the employer report to the local OSHA area office any accident that results in one or more deaths or in the hospitalization of five or more employees. This report may be oral or in writing, but must be made within 48 hr of the accident. In states with approved state plans, the report shall be made to the state agency with enforcement authority for occupational health and safety. It is advisable to have positive evidence that all required reports of this type are made. Telegrams or prompt written confirmation are good pieces of evidence.

Violations of the foregoing are subject to a penalty of up to $1000 per violation. Failure to maintain the log or supplemental record (or the equivalent) during the period of a reportable occurrence warrants a proposed penalty of $100 per form. If the annual summary is not compiled and posted as required, the proposed penalty will be $200. A $400 penalty will be proposed for each failure to report (within the above time limit) serious injuries and deaths.

On October 16, 1979, OSHA proposed in the *Federal Register* (44 FR 59561) that the 48-hr reporting period be reduced to 8 hr. As of this writing, this proposal is undergoing the public-review procedure.

SAFETY AND RISK MANAGEMENT

Paul E. Stanley and Eleanor R. Wagner

INTRODUCTION

The preceding chapters have been presented with the basic intent that the principle laid down by Hippocrates (and later by Florence Nightingale) might be fulfilled: *Primun non Nocere* — do no harm. In modern terms, the Joint Commission on Accreditation of Hospitals writes in its manual: "The patient has the right to expect reasonable safety in so far as the hospital practices and environment are concerned."[1] It is the intent of this chapter to point out a few reasons why the safety practices have been detailed and to summarize how they may be implemented.

In an effort to assure that safety for the patient (and the staff) is provided as fully as possible, as many as 28 or 30 standards-making organizations (including governmental agencies) have promulgated over 1000 regulations, codes, standards, and laws dealing with the subject. The National Fire Protection Association alone has more than 25 publications covering topics ranging from fire safety and building design to electrical safety and the safe use of anesthetic gases.[2] It has been estimated that nearly 25% of the cost of operating a hospital comes from meeting the many codes, standards, and regulations imposed on the health care industry.[3,4]

In spite of the heavy regulation of hospital operation, the rise in the number and costs of malpractice suits against medical practitioners and hospitals has been all but overwhelming. Before 1930, the average award in the almost rare malpractice suit was about $5,000. By 1950, the figure was above $25,000 and had risen to $50,000 by 1960. In the 1970s, the level was above $250,000 and is in fact approaching $500,000. The number of cases is also rising; not a few million-dollar awards have been approved by the courts.[5]

The reasons are many and complex. In the past, the medical profession was held in such high esteem that no one thought of taking legal action against a physician, nurse, or hospital. Medicine was considered a charitable and necessary service; if a mistake was made or even if a life was lost, the cost was not high compared to the enormous good that was done for most. More recently, the attitude has changed. An informed or, perhaps, misinformed public has come to regard the health care field with its rising costs of health care as part of the big-business establishment — very affluent. The public has come to demand that "the difficult must be routine, the impossible frequent, and the miraculous only slightly less than frequent."[6]

To this must be added the fact that health care has become increasingly complicated, especially since the introduction of electronic instrumentation after World War II. In the not-too-distant past, medical practice was a one-on-one event. The physician examined the patient with only a stethoscope and thermometer to aid his own physical senses. Besides, he knew his patient personally and could judge his health on an almost subjective basis. Today, the plethora of devices, tests, and computer-aided processes have often reduced the physician-patient relationship to such an impersonal level that there has been a deterioration of satisfaction on the part of the patient, causing him to feel that he has received little, if any, care. Such a feeling of less-than-optimum medical treatment, coupled with the patient's awareness of the availability of legal redress, has led, it is believed, to the flood of malpractice suits.[7]

MALPRACTICE AND NEGLIGENCE LAW

While malpractice is a term formerly applied to improper medical practice in the limited sense of professional misconduct, recent changes in the public attitude toward health care have extended the term in the mind of the public to include almost all areas of hospital operation. It is estimated that from 2 to 5% of malpractice suits involve the allegation that one or more pieces of apparatus had been involved and that harm occurred because such apparatus failed to perform effectively and safely.[8] The failure may be alleged to have been because of poor design, poor maintenance, improper use of a device, or other negligent practices.

Negligence is defined as failure to exercise reasonable care. Any professional, whether physician, nurse, engineer, or other practitioner, may be liable for any harm to the patient when it can be shown that he/she failed to do that which can be reasonably expected of such a professional under the same or similar circumstances. This may mean that negligence can be alleged when the side rails of the bed are not raised and the patient falls out of bed, or any of hundreds of similar failures to perform in what may be considered a reasonable manner. For negligence to be shown in any case, four conditions must exist: (1) a legal duty or obligation on the part of the defendant to exercise a certain standard of care, (2) a failure on the part of the defendant to discharge that duty, (3) an injury or loss sustained by the plaintiff as a result of the defendant's failure, and (4) a reasonably close connection between the defendant's failure and the plaintiff's injury, or, in legal terminology, proximate cause.[9]

Liability may be incurred, in another sense, under breach of warranty rules. In this case, the defendant may be held responsible for implying or expressing an opinion asserting the propriety or fitness for the purpose of a device or procedure affecting the patient. For example, the clinical engineer may indicate that a piece of electromedical instrumentation is safe as far as electrical shock is concerned. Should a patient receive a shock from the device, the engineer may conceivably be held liable for any resultant injury. Under the concept of strict liability, all persons in the line of distribution of a product from the manufacturer to the ultimate user (the patient) may be held liable for harm to the patient even though the cause may have been poor design or poor manufacturing practices on the part of the original supplier.[10]

Risk Management

The medical community as a whole has responded to the criticism that it has, in some sense, failed to achieve its full potential of providing quality health care by the implementation of programs aimed at assuring the safety the patient expects. Safety programs or risk-management programs exist to minimize the probability of harm and maximize the quality of health care in general. Put simply, risk management is a program designed to identify situations, methods, devices, policies, and procedures everywhere in the hospital that could result in harm to the patient, staff, or public, and to implement means by which such situations, methods, devices, policies, and procedures can be changed. The program must include all of a number of vitally important steps and must be conducted in a systematic manner or systems-analysis procedure. The hospital is an exquisitely complex system with many interconnecting and feedback loops. Its analysis from the risk viewpoint can be achieved only by attending to every detail.

The first major step in establishing and carrying out a risk-management program is full commitment to the concept.[11] As the first standard for functional safety set forth by the Joint Commission on Accreditation of Hospitals contemplates a multidisciplinary safety committee in the hospital, and since most hospitals have such a committee, this provides a good basis for the risk-management team. However, all too often appointment to the safety committee may be treated rather casually, and as a bit of extra bother. Recognition of both the importance of risk management by the administration and the work of the safety-committee (or risk-management team) members in a special way may be the most important step in the process. Enthusiasm for providing reasonable safety for the patient in all areas of his care can be engendered throughout the staff by a fully committed, dedicated risk-management team. The alternative of a risk-management consultant with supporting staff (either in-house or contracted for) may be considered.

THE AUTHORITY OF THE RISK-MANAGEMENT TEAM

If the safety committee or risk-management team is to be effective, it must have the authority to take action whenever and wherever it feels that action is called for. To the extent permitted by law, it must have access to hospital records (including medical records, if necessary) and other documents, and be authorized to interview key members of the staff when such is deemed advisable. In order that it can gracefully carry out its studies, it must have a management-level cadre and be broadly interdisciplinary, including physicians, nurses, department heads, and administrative personnel.

The risk-management team must owe its existence to action by the chief executive officer of the hospital and the approval of the medical staff and the governing board of the facility. Its scope of operation should be well defined (in writing) by the administration of the hospital, and be approved by the medical staff.[12] Its authority should extend to the enablement of procedures allowing the clinical engineer to remove from service apparatus of questionable safety or efficacy, and to the impounding of equipment involved in an incident in which injury could possibly be alleged.

THE RESPONSIBILITIES OF THE RISK-MANAGEMENT TEAM

The primary responsibility of the safety committee or risk-management team is to establish and operate a safety program for the hospital.[11,12] The principles involved in this activity are discussed in detail in Chapter 4 of this handbook and are set forth for particular sections of the hospital in other chapters. Here, they are repeated briefly in somewhat different order and emphasis.

Enumeration and Evaluation of Risks

Once a risk-management team is established, it needs to begin an evaluation of risks existing within the hospital. All too often a hospital has an incident-reporting procedure in which each event is treated as an isolated occurrence or simply an accident. No effort is made to evaluate and correlate the data collected in order to determine patterns or interrelationships between divisions or subsystems of the hospital, including the human operator. The risk-management team should make certain that such is not the case in its hospital. In fact, all indications of patient dissatisfaction (reports from the joint commission, state health and fire marshall inspection reports and insurance carrier evaluations, every incident report whether or not injury has resulted, and all claims against the hospital) should be intergrated—with the advice and assistance of the hospital legal and insurance counsel—into the analysis of the degree of safety or risk control within the hospital. The analysis should be in keeping with the policies, procedures, and standards discussed elsewhere throughout this handbook.

The analysis of the data accumulated in this process must be guided by several criteria. Financial loss due to damage to equipment or facility and subsequent "down time" is important, but so also is the possibility of injury or death of hospital employees. These must be carefully weighted and included in the algorithm that defines the risks existent in the hospital. However, above these is the measuring of the quality-assurance coefficient of the care given to the hospital patients. Quality assurance implies that the care of the patient, in all aspects, strives to be as near perfect (excellent) as possible.[13] In turn, this requires the development of special criteria for the measurement of the degree of excellence of the care. Since such criteria will involve the technicalities of the medical and nursing professions, a peer review process is implied as being a necessary part of the work of the risk-management team.

Even the reputation of the hospital as a caring institution is affected by most of the parameters discussed above, and the overall operating success of the hospital is very dependent upon the public opinion of the service rendered.

Educational Programs

No matter how committed the risk-management team and the entire staff may be to the task of providing a safe hospital, and no matter how carefully a complete catalog of potential risks is prepared, nor how precisely the analysis of these risks is carried out, nothing will be accomplished unless there is a full staff commitment to provide corrective measures wherever they are needed. The development of this commitment is in the province of an educational program conducted by the team or some segment of it. The educational activity must include every member of the hospital staff — physicians, nurses, administrators, and physical facility employees. It should be part of the orientation instruction given to new employees and may be extended to a public information program. The purpose of this handbook is to provide some of the material for such a program. It can be enhanced by publications from the American Hospital Association, the National Safety Council, and the National Fire Protection Association, as well as guides to safety published by state boards of health and other organizations.

Policies and Procedures

Already referred to is the review of the written policies and procedures of the hospital. It should be the responsibility of the risk-management team to propose changes in these matters and to assist the affected sections of the hospital in the rewriting of the manuals for safe operation. These may well extend into the personnel department employment procedures in an effort to assure the hiring of adequately prepared personnel at all staff levels.

The risk-management team should further the preparation of documentation of hospital activities including incident reporting, inspection and testing of facilities and equipment reporting, and even the medical records system. Good records may provide excellent protection in the event of a suit against the hospital.

CONCLUSIONS

An overall safety- or risk-management program encompassing the principles set forth throughout this handbook is essential to successful hospital operation. However, the program must be designed to fit the particular needs and methods of the hospital. It must be fully implemented in the effort to provide safety for all of the hospital population, thereby securing for the hospital maximum protection against the risks attendant to its basic mission.

REFERENCES

1. Joint Commission on Accreditation of Hospitals, Accreditation Manual for Hospitals, Chicago, 1979, xiii.
2. Basic Library of Health Care Safety, National Fire Protection Association, Boston, continuously updated.
3. P/K Associates, Cost containment: how's it working, *J. Am. Hosp. Assoc.*, 53(2), 53, 1979.
4. **McCarthy, C. M.**, New York study shows regulatory costs unreasonably high, *J. Am. Hosp. Assoc.*, 53(2) 89, 1979.
5. **Wagner, E. R.**, Personal liability of the clinical engineer, notes for a seminar at Purdue University, Lafayette, Ind., November 30, 1977.
6. **Porterfield, J. D., III**, To the defense of the system, *J. Am. Hosp. Assoc.*, 48, 49, 1974.
7. Report of the Secretary's Commission on Medical Malpractice, Publ. No. 78-88, U.S. Department of Health, Education and Welfare Government Printing Office, Washington, D.C., 1973.
8. **Ridgway, M.**, The role of biomedical instrumentation in malpractice, Annual meeting of the Association for the Advancement of Medical Instrumentation, Las Vegas, 1979.
9. **Wagner, E. R.**, Liabilities for improper use of equipment, *J. Am. Hosp. Assoc.*, 48, 1974.
10. **Favoriti, R. E.**, Legal and practical problems facing the clinical engineer, *J. Assoc. Adv. Med. Instrum.*, 12, 134, 1978.
11. **Brown, J. C.**, Establishing a risk management program, Annual meeting of the Association for the Advancement of Medical Instrumentation) Las Vegas, May 20-24, 1979.
12. **Van Sluyter, C. K. and Hays, P. G.**, Interdisciplinary task force designs risk management program, *J. Am. Hosp. Assoc.*, 52, 87, 1978.
13. Quality Assurance Program for Medical Care in the Hospital, American Hospital Association, Chicago, 1972.

Index

INDEX

A

B

C

D

E

F

J

K

L

M

N

R

S

T

U

V

W

X

Y